METABOLIC ACTIVATION OF DRUGS AND
OTHER XENOBIOTICS IN HEPATOCELLULAR CARCINOMA

Metabolic Activation of Drugs and Other Xenobiotics in Hepatocellular Carcinoma

Grace S. N. Lau

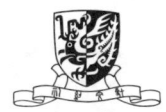

The Chinese University Press

ISBN 962–201–744–4

THE CHINESE UNIVERSITY PRESS
The Chinese University of Hong Kong
SHA TIN, N. T., HONG KONG
Fax: (852) 2603 6692
      (852) 2603 7355
E-mail: cup@cuhk.edu.hk
Web-site: http://www.cuhk.edu.hk/cupress/w1.htm

Printed in Hong Kong

Table of Contents

Foreword

The Chinese University of Hong Kong is committed to training students of the highest calibre for the increasingly sophisticated needs of society. In pursuance of this goal, the University has, from its inception in 1963, attached great importance to research and to the development of postgraduate programmes. A large number of research postgraduate programmes are now offered, spanning a broad spectrum of disciplines, and nearly a thousand students are now enrolled. Doctoral programmes were launched in 1980, and since then some 120 doctorates have been awarded; this number is set to increase very significantly in the near future, reflecting the larger intake in recent years.

The theses, which report the findings of research, represent the fruit of the students' work. Much of the material in these theses have already found their way into journals and conference presentations, from which fellow researchers world-wide can have access. However, it would be of interest to the wider public, and also a source of encouragement to aspiring doctoral students, if some of these theses could be published in the form of monographs. It is therefore a matter of much delight that this idea can be realized with the generous support of The Chinese University of Hong Kong Alumni Fund. Under the *Young Scholars Dissertation Awards* scheme, Ph.D. students graduating from 1993 onwards may apply, or may be nominated by their Faculty Deans, to have their theses published by The Chinese University Press. The theses are scrutinized by external assessors of high international standing, and three of the best theses each year are then selected for the award. This monograph is one of the 1994 theses so selected. It is hoped that, through this book, readers may share the research results of the student, and also get a glimpse of both the toil that went into the work, and the joy of bringing novel ideas and results to light. We hope that the thesis will be found to be intellectually stimulating, and will provoke further discussions on the topic, and further in-depth research in related areas.

I take this opportunity to congratulate Dr. Grace S. N. Lau on her work. The University also wishes to express its deepest gratitude to the CUHK Alumni Fund, without whose generous support this publication would not be possible. The Chinese University Press has rendered most useful advice and assistance in the assessment, editing and publication.

Kenneth Young
Dean, Graduate School

Acknowledgements

I would like to thank the following people without whom this thesis could not have materialised:

My supervisor, Dr. Julian Critchley, Reader and Chairman, Department of Clinical Pharmacology, The Chinese University of Hong Kong, for his constant support and encouragement.

Dr. Don Neal, who kindly arranged for me to work in the Toxicology Unit, Medical Research Council, Carshalton, Surrey, England, to complete part of the experimental work for this thesis and also for his supervision on all aspects of the aflatoxin work, throughout the six-month period I spent there.

Friends and colleagues in The Chinese University of Hong Kong, especially those in the Department of Clinical Pharmacology and The Lee Hysan Laboratory, for their help and support in too many ways to mention.

Friends in the Medical Research Council, Carshalton, who made my time there enjoyable and helped me use it productively.

My parents and my husband for their loving support and understanding in everything I do. Without them, I could not have come so far.

Grace S. N. Lau

List of Abbreviations

AAP	2-acetamidophenol
AFB_1	Aflatoxin B1
AFB_1-8,9-epoxide	Aflatoxin-8,9-epoxide
AFB_1-dihydrodiol	8,9-dihydro-8,9-dihydroxy-AFB_1
AFB_1-GSH	Aflatoxin-glutathione
AFB_1-lysine	Aflatoxin-lysine adduct
AFB_1-N^7-Gua	8,9-dihydro-8-(N^7-guanyl)-9-hydroxy AFB_1
AFB_{2a}	8,9-Dihydro-8-hydroxy aflatoxin B_1
AFM_1	Aflatoxin M_1
AFP_1	Aflatoinx P_1
AFQ_1	Aflatoxin Q_1
ANOVA	Analysis of variance
AUC	Area under plasma concentration versus time curve
BSA	Bovine serum albumin
BSA-AFB_1	Aflatoxin B_1-modified bovine serum albumin
Cl	Plasma clearance
C_{max}	Peak plasma concentrations
CV	Coefficient of variation
DMSO	Dimethyl sulphoxide
ELISA	Enzyme-linked immunosorbent assays
FRM ANOVA	Friedman repeated measures analysis of variance
GSH	Reduced glutathione
GST	Glutathione S-transferase
HAT	Hypoxanthine Aminopterin Thymidine
HBcAg	Hepatitis B virus core antigen
HBsAg	Hepatitis B virus surface antigen
HBV	Hepatitis B virus
HCC	Hepatocellular carcinoma
HGPRT	Hypoxanthine guanine phosphoribosyl transferase
HPLC	High performance liquid chromatography
IARC	International Agency for Research on Cancer

MRT	Mean residence time
NADPH	Reduced nicotinamide adenine dinucleotide phosphate
NAAPQI	N-acetyl-p-benzoquinoneimine
PBS	Phosphate buffered saline
PBS-gelatin	PBS with 0.25% gelatin
PBS-Tween 20	PBS with 0.05% Tween 20 (Polyoxymethylenesorbitan monolaurate)
ppb	Parts per billion
r	Product moment correlation coefficient
R	Intraclass correlation coefficient of reliability
RIA	Radioimmunoassay
RM ANOVA	Repeated measures analysis of variance
SD	Standard deviation
SNK	Student-Newman-Keuls test
t_{max}	Time to reach peak plasma concentration
TMB	3,3',5,5'-tetramethylbenzidine
$t_{1/2}$	Half-life
V_d	Volume of distribution
WHO	World Health Organisation

Abstract

The metabolic activation of many drugs and xenobiotics *in vivo* is effected through the large family of cytochrome P450s enzymes that catalyse a diverse spectrum of reactions including the metabolism of both endogenous and exogenous compounds. There is considerable evidence suggesting that changes in P450 activities can affect the *in vivo* toxicity of drugs in both animals and humans. Oxidative metabolism by cytochrome P450 enzymes has been implicated in the pathogenesis of cancer, through the formation of toxic intermediates and carcinogenic metabolites are formed from drugs and xenobiotics. A marked overall increase in the metabolic activation of the commonly used analgesic agent, paracetamol, was found in patients with hepatocellular carcinoma, as indicated by a much higher percentage recovery of the oxidative metabolites cysteine and mercapturate conjugates, compared to healthy controls and patients with chronic hepatitis B infection. It was thought that metabolic activation of some drugs and xenobiotics through the actions of specific cytochrome P450s may be enhanced in patients with hepatocellular carcinoma.

The *in vivo* metabolic activation of two xenobiotics, namely paracetamol and aflatoxin B_1, using different approaches, were studied in human subjects in this project. The first study involved a full pharmacokinetic study of paracetamol, whose hepatotoxicity is dependent on its *in vivo* metabolic activation. It was carried out in 5 different groups of subjects: healthy subjects, patients with alcoholic liver disease, chronic hepatitis B infection, patients with impaired renal function and patients with hepatocellular carcinoma.

An HPLC method for the measurement of paracetamol and its metabolites in both plasma and urine was developed and validated. It involved minimum sample preparation and had excellent precision, accuracy and recovery. Pharmacokinetic modelling was carried with the aid of the SIPHAR pharmacokinetic programme (version 4.0) and parameters estimated for each subject include the area under the plasma concentration-time curve, clearance, elimination half-life, mean residence time and volume of distribution of paracetamol. In addition, urinary recovery data and metabolic clearances to each metabolite were also calculated. The aim of this part of this project was to elucidate the mechanisms of altered metabolism of paracetamol in patients with hepatocellular carcinoma. Following administration of a 20 mg kg^{-1} body weight dose of paracetamol, the only statistically significant difference in the pharmacokinetics of paracetamol between subjects with hepatocellular carcinoma and subjects in other study groups was an enhanced oxidative metabolic pathway and thus increased metabolic clearance to the cysteine and mercapturate conjugates. The metabolic activation of paracetamol to the toxic intermediate, seemed to be genuinely enhanced among patients with hepatocellular carcinoma and a small proportion of patients with chronic liver diseases, and was not due to an impairment of other metabolic pathways. This enhanced metabolic activation by cytochrome P450s might also be involved in the formation of carcinogenic substances from other xenobiotics such as the mycotoxins aflatoxins with some implications in the pathogenesis of hepatocellular carcinoma.

The other xenobiotic whose metabolic activation was studied in this project was the mycotoxin aflatoxin B_1 (AFB_1). There is considerable evidence indicating an association between AFB_1 ingestion and liver cancer in humans but there is no published data on the possible human exposure and association with hepatocellular carcinoma in Hong Kong. In this study, an enzyme linked immunosorbent assay technique, using a rat monoclonal antibody raised against AFB_1, was developed for monitoring the levels of the major AFB_1-albumin adduct, AFB_1-lysine, in human serum. The study procedure included a hydrolysis step of the serum albumin, clean up steps using Sep-Pak C_{18} cartridges and specific immunoaffinity columns. The method was validated using animals treated with ^{3}H-AFB_1. The overall recovery of the method was 23.3% and the absolute detection limit was about 2 pg AFB_1 per mg of albumin. This detection limit translates to a daily intake of approximately 2 ng AFB_1 and compares favourably with other published methods.

Serum samples from 147 subjects were studied including patients with hepatocellular carcinoma, other liver diseases and individuals without evidence of any liver disease. As the formation of the albumin adduct must be preceded by the in vivo metabolic activation of AFB_1 to its reactive immediate, the measurement of the albumin adduct also serves as an index of metabolic activation. Nevertheless, despite the very low detection limit offered by our assay, none of the serum samples studied showed a measurable level of the adduct. Previous validations on this assay indicate that it is unlikely that these results were false negatives. It is thus concluded that if AFB_1-albumin adducts existed in the serum of the study subjects at all, they were at extremely low levels, and the in vivo metabolic activation of AFB_1 is unlikely to play a major role in the aetiology of hepatocellular carcinoma in Hong Kong.

CHAPTER 1

General Introduction and Study Objectives

1.1 Metabolic activation — role in drug toxicity and carcinogenesis

The biotransformation of relatively inert chemicals to highly reactive metabolites is commonly referred to as 'metabolic activation', and is now recognised to be an initial event in several kinds of chemical-induced toxicities. One of the most well-known and classic example is paracetamol toxicity. Therapeutic doses of the common and widely-prescribed antipyretic analgesic paracetamol, are very safe and virtually completely eliminated by hepatic metabolism and renal excretion within 24 hours. In normal healthy individuals, 5–10% of a therapeutic dose undergoes oxidative metabolism by cytochrome P450 dependent microsomal enzymes with the formation of a potentially hepatotoxic intermediate, probably N-acetyl-p-benzoquinoneimine (Jollow, Mitchell, Potter, Davis, Gillette & Brodie, 1973; Mitchell, Jollow, Potter, Davis, Gillette & Brodie, 1973a; Mitchell, Jollow, Potter, Gillette & Brodie, 1973b) (see Chapter 2 for details on the metabolism of paracetamol). This reactive intermediate is normally conjugated with hepatic reduced glutathione and excreted as inactive mercapturate and cysteine conjugates. In overdosage or when the hepatic glutathione store is depleted, the reactive intermediate can attack vital cell organelles and macromolecules, causing hepatic necrosis. Fig. 1.1 is a simplistic scheme for the role of metabolic activation in cellular toxicity. It is known that in some cases a single enzymatic reaction is involved in the metabolic activation of a chemical while in others, several enzymatic

Figure 1.1   Role of metabolic activation in cellular toxicity

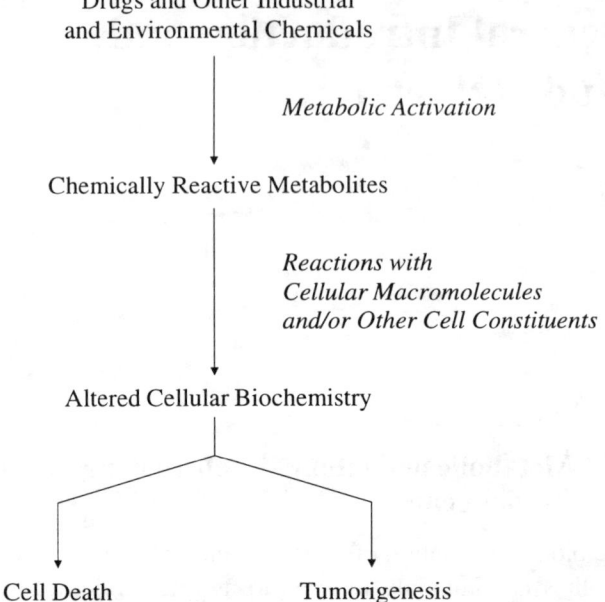

Nelson, SD, *Journal of Medicinal Chemistry* 1982;25:753–65.

and/or chemical reactions are involved in the generation of a chemically reactive metabolite. For example, there is evidence for the involvement of multiple forms of cytochrome P450 in the generation of the reactive 8,9-epoxide from the hepatotoxic mycotoxin aflatoxin B_1 (AFB_1) (Forrester, Neal, Judah, Glancey & Wolf, 1990).

Apart from paracetamol, other examples of drugs that are metabolised to reactive products include the hydrazines (isoniazid, iproniazid, procarbazine and hydralazine), procainamide, the benzenoid aromatics (thalidomide, phenytoin), the nitroaromatics (nitrofurantoin, chloramphenicol and metronidazole) and a whole host of other commonly used drugs. A review on the metabolic activation of these agents has been provided by Nelson (Nelson, 1982).

The metabolism of xenobiotics (foreign substances to the body including drugs and chemcials) *in vivo* has been classified broadly into two phases. Phase I reactions include oxidations, reductions and hydrolyses;

whereas Phase II reactions are defined as conjugation reactions including glucuronidation, sulphation, acylation, methylation and conjugation with glutathione. Most drugs and other xenobiotics are metabolised into more polar compounds that can be rapidly removed from the body while others (pro-drugs) are transformed to therapeutically active metabolites. Since these are the same enzymes that catalyse the formation of reactive, toxic metabolites from some drugs, it seems clear that the structural features of drug molecules and their metabolites determine whether the metabolic reaction produces a detoxification product or a potentially toxic metabolite, and not differences in the nature of the catalytic reaction (Nelson, 1982). Two mechanisms are involved in the initiation of the chain of reactions that ultimately lead to toxicity:

1. Covalent binding of reactive metabolite to tissue macro-molecules
2. Reactive metabolite-induced oxidative stress

Covalent binding is considered an experimental parameter which serves as an index of metabolic activation or the formation of highly reactive metabolites which are often difficult to measure or even isolate. Very often radiolabelled drug is administered to animals or used as substrate in enzyme studies. The amount of radiolabel retained by various macro-molecules including proteins and nucleic acids is then assayed after various steps of extraction. Another method is to subject these modified macromolecules to a digestion process and determine the structure of the ultimate adduct(s). This method poses many problems as it is difficult to ensure that some changes have not occurred during the digestion and workup process, therefore, it has not been possible to apply it widely to the study of a large number of drugs and chemicals. AFB_1 is one such toxic chemical whereby the chemical structure and properties of its major serum albumin and DNA adducts have been successfully elucidated (see Chapter 3 for detail review).

Covalent binding studies have also been a useful tool during the investigation of the role of metabolic activation in the initation of the hepatic toxicity of paracetamol. Apart from demonstrating that a reactive intermediate was involved in the causation of hepatic toxicity, dose dependency of the toxicity of paracetamol was also shown. In general, the severity of drug/chemical toxicity involving metabolic activation as an intermediate step depends on:

a. the proportion of the dose that is converted to reactive metabolite

b. the proportion of reactive metabolite that becomes covalently bound

c. the proportion of covalently bound metabolite that is attached to critical macromolecules and

d. the proportion of (c) that cannot be replaced or repaired that leads to toxicity

These factors can potentially be modified by endogenous or exogenous modalities and thus contribute to inter-individual variation in the susceptibility to the toxicity of various xenobiotics. These may include genetic predisposition, metabolising enzyme induction or inhibition by other environmental agents and the activity/capacity of other detoxification pathways.

The other mechanism involved in the initiation of the chain of reactions that ultimately lead to toxicity is oxidative stress caused by the reactive metabolite. It requires redox cycling of a compound through radical intermediates that can reduce molecular oxygen to superoxide anion, then to hydrogen peroxide and hydroxyl radical, all of which are believed to be involved in the initiation of membrane lipid perioxidation, leading subsequently to cell death. Thus, deficiency of vitamin E, a known free radical scavanger, and selenium, required for the synthesis of most glutathione peroxidases (enzymes that destroy hydrogen perioxide), should enhance *in vivo* toxicity of drugs that appear to involve this mechanism. Examples of drugs causing toxicity by such mechanism include nitroaromatics and anthraquinone anticancer agents.

The cytochrome P450 is a large family of enzymes that catalyse a diverse spectrum of reactions, including the metabolism of endogenous compounds such as cholesterol, fatty acids and steroids and exogenous compounds such as drugs and environmental chemicals. Many different P450 isoenzymes have been purified from human liver and their corresponding cDNAs cloned and classified into families and subfamilies (Nebert, Nelson, Coon, Estabrook, Feyereisen, Fujii-Keriyama, Gonzalez, Guengerich, Gunsalus, Johnson, Loper, Sato, Waterman & Waxman, 1991; Gonzalez, 1992). They are responsible for the metabolism of a wide range of endogenous and foreign compounds, and in man the transformation of many drugs and chemical carcinogens is mediated by the P450 system. Oxidative metabolism by cytochrome P450 has been implicated in the pathogenesis of cancer and is known to form carcinogen metabolites from xenobiotics such as polycyclic aromatic hydrocarbons e.g.

benzo[a]pyrene and the mycotoxin AFB_1 see (Guengerich, 1988). Since the activation of potentially toxic substances and procarcinogens to their respective reactive forms is mediated by specific form(s) of the cytochrome P450 enzymes, their relative expression will affect the amount generated or the rate of generation of the reactive intermediates.

Considerable evidence suggests that changes in P450 composition can affect *in vitro* and *in vivo* metabolism of drugs in both animals and humans, but the evidence is less clear in the case of carcinogens. Supporting data have come from different lines of research. Animals with genetic predisposition for an altered cytochrome P450 composition enhanced tumour formation when challenged with some carcinogens. These tumours include lung tumour associated with 3-methylcholanthrene, leukaemias (benzo[a]pyrene, 3-methylcholanthrene), brain tumour (3-methylcholanthrene) and lymphomas (dimethylbenz[a]anthracene) (Nebert, Atlas, Guenthner & Kouri, 1978; Levitt, Fysh, Jensen & Nebert, 1979; Nebert, 1981). Evidence for the association of cancer risk with P450 composition in humans is less well developed. A major line of investigation involved correlation of cancer risk with drug oxidation polymorphisms in humans. Idle *et al.* reported a possible relationship between the *in vivo* rate of debrisoquine 4-hydroxylation and the incidence of liver cancer in Nigerians, suggesting an aetiological role involving the metabolic activation of AFB_1 (Idle, Mahgoub, Sloan, Smith, Mbanefo & Bababunmi, 1981), but the role of debrisoquine 4-hydroxylase in AFB_1 activation has not been established or supported. Extensive metabolisers of debrisoquine were also shown to have a significantly elevated risk of lung cancer (Idle, 1989). On the other hand, in a more recent study, increased risk of lung cancer was not seen in extensive metabolisers of debrisoquine, but paradoxically a significantly increased proportion of poor metabolisers was seen in leukaemia, bladder cancer and melanoma patients (Wolf, Smith, Gough, Moss, Vallis, Howard, Carey, Mills, McNee, Carmichael & Spurr, 1992). These associations suggest CYP2D6 (nomenclature according to Nebert (Nebert *et al.*, 1991)), the cytochrome P450 enzyme catalysing the 4-hydroxylation of debrisoquine, is either directly involved in carcinogen detoxification and carcinogenesis or that the gene encoding this protein is in linkage with another cancer-causing gene. Recent studies revealed that the recovery of the oxidative metabolites of paracetamol in the 24 hour urine collection was much increased among patients with hepatocellular carcinoma, compared to healthy subjects and other patients with chronic liver diseases (Leung & Critchley, 1991), and among patients with bladder carcinoma (Dolara, Lodovici, Salvadori, Saltutti, Delle Rose, Selli & Kriebel, 1988). It was thought that an increased capability of forming the reactive intermediate of paracetamol, through the catalytic actions of specific cytochrome P450s, might predispose an individual to these cancers. A major challenge still lies ahead in the research of P450 isoenzymes in order to understand their role in chemical carcinogenesis, and to determine the relative contribution of genetic and environmental factors in an individual's capacity to metabolize and activate carcinogens. Biochemical and immunological methods and molecular genetic approaches have been suggested to be the tools that can be employed today for pursuit in this area (Miles & Wolf, 1991).

1.2 Hepatocellular carcinoma

1.2.1 Epidemiology

Benign and malignant tumours may arise in the liver from the hepatocytes, bile duct epithelium or the supporting mesenchymal tissue. All are rare except hepatocellular carcinoma (HCC) (Christopherson & Mays, 1987). HCC occurs either as a single mass or as scattered nodules of tumours. Around 80% have pre-existing cirrhosis. The tumour tends to invade the portal and hepatic veins and spreads to the abdominal lymph-nodes and bones. Histologically, the tumour is typically composed of cells resembling hepatocytes.

HCC is uncommon in the United States, United Kingdom and the countries of North Europe. But in other geographic areas, it ranks as one of the most common of all malignant neoplasms, at least in the male population. Areas of high incidence include Southeast Asia, the Western Pacific and Sub-Saharan Africa. Worldwide it has been estimated that over 1,000,000 new cases occur each year (London, 1981). The estimates of the frequency of HCC and its epidemiology have probably been underestimated due to by the difficulties in definitive diagnosis and correct classification of the cancer.

There are striking geographic and racial variations in the occurrence of HCC and it is found most commonly in developing countries. The global picture is best defined by the grouping of countries or populations into:

(1) very high rates (> 20 per 100,000 males per year)
(2) intermediate rates
(3) low rates (< 5 per 100,000 males per year)

The occurence of HCC, according to different incidences, reported from different countries is list in Table 1.1. Another feature to illustrate this range of occurrence is that HCC is the most common cancer seen in Mozambique and Taiwan, the third most common in China and Hong Kong, but ranks only 22nd in the U.S.A.

Table 1.1   Global distribution of hepatocellular carcinoma

1. Very high rate (> 20/100,000 males per year)
   China
   Southeast Asia
   West and Southern Africa
   Chinese population in Hong Kong
   Taiwan
   Singapore
2. Intermediate rate (5–20/100,000 males per year)
   Japan
   Southern Europe
   Bulgaria, Poland, Yugoslavia, France, Hungary,
   Czechoslovakis, Belgium and Austria
   New Zealand Maoris
   Hawaiians
   Chinese in the U.S.
3. Low rate (< 5/100,000 males per year)
   U.K.
   U.S.A.
   Canada
   Australia
   Israel
   Scandinavia
   Latin America
   India
   New Zealand non-Maori

(Adapted from Linsell, 1987).

There is also considerable within-country variation, particularly in large countries such as China. Here the incidence is much higher in the northeast, east coastal area and southeast areas.

Worldwide there are more males with HCC than females. Among Chinese and Africans, the ratio is about 4:1, but in Caucasians, there is only at most a twofold difference. Chinese immigrants in the U.S.A. retain this male excess risk. It is of patho-aetiological interest that immune response to infections by the hepatitis B virus (HBV), as measured by the presence of antigens and antibodies does not demonstrate such a marked sex difference. Females generally remain carriers for a shorter period of time compared to males suggesting they deal more efficiently with the viral infection (Linsell, 1987).

In all populations, the incidence increases with age. In countries of high incidence, there is a marked shift to the younger age groups. In Africa the average age is around 40 years of age and in Asia around 50 years of age. In Mozambique, the incidence in 25–34 year old males was 500 times the equivalent white population in the U.S.A. or the U.K.. However, in the 65-plus group, this excess decreased to 15 times (Linsell, 1987).

Hong Kong is also considered an endemic area for HCC where it is currently the 2nd commonest cancer death in Hong Kong, after lung cancer. According to the 1984 Cancer Registry published by the Hong Kong Government, there are more than 1,000 new cases of HCC registered the incidence rate was 28.6/100,000 for the male and 7.7/100,000 for the female (Medical and Health Department Hong Kong Government, 1984). A total of 1,000 cases were registered in the year with a male to female ratio of 4 to 1 and it accounted for 7.5% of all the cancer cases seen in Hong Kong. The incidence has nearly doubled in just over 20 years from 16.9/100,000 per year for males in 1965 to 28.4/10,000 in 1987 (The Federation of Medical Societies, 1989) (see Table 1.2).

Hong Kong lies in an endemic area of HCC along with the southeast coast of China, where the incidence is particularly high in the provinces Shanghai, Guangxi, Fujian, Jiangsu and Guangdong. In Hong Kong, the median age of presentation is around 50, a relatively young age compared to other cancers such as colon and lung cancers and the mortality rate tends to level out in the older age group. Most patients present late with hepatomegaly with an overall median survival of about 8 weeks if treatment cannot be instituted. If some treatment can be offered, including surgery and chemotherapy, the median survival can be prolonged to 18 weeks (Shiu, Dewar, Leung, Leung, Chan, Tao, Lui, Chan, Lau & Metreweli, 1990).

1.2.2   Aetiological factors

Although the exact mechanisms of neoplastic transformation in HCC are still far from being fully understood, several factors have been strongly associated with the incidence of HCC and incriminated as aetiologic factors. These include:

Table 1.2   Incidence of hepatocellular carcinoma in Hong Kong

> 1,000 new cases per year

2nd commonest cancer death

♂ ♂ ♂ ♂   ♀

Median age   50

Median survival   8 weeks

	per 100,000 (male)/year
1965	16.9
1978	27.2
1984	27.9
1987	28.4

1. HBV infection
2. Cirrhosis
3. Aflatoxins
4. Cigarette smoking
5. Alcohol
6. Non-A Non-B hepatitis infection

1.2.2.1 Hepatitis B virus infection

Much evidence has accumulated during the last two decades in support of a aetiological role of HBV in the development of HCC. The most important data came from epidemiology studies and research in the molecular biology area.

Epidemiology

There is a geographic correlation between the incidence of HCC and the prevalence of chronic HBV infection. The global pattern of the carriage of HBsAg follows closely the division of HCC into high, intermediate and low areas (Linsell, 1987). There are estimated to be around 300 million chronic hepatitis B surface antigen carriers in the world. Correlation studies have demonstrated that there is a strong positive correlation between the incidence of HCC with the prevalence of the carrier state of the HBV surface antigen (HBsAg). Southeast Asia and sub-Saharan Africa which have very high HBsAg prevalence rates (over 10%), also have the highest incidence of HCC. On the other hand, the low incidence of HCC in Northern Europe, N. America and Australia correspond with a low HBsAg carrier rate in these areas (Lau & Lai, 1990). This is depicted in Table 1.3.

This close association between HCC and HBsAg carriers also applies to areas within a single country. In China, provinces south of the Yangtze river have a higher incidence of HBsAg carriage and HCC than those north of the river. However, this relationship is not consistently found in countries where HCC has a low overall incidence. In the U.S.A. and Australia, the HCC rates are higher than the overall HBsAg carrier rates. It

Table 1.3 Death rates from hepatocellular carcinoma, and incidence of HBsAg in healthy carriers and in cases of HCC by countries/places

Country/Place	Standardised death rate of HCC per 100,000 in males	HBsAg carrier (%)	HBsAg in HCC (%)
Hong Kong	38.9	10.0	82.0
Singapore (Chinese)	31.0	6.6	35.3
Philippines	—	15.5	70.0
China	19.6	14.5	86.0
Taiwan	—	12.5	70.3
Japan	12.5	2.6	40.3
Thailand	4.1	9.8	71.4
India	3.1	3.2	41.2
S. Africa (Bantu)	19.2	9.0	61.6
Uganda	6.5	6.5	55.2
Senegal	—	11.7	61.2
Greece	16.8	4.7	63.1
Italy	10.7	3.0	66.0
Spain	10.4	0.3	35.0
Britain	2.0	1.4	47.4
Greenland	2.4*	10.0[+]	—
U.S.A.	1.4	0.3	17.0
Australia	1.4	0.2	40.0

* standardised death rate for primary liver cancers which include hepatocellular carcinomas, cholangiocarcinoma and hepatoblastomas.
[+] between 10–20 years old
(Adapted from Lau and Lai, 1990).

was suggested that this may be related to high risk ethnic immigrants such as Chinese in the U.S.A. (Lau & Lai, 1990). Greenland and Chile, on the other hand, have high HBsAg carrier rates but much lower than expected incidence of HCC. In the global sense, the incidence of HBV markers is consistently higher in HCC patients than in control populations from the same areas. This is also shown in a number of case control studies where the relative risks and attributable risks were estimated to be much increased (Table 1.4). A large cohort study involving 22,707 subjects from Taiwan showed a relative risk of 217 for HBsAg carriers and a attributable risk of 93.9% (Beasley, Huang & Lin, 1981). The lack of association between HBV with other cancers and metastatic liver cancer suggests that this association is also specific.

Table 1.4   Case-control studies on HBsAg and HCC

Study population	No. of subjects		HBsAg + (%)		Relative risk	Attributable risk (%)
	HCC	Controls	HCC	Controls		
Hong Kong	107	107	82.0	18.0	21.3	78.5
China	50	50	86.0	22.0	17.0	77.9
Philippines	104	84	70.0	18.0	10.8	63.9
Greece	184	451	45.9	7.3	10.7	41.6
Senegal	165	328	61.2	11.3	12.4	56.3
S. Africa	289	213	61.6	11.3	12.6	56.7
U.S.A.	86	161	17.9	0.0	17.0	—

(Adapted from Lau and Lai, 1990).

Molecular biology

According to Zuckerman (Zuckerman, 1974), five criteria should be fulfilled for the establishment of the oncogenic role of a virus:

(i)   the infection must precede oncogenesis
(ii) the tumour cells must contain antigens specific for the virus
(iii) the tumour cells can produce the viral agent
(iv) the virus can cause malignant transformation
(v)   active immunization against the virus will reduce the incidence of the tumour

Evidence in support of these criteria has accumulated for the oncogenic role of HBV in the development of HCC from different aspects of research. The epidemiology data presented above indicated that in endemic areas, HBV infection preceded the development of HCC.

In patients with HCC, HBsAg can commonly be demonstrated with histochemical stains or immunological techniques in the cytoplasm of non-malignant hepatocytes (Wu, 1978), sometimes core antigen (HBcAg) is also identified in the nuclei (Nayak, Dhar, Sachdeva, Mittal, Seth, Sudarsanam, Reddy, Wagholikar & Reddy, 1977). In a study done on 566 patients with liver disease from Hong Kong, HBsAg was identified in the liver in 50% of the patients with cirrhosis alone, 39% of HCC alone but 83% with HCC and cirrhosis (Gibson, Wu, Ho & Lauder, 1980).

Hepatoma cell lines have been derived from HBV carriers with HCC. They are found to secrete HBsAg and were shown to have integrated HBV DNA (Ho, Wu & Mak, 1981). Integrated HBV DNA were also found in the liver of patients with chronic hepatitis and HCC. This was demonstrated in HCC patients from China, southern and west Africa, France, Greece and the U.S.A.. These data are consistent with the intepretation that integration of HBV DNA into the liver cell genome preceded the development of HCC (Linsell, 1987). HBV DNA was found in tumour tissue of HCC patients, even when they have no detectable HBV marker in their serum (Bréchot, Degos, Lugassy, Thiers, Zafrani, Franco, Bismuth, Trepo, Benhamou & Wands, 1985). These further support other points in Zuckerman's criteria that the tumour cells *can* produce the viral agent and it can cause malignant transformation. A number of endemic countries, including Hong Kong and Taiwan, are carrying out vaccination programmes for high risk people and all newborn infants. These programmes will hopefully provide further support for the oncogenic role of HBV if the incidence of HCC turns out to be reduced by active immunization.

Animal models

The association of HBV with the development of HCC is also seen among other animal species. Hepatitis B-like viruses have been identified in animals, including Eastern woodchucks, ground squirrels and Pekin ducks. These viruses have the same morphology and genomic organisation as human HBV but do not infect human. In the woodchuck, acute and chronic hepatitis as well as HCC have frequently been observed. In one study, woodchucks raised in the absence of external cocarcinogens were found to develop HCC as well (Popper, Roth, Purcell, Tennant & Gerin, 1987).

The following comment was issued by the World Health Organisation and illustrate the strong association of HBV with HCC: *"All the published evidence is consistent with the interpretation that integration of HBV DNA into the genome of the hepatocyte precedes the development of hepatocellular carcinoma by months or years. Although these studies do not prove that HBV is oncogenic, the finding of HBV DNA in many patients with HCC and in all patients with HCC with markers of the virus is highly suggestive."*

Although the above points are highly supportive of the causal role of HBV in HCC, there are data from other studies indicating that other factors are involved:

1. Some geographical areas with a high HBsAg positive rate do not have a correspondingly high HCC rate e.g. Greenland Eskimos (Melbye, Skinhoj, Nielsen, Vestergaard, Ebbesen, Hansen & Biggar, 1984). Furthermore, in Nigeria, the prevalence rates of HBV carriers are nearly identical in males and females, yet HCC occurs 5 times more frequently in the male than in the female, indicating some other factors are likely to be at relevant in this population (Ayoola, 1984).

2. A small proportion of HCC patients is negative for all HBV serologic markers and no HBV DNA integration can be demonstrated in the genome of their HCCs.

3. In Japan, the prevalence of HBsAg is declining but the frequency of HCC has tripled during the last 15 years. Non-A Non-B hepatitis virus has been suggested as a causative agent (Okuda, Isaburo, Hanai & Urano, 1987).

4. HCC in Africa presents at comparatively young age when compared to Asians. The role played by environmental factors e.g. other carcinogens in rural areas seems to be contributory.

5. In the U.K., a prospective study of 613 HCC patients showed that cirrhosis, but not HBsAg positivity was the major risk factor (Zaman, Melia, Johnson, Portman, Johnson & Williams, 1985).

6. No oncogenes have yet been incriminated despite active research.

1.2.2.2 Cirrhosis

Cirrhosis is a common accompanying feature of HCC, occurring in 60–90% of HCC cases. It has been shown that different forms of cirrhosis carry varying risks in the development of HCC. In a prospective study of

613 HCC patients carried out in the U.K., cirrhosis was shown to be the major risk factor for the development of HCC and that HBsAg carriage was only important because it was a cause of cirrhosis. In this group, alcoholism was a more important cause of cirrhosis than HBV infection (Zaman *et al.*, 1985). However, it was commented that since patients without previous symptomatic cirrhosis were not included in this study, the validity of the conclusions should be taken with reservation as it is well documented that the majority of HCC is associated with asymptomatic cirrhosis (Lau & Lai, 1990). However, from two other studies, it was shown that the presence of cirrhosis increased the relative risk of the development of HCC in HBsAg-positive patients (Gibson *et al.*, 1980; Beasley *et al.*, 1981).

Several mechanisms have been suggested for the role played by cirrhosis in the development of HCC. It has been suggested that due to various aetiologies including viral infection and hepatocarcinogens, resistant hepatocytes undergo proliferation and regeneration accompanying the chronic necroinflammatory changes, leading to cirrhosis. These resistant hepatocytes become preneoplastic or neoplastic and undergo selective clonal cell expansion (Harris & Sun, 1984). This is supported by the finding in woodchucks that necroinflammation precedes the development of HCC (Popper *et al.*, 1987). An alternative mechanism is that the metabolic activation of hepatocarcinogens may be enhanced or their detoxification impaired in cirrhotic liver tissues, predisposing the individual to the carcinogenicity of these environmental agents (Lau & Lai, 1990).

1.2.2.3 Aflatoxins

Many chemicals both naturally occurring and synthetic, have been shown to produce HCC in animal experiments but man is exposed to only a few of these potential carcinogens. Mycotoxins are produced by fungi on cereals and other foods which have been harvested and stored under hot and humid conditions. It is now clear that aflatoxins are the only members of this group for which there is sufficient evidence of hepatocarcinogenesis in man. Amongst the four major members of this group of mycotoxins, AFB_1 is the most toxic and carcinogenic. Its hepatotoxicity and hepatocarcinogenicity are well documented in many animal models and in humans (see Section 3.1.4). Evidence of aflatoxin induced cancer risk in man has been issued by various institutions including the International Agency for Research on Cancer (IARC) and World Health Organisation (WHO)

(IARC, 1976; World Health Organization Task Group on Environmental Health Criteria for Mycotoxins, 1979; IARC, 1987).

Correlation studies between the dietary intake of AFB_1 and the incidence of HCC have been done (Table 1.5). Although comparisons between these studies is not directly relevant as the methods employed for the analyses were different, these studies all showed a direct positive correlation between AFB_1 exposure and the incidence of HCC. Biochemical and molecular epidemiological data in support of AFB_1 as a human hepatocarcinogen have been obtained from a number of countries including The People's Republic of China, Swaiziland and Kenya (see Section 3.1.5 for detail review).

1.2.2.4 Other factors

Some studies have shown increased incidence of HCC amongst smokers but no dose-response relationship has yet been demonstrated (Garfinkel,

Table 1.5 Epidemiological data supporting a dose-dependent relationship between aflatoxin and hepatocellular carcinoma incidence

Country	Area	Aflatoxin intake $(ng\ kg^{-1}\ day^{-1})$*	Hepatoceullar carcinoma	
			Number of cases	Incidence $(no./10^5$ population per year)[+]
Kenya	High altitude	3.5	4	1.23
Thailand	Songkhla	5.0	2	2.00
Swaziland	High veld	5.2	11	2.18
Kenya	Middle altitude	5.9	33	2.51
Swaziland	Mid veld	8.9	29	3.83
Kenya	Low altitude	10.0	49	4.01
Swaziland	Lebombo	15.4	4	4.27
Thailand	Ratburi	45.0	6	6.00
Swaziland	Low veld	43.1	42	9.18
Mozambique	Inhambane	222.1	101	16.1–25.4

Study period: 1 year in Thailand, 3 years in Mozambique and 4 years in Kenya and Swaziland.
* Estimated average daily intake expressed as ng of aflatoxin per kg of body weight.
[+] Incidence expressed as number of new cases per 100,000 population per year.
(Adapted from Peer and Linsell, 1977).

1980; Oshima, Tsukuma, Hiyama, Fujimoto, Yamano & Tanaka, 1984). A report from Hong Kong indicated a relative risk of 3.3 of developing HCC among heavy smokers who are non-HBsAg carriers, compared to light and non-smokers (Lam, Yu, Leung & Henderson, 1982). This was taken to indicate that HBV infection and cigarette smoking were independent risk factor for HCC. However, other reports have showed no correlation between cigarette smoking and HCC incidence (Stemhagen, Slade, Altman & Bill, 1983; Austin, Delzell, Grufferman, Levine, Morrison, Stolley & Cole, 1986).

Conflicting reports on the correlation between alcohol consumption and incidence of HCC are also found. There is no experimental evidence that alcohol is carcinogenic but some retrospective studies did show that a dose-dependent trend exists (Stemhagen *et al.*, 1983; Austin *et al.*, 1986). Nevertheless, the fact that only a proportion of alcoholics develop chronic liver disease and an even smaller proportion of them develop HCC seems to indicate that ethanol consumption alone is not a strong aetiologic factor in HCC. It is likely that alcohol is related to the development of HCC through hepatic cirrhosis and/or when there is coexisting chronic HBV infection (Lau & Lai, 1990).

In Japan, prevalence of HBsAg is declining but the frequency of HCC has tripled during the last 15 years. Non-A Non-B hepatitis virus has been suggested as a causative agent (Okuda *et al.*, 1987). Infection by Non-A Non-B hepatitis virus typically occurs following blood transfusion. The time interval between the acute hepatitis to the development of HCC was found to be around 15–18 years. About 40% of the HCC cases in Japan had a history of past blood transfusion with an average time lapse of 20 years.

It is now known that most of the post-transfusional Non-A Non-B hepatitis are caused by Hepatitis C. The disease progresses to chronic hepatitis in up to 50% of patients acutely infected and 20% to cirrhosis. Advances in molecular biology have improved the accuracy of diagnosis and an assay for antibody to HCV has been developed (Choo, Kuo, Weiner, Overby, Bradley & Houghton, 1989). Its aetiologic role in HCC was discussed and reviewed in recently (Tabor & Kobayashi, 1992).

1.2.2.5 Summary

The mechanism of hepatocarcinogenesis is still far from clear but there are certain identifiable aetiologic factors associated with the development of

HCC. These include infection by HBV, possible hepatocarcinogens with AFB_1 being most frequently implicated, liver cirrhosis, alcohol consumption and other hepatitis viruses. A multi-factorial aetiology is favoured whereby synergism between such factors is important (Ayoola, 1984; Harris & Sun, 1984). Following insult to hepatocytes viruses, alcohol and/ or carcinogens, infected or injured cells will be eliminated rapidly. However, during transition to chronicity, resistant cells become preneoplastic/ neoplastic with integrated HBV genetic material or mutated due to adduct formation with carcinogens e.g. AFB_1, leading to mutational hot spots (Bressac, Kew, Wands & Ozturk, 1991; Harris, 1991; Hsu, Metcalf, Sun, Welsh, Wang & Harris, 1991). Cirrhosis often accompanies the proliferative stage of cellular repair and may cause more random viral integration and cellular gene expression (Lau & Lai, 1990). This may also predispose the hepatocytes to hepatocarcinogens due to altered metabolic activation of these agents or an impairment of their detoxification.

1.3 Study objectives

The theme of this PhD thesis is on the metabolic activation of drugs and carcinogens in relation to toxicity and carcinogenesis. The interest in this area in The Department of Clinical Pharmacology stemmed from the findings of a previous study that showed a significantly increased percentage of oxidative metabolites of an oral 1.5 g dose of paracetamol in the 24 hour urine from patients with hepatocellular carcinoma (Leung & Critchley, 1991). The percentage recovery of these oxidative metabolites, the mercapturate and cysteine conjugates of paracetamol, is an index of the metabolic activation of paracetamol *in vivo*. A small proportion of patients with chronic hepatitis also had evidence of increased metabolic activation of paracetamol and this complemented earlier work which showed increased metabolic activation in some Caucasian chronic alcoholics (Critchley, Cregeen, Balali-Mood, Pentland & Prescott, 1982). Although the most likely explanation for the increased fractional recovery of oxidative metabolites is increased activity of the cytochrome P450 enzymes, another possibility is impairment of the major pathways of metabolism i.e. glucuronide and sulphate conjugation. Reduced capacity for conjugation would slow up the elimination of paracetamol from the blood maintaining high concentrations for longer and promote paracetamol clearance through the cytochrome P450 pathway. However, if the latter explanation for increased oxidative metabolism was the case, then plasma paracetamol half lives would be correspondingly longer in patients with high urinary recoveries of oxidative metabolites. In our studies based solely on 24 hour urine collections, we could not not calculate plasma paracetamol half lives directly whether they were significantly altered in the HCC patients, but they could be estimated indirectly. For subjects with normal renal function, the renal excretion of unchanged paracetamol will be a direct function of the area under the plasma concentration-time curve (AUC) which in turn is a direct function of the plasma paracetamol half-life. There was no evidence of a significantly increased fractional urinary recovery of unchanged paracetamol in the HCC patients in our study with increased recoveries of the oxidative metabolites. Thus, the increased formation of oxidative metabolites does not appear to be due to impairment of the major conjugation pathways with an associated prolongation of plasma paracetamol half life.

However, studies were clearly required involving measurement of plasma concentrations as well as urinary recoveries in order to confirm (or refute) the above assumptions. We would hope to show whether patients with evidence of increased metabolic activation have normal or prolonged plasma paracetamol half-lives and also confirm that there is a close relationship between plasma paracetamol half life, the AUC and the urinary recovery of unchanged paracetamol. One of the areas of interests we would like to address is thus the full pharmacokinetics of paracetamol in these patients with HCC and the differences, if any, from healthy subjects and patients with other liver diseases. The results from this pharmacokinetic study will help explain the mechanism of the increased metabolic activation of paracetamol in HCC patients and hopefully may shed light on the cause and significance of this finding.

The aflatoxins, especially AFB_1, have been implicated as human carcinogens which play an aetiologic role in HCC. Although there is little information on the dietary exposure to AFB_1 in Hong Kong, our neighbouring provinces in China along the southeast coast, particularly Guangdong, Fujian, Jiangsu, Guangxi and Shanghai, have a high incidence of both HCC and dietary AFB_1 exposure. It is also of great interest that metabolic activation is a prerequisite for the toxicity and carcinogenicity of AFB_1. Another objective of this project to make an attempt to demonstrate any difference in the metabolic activation of AFB_1 by subjects with and without liver diseases, including chronic HBV infection, and patients with HCC. It may provide some clarification on the possible aetiologic role of AFB_1 in HCC in Hong Kong. Since there is no information available on the biochemical or molecular epidemiology of aflatoxins in Hong Kong, a study method that would provide information on both AFB_1 exposure and its *in vivo* metabolic activation was favoured. The other main task of this project was the development of a method to monitor AFB_1-albumin adducts in human serum. If findings reveal modified metabolic activation of AFB_1 by patients with liver diseases or HCC, it is hoped that further research can be pursued to elucidate any correlation with the increased metabolic activation of paracetamol in these same groups of patients.

CHAPTER 2

The Metabolism of Paracetamol in Healthy Subjects and in Patients with Liver Diseases and Hepatocellular Carcinoma

2.1 Introduction

2.1.1 History of paracetamol

Derivatives of aniline were first used in the mid 19th century for their antipyretic effect. Acetanilide was produced from the acetylation of aniline and its introduction into medicine was the result of serendipity (Insel, 1992). It was believed that naphthalene, under investigation for the treatment of intestinal parasites, was substituted by mistake with acetanilide and its antipyretic properties revealed. Within a short time, acetanilide was introduced for clinical use as an antipyretic which stimulated interest in other aniline derivates and phenacetin was introduced the following year in 1887 (Spooner & Harvey, 1976).

The use of paracetamol (N-acetyl-p-aminophenol) was first reported in 1893 by von Mehring (Spooner & Harvey, 1976) who concluded that because of its haemotological side effects of methaemoglobinaemia, it could not be recommended despite prompt antipyretic and analgesic actions. Thus acetanilide and phenacetin were the preparations predominantly used for the relief of fever well into the 20th century and by which time they were also being used for the relief of mild to moderate pain.

It was not until the late 1940's when Brodie and his colleagues started to investigate the metabolism of acetanilide (Brodie & Axelrod, 1948) and phenacetin (Brodie & Axelrod, 1949) that the interest in paracetamol was revived. Their investigations showed that both acetanilide and phenacetin were metabolised into paracetamol and to which they owed their antipyretic and analgesic properties. The chemical structures of paracetamol and related compounds are shown in Fig. 2.1. It was found that the methaemoglobin forming side effects initially associated with paracetamol was due to contamination with p-phenetidine, another meta-bolite of phenacetin, and paracetamol was devoid of this side effect (Brodie & Axelrod, 1949). Thus, it was concluded that paracetamol was an effective analgesic and antipyretic agent which did not have the haematological side effects of acetanilide and phenacetin.

Figure 2.1   Chemical Structure of Paracetamol and Related Compounds

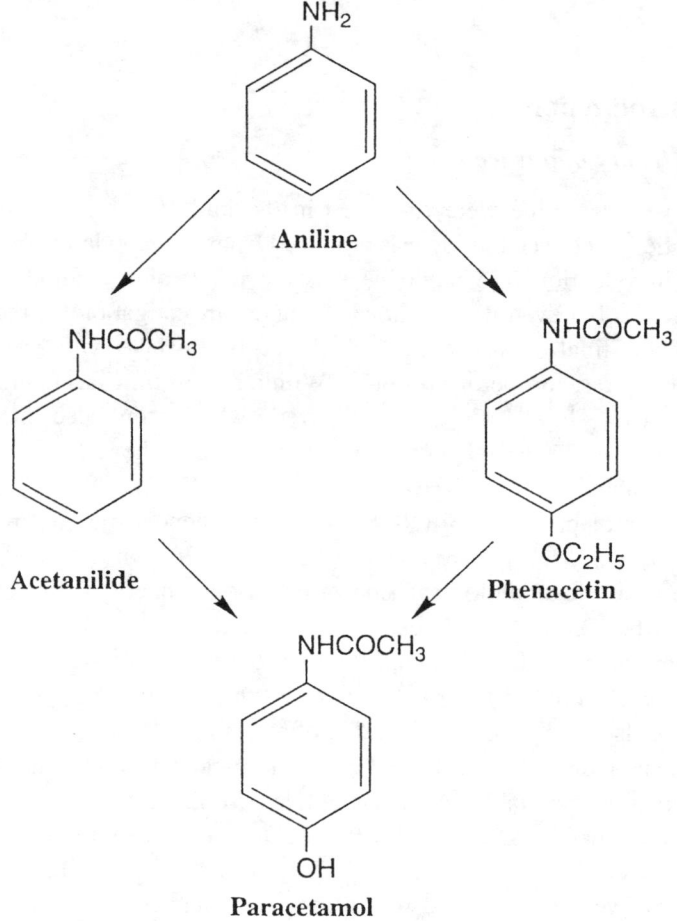

Paracetamol was first introduced in Britain in 1956 as the branded product Panadol, each tablet containing 500 mg of paracetamol. It slowly gained acceptance and was first included in the British Pharmacopoeia in 1963. Ever since, the consumption of paracetamol has steadily risen annually, at the expense of the use of aspirin preparations. Phenacetin was condemned as the causative agent of analgesic nephropathy (Prescott, 1982) which combined with an apparent lack of therapeutic advantage over paracetamol lead to its virtual commercial demise (Clissold, 1986). Branded combination products of paracetamol with codeine, dihydrocodeine, dextropropoxyphene and pentazocine were also introduced, as well as a large number of generic paracetamol preparations. The extent of the use of paracetamol and its world-wide acceptance reflects its safety and effectiveness in normal and proper therapeutic use.

When used in the recommended therapeutic dosage, paracetamol is a safe and effective analgesic for mild to moderate pain and also possesses an antipyretic action. It is well tolerated and produces few side effects (BNF, 1993). The most commonly reported adverse effect is hepatotoxicity which occurs following an acute overdosage. It damages the liver through the formation of a reactive intermediate. The mechanism by which paracetamol exerts its hepatotoxicity was elucidated by Mitchell and colleagues (Jollow, Mitchell, Potter, Davis, Gillette & Brodie, 1973; Mitchell, Jollow, Potter, Davis, Gillette & Brodie, 1973a; Potter, Davis, Mitchell, Jollow, Gillette & Brodie, 1973). A small proportion of paracetamol is metabolised by the mixed function oxidases, cytochrome P450, to an electrophilic reactive intermediate. Normally this is inactivated by conjugation with reduced glutathione and further metabolised and excreted as the cysteine and mercapturate conjugates in the urine. When the store of glutathione is exhausted, such as following overdosage, this toxic reactive metabolite binds covalently to other nucleophiles such as vital cell elements resulting in liver necrosis.

The elucidation of the metabolic pathways of paracetamol and its mechanism of hepatotoxicity allowed a rational approach to the treatment of paracetamol poisoning. Glutathione precursors and other sulphydryl compounds have been used with success in this respect (Prescott, 1983).

2.1.2 *Pharmacology of paracetamol*

Paracetamol has analgesic and antipyretic effects and an efficacy similar to aspirin. It is indicated for mild to moderate pain and is well tolerated in both adults and children. However, it has weak anti-inflammatory effects which can only be demonstrated in animal models at doses considerably in excess of those required for analgesia (Insel, 1992). It has not been satisfactorily established why paracetamol is an effective analgesic but only a weak anti-inflammatory agent. The exact mechanisms of pain, fever and inflammation are not fully understood and the explanations for the actions of antipyretic analgesics are also incomplete. It has been suggested that both the release of CNS prostaglandins, involving central pain circuits, as well as sensitisation of peripheral pain receptors by locally released prostaglandins are involved in inflammatory hyperalgesia. There is some evidence suggesting that paracetamol has a weak inhibitory influence on peripheral prostaglandin biosynthesis but that it is a potent inhibitor of prostaglandin production within the central nervous system; therefore, it lacks substantial anti-inflammatory activity but the inhibition of CNS prostaglandins makes paracetamol an effective analgesic and antipyretic agent (Ferreira & Vane, 1974; Flower, 1974). However, it is not known why central nervous system cyclo-oxygenase is more sensitive to paracetamol than peripheral cyclo-oxygenase.

2.1.3   *Absorption, Distribution, Metabolism and Excretion*

2.1.3.1   Absorption

Paracetamol (molecular weight 151.2) is a moderately water and lipid soluble weak organic acid, with a pKa 9.5. It is largely un-ionised over the physiological range of pH. It is invariably taken by mouth though rectal dosage forms are also available. After oral administration, paracetamol is absorbed rapidly and almost completely (Rawlins, Henderson & Hijab, 1977) from the upper gastro-intestinal tract by passive diffusion. It is only minimally absorbed from the stomach and the more rapid absorption from the small intestine is presumably due to the greater relative surface area. The rate of absorption largely depends on gastric emptying, which can be affected by the presence of food, posture, disease state and the effect of other drugs.

Gastric emptying influences paracetamol absorption directly by controlling the rate at which the drug is delivered to the small intestine (Heading, Nimmo, Prescott & Tothill, 1973). The rate of absorption has been shown to be more rapid in fasting subjects but the concomitant administration of food produces little effect on the extent of absorption, as reflected by the comparable area under the plasma concentration versus time curve

(AUC) (McGilveray & Mattok, 1972). The effect on gastric emptying of food may also be attributed to dilution and possibly adsorption of drug onto food constituents (Prescott, 1974). Posture may inherently affect the gastric emptying rate. Paracetamol absorption seems to be slower during sleep (McGilveray & Mattok, 1972) and has been found to be delayed in subjects lying on the left side, due to slower gastric emptying in this position, compared to standing or lying on the right side (Nimmo, Heading, Tothill & Prescott, 1973; Renwick, Ahsan, Challenor, Daniels, Macklin, Waller & George, 1992). Although t_{max} values are lower, the total amounts absorbed do not differ.

Pharmacological agents have also been demonstrated to affect the rate of paracetamol absorption. Agents which modify gastric emptying including propantheline, metoclopramide and opioids have been shown to have significant effects on its rate of absorption (Nimmo *et al.*, 1973; Nimmo, Heading, Wilson, Tothill & Prescott, 1975). The effect of other disease states, including pyloric stenosis, achlorhydria, coeliac disease and thyroid dysfunction, on paracetamol absorption rate was reviewed by Forrest *et al.* (Forrest, Clements & Prescott, 1982). Gastric emptying has not been shown to be significantly different between young and old volunteers and age did not seem to alter this rate-limiting step in paracetamol absorption (Gainsborough, Maskrey, Nelson, Keating, Sherwood, Jackson & Swift, 1993).

In fasting healthy subjects, the absorption of paracetamol in solution is very rapid with peak plasma concentrations reached within 15-30 minutes (Prescott, 1980). Absorption from tablets is usually slower and the formulation may also influence the rate of absorption (Richter & Smith, 1974; Ameer, Divoll, Abernethy, Greenblatt & Shargel, 1983; Dougall, Cunningham & Nimmo, 1983). Inter-individual variation in paracetamol absorption, possibly governed by the rate of gastric emptying, can be a consideration (McGilveray & Mattok, 1972; Prescott, 1974; Nash, Stein, Penno, Passananti & Vesell, 1984).

Following absorption, the systemic availability is incomplete, a variable proportion being lost through first-pass metabolism. It seems to be dose-dependent, decreasing from nearly 90% after a dose of 1–2 g, to 63% following 0.5 g (Rawlins *et al.*, 1977), although Clements *et al.* found that oral systemic availability was 80% and independent of dose (Clements, Critchley & Prescott, 1984). A gastric emptying study by Clements *et al.* showed that mono-exponential emptying was often preceded by a short period during which a proportion of the dose passed rapidly through the pylorus as a bolus or 'squirt' (Clements, Heading, Nimmo & Prescott, 1978). A pharmacokinetic model was described which takes into account the influence of various rates and patterns of gastric emptying on paracetamol absorption. It describes the biphasic gastric emptying pattern most commonly seen in study subjects, in which a fraction of the total administered dose leaves the stomach rapidly within the first 10–15 minutes, followed by a monoexponential decrease of the remaining fraction. The commonly observed occurrence of two peaks early in the plasma concentration-time curve was said to be due to an interruption in gastric emptying. The first rapid decline in plasma concentration starts at the time when emptying from the stomach temporarily ceases.

2.1.3.2 Distribution

After absorption, paracetamol is rapidly and relatively uniformly distributed throughout most body tissues, achieving a tissue to plasma concentration ratio of near unity (Forrest *et al.*, 1982; Clissold, 1986). In a group of healthy subject, the plasma concentration-time curves following intravenous administration are multiexponential and the initial short half-life (3–19 minutes) indicates a rapid distribution phase (Prescott, 1980). In the same group of subjects, paracetamol was administered orally and after the initial distribution phase, plasma concentrations declined in parallel with those after intravenous administration. The apparent volume of distribution increases from 0.5 l/kg bodyweight immediately after intravenous injection to about 0.9 l/kg after distribution is complete. Generally, this value is similar in healthy subjects, the elderly and various patient groups including patients with epilepsy, Gilbert's syndrome and in anephric patients.

There is no appreciable binding to erythrocytes in man or pigs over the range of plasma concentration of 50–300 g ml^{-1}. Plasma protein binding only occurs at paracetamol concentrations greater than 60 g ml^{-1}. At much higher concentrations, similar to those observed after toxic dose ingestion in man, the drug is bound 15–21% to plasma proteins. The glucuronide and sulphate conjugates of paracetamol do not bind to plasma proteins either (Gazzard, Ford-Hutchinson, Smith & Williams, 1973; Lowenthal, Øie, Van Stone, Briggs & Levy, 1976; Morris & Levy, 1984).

2.1.3.3 Metabolism

Paracetamol is extensively metabolised by the liver and only 2–5% of a therapeutic dose is excreted as the unchanged drug in the urine. As has already been pointed out, this fraction is directly related to the plasma paracetamol AUC. Although metabolism in the gastrointestinal tract has also been observed in rats (Josting, Winne & Bock, 1976) and in man (Rogers, Back & Orme, 1987a), this seems to be an insignificant site of metabolism as the percentage urinary recoveries of both paracetamol and its metabolites following oral and intravenous administration are similar (Clements *et al.*, 1984).

Although paracetamol is almost completely absorbed from the upper gastrointestinal tract, its bioavailability is only about 70–80% (Rawlins *et al.*, 1977; Perucca & Richens, 1979; Clements *et al.*, 1984), being limited by first pass metabolism by the liver. The bioavailability seems to be dose dependent, decreasing from about 89% after a 1 g dose to 63% after a 0.5 g dose (Rawlins *et al.*, 1977), but this was not confirmed by a more recent study (Clements *et al.*, 1984).

The major route of paracetamol metabolism is by conjugation at the hydroxyl group. After a therapeutic dose, the glucuronide and sulphate metabolites account for over 80% of the metabolism. A minor fraction is converted by cytochrome P450-dependent hepatic mixed function oxidases to a highly reactive alkylating metabolite, probably N-acetyl-p-benzoquinoneimine (NAPQI) (Miners & Kissinger, 1979; Dahlin, Miwa, Lu & Nelson, 1984). This metabolite is usually rapidly inactivated by conjugation with reduced hepatic glutathione (GSH), and is eventually eliminated as the cysteine and mercapturate metabolites in the urine.

Unlike glucuronide conjugation, sulphate conjugation of paracetamol is dose dependent and becomes saturated within the therapeutic dose range. The limited capacity of this metabolic route is evident following both oral and intravenous administration (Levy & Yamada, 1971; Clements *et al.*, 1984). The decreased formation of the sulphate conjugate at higher doses of paracetamol is accompanied by a corresponding increase in the extent of glucuronide conjugation. In comparison the percentage recoveries of unchanged paracetamol, its cysteine and mercapturate conjugates are relatively constant within a subject, though there is large inter-subject variation. These metabolic pathways seem relatively unaffected by the dose administered and the route of administration when the dose is within the therapeutic range.

When the dose of paracetamol greatly exceeds the therapeutic range, the ability to inactivate the reactive metabolite by conjugation with GSH becomes limited. Normally, with therapeutic doses, the reactive metabolite is deactivated by conjugation with GSH (Jollow *et al.*, 1973; Mitchell *et al.*, 1973a; Mitchell, Jollow, Potter, Gillette & Brodie, 1973b; Potter *et al.*, 1973). The conjugate is then converted to the cysteine conjugate of paracetamol by loss of glutamyl and glycine moieties, catalysed by glutamyl transferase and dipeptidase respectively. The cysteine conjugate is then acetylated by N-acetyl transferase to form the mercapturate conjugate of paracetamol (Speirs, 1989). After overdosage, the hepatic GSH stores become depleted and the electrophilic reactive intermediate NAPQI, attacks other nucleophiles. The resulting hepatic necrosis is caused by the covalent binding of this reactive species to vital hepatic macromolecules. The major metabolic pathways of paracetamol are summarised in Fig. 2.2.

Other minor metabolites including 3-hydroxy and 3-methoxyparacetamol (Andrews, Bond, Burnett, Saunders & Watson, 1976) and 3-thiomethylparacetamol (Klutch, Levin, Chang, Vane & Conney, 1978) have also been detected in man after therapeutic doses. The 3-methoxyparacetamol metabolite was only found following overdosage (Knox & Jurand, 1977; Knox & Jurand, 1978).

After a therapeutic dose of 20 mg/kg, the excretion of unchanged paracetamol and its metabolites is almost complete within 24 hours. The precentage recoveries of the various metabolites calculated as the percentage of the administered dose of the various metabolites were as follows: unchanged paracetamol 4%, glucuronide 55%, sulphate 30%, cysteine and mercapturate, both 4% (Prescott, 1980). This excretion pattern is altered in overdose patients with only about 10–20% of the total ingested amount being excreted as the sulphate. There is a corresponding increase in the percentage recovery of glucuronide conjugate and unchanged drug in the urine which reflects the limited capacity of the sulphate conjugating metabolic pathway. As the amount of drug remaining in the body decreases, the fractional recovery of paracetamol sulphate progressively increases.

The excretion patterns of the cysteine and mercapturate conjugates remained unchanged in a group of paracetamol overdose patients who did not develop liver damage, irrespective of the antidotal treatments given. These treatments were cysteamine, methionine, N-acetylcysteine and supportive care only. In another group of poisoned patients who developed severe liver damage, there was a significantly increased excretion of cysteine and mercapturate conjugates. The percentage recovery of these two metabolites was twice that from patients without liver damage. This reflects an increased proportion of the dose being converted to the toxic intermediate. At the peak of the excretion of these oxidative metabolites,

Figure 2.2 The Major Metabolic Pathways of Paracetamol

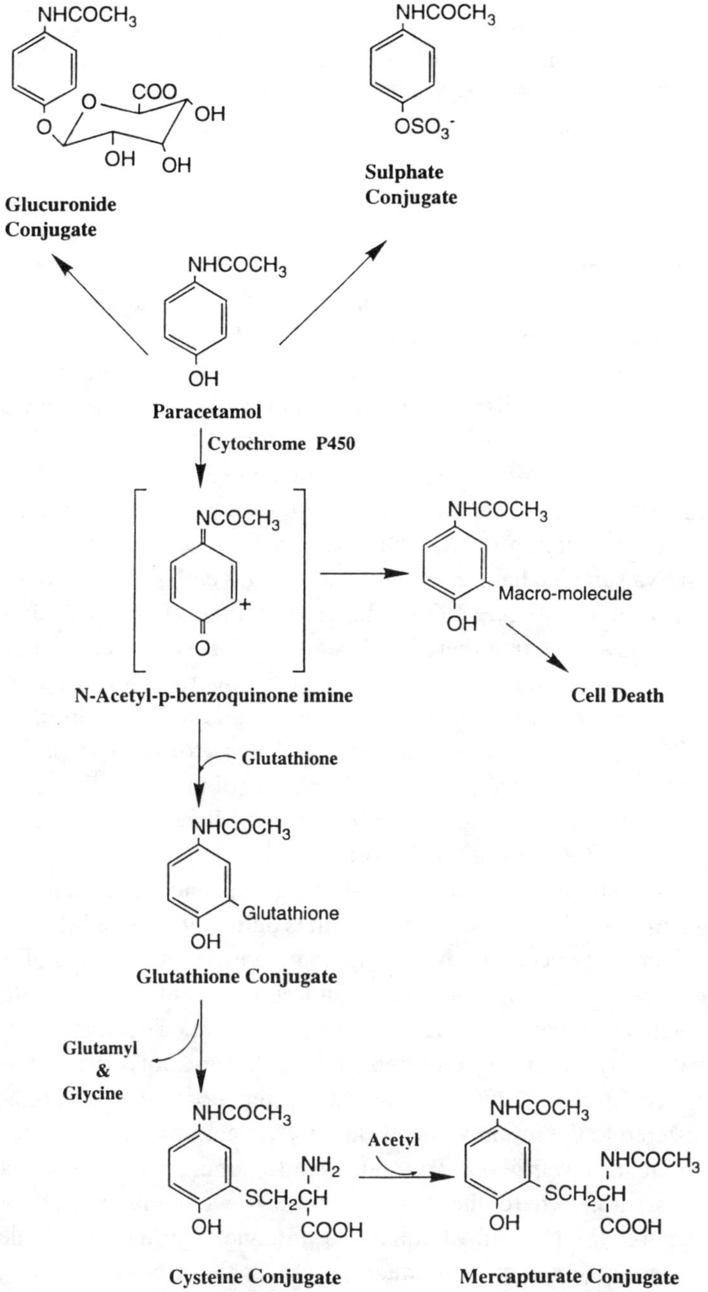
NHCOCH3
COO
O
OH
O
OH
OH
Glucuronide
Conjugate
NHCOCH3
OSO3-
Sulphate
Conjugate
NHCOCH3
OH
Paracetamol
Cytochrome P450
NCOCH3
+
O
N-Acetyl-p-benzoquinone imine
NHCOCH3
Macro-molecule
OH
Cell Death
Glutathione
NHCOCH3
Glutathione
OH
Glutathione Conjugate
Glutamyl
&
Glycine
NHCOCH3
NH2
SCH2CH
OH
COOH
Cysteine Conjugate
Acetyl
NHCOCH3
NHCOCH3
SCH2CH
OH
COOH
Mercapturate Conjugate

which is usually about 30 hours after overdose, they account for up to 20–50% of the total amount of metabolites and unchanged paracetamol excreted (Prescott, 1980).

The mean terminal elimination half-life of paracetamol has been reported to be within 1.5–2.5 hours after therapeutic doses given intravenously (Clements & Prescott, 1976; Rawlins *et al.*, 1977; Perucca & Richens, 1979; Prescott, 1980). Clements and Prescott commented that, depending on the method of weighting of individual data points, there could be wide variations in the value obtained by non-linear regression analysis (Clements & Prescott, 1976). Beyond the absorption phase in oral administration, the plasma concentration of paracetamol decreases in parallel with that beyond the distribution phase after intravenous administration (Prescott, 1980). Rawlins *et al.* reported no difference in the plasma half-life after different oral doses nor between oral and intravenous dosing (Rawlins *et al.*, 1977). The reported total body clearance values are about 5 ml kg^{-1} min^{-1}. The physicochemical properties and pharmacokinetic parameters of paracetamol are shown in Appendix 2.1.

The determination of the pharmacokinetic properties of paracetamol using saliva samples has been evaluated by Lowenthal *et al.* and Maddern *et al.* (Lowenthal *et al.*, 1976; Maddern, Miners, Collins & Jamieson, 1985). It was shown that there is a linear correlation between paracetamol concentrations in saliva and plasma except for the first 1-3 hours when the concentrations in saliva are relatively higher due to retention of some of the orally ingested drug in the oral cavity. The use of salivary paracetamol levels has been widely applied in other pharmcokinetic studies (Mucklow, Fraser, Bulpitt, Kahn, Mould & Dollery, 1980; Miners, Attwood & Birkett, 1983; Miners, Robson & D.J., 1986).

The metabolism of paracetamol is age dependent. In neonates and young children, glucuronide conjugation is deficient. The 'adult' pattern of metabolism of paracetamol was found to be present by 12 years of age, but in children up to the age of 9 years and newborn infants, paracetamol is eliminated principally as the sulphate conjugate. The overall rates of elimination by neonates, children and adults are not different (Miller, Roberts & Fischer, 1976). In this study the dose of paracetamol was administered to the infant subjects directly via a nasogastric tube to ensure an accurate dose was given. In another study, infants received paracetamol via breast milk where the nursing mothers were given oral doses of paracetamol (Notarianni, Oldham & Bennett, 1987). The dose of paracetamol received by individual infant was thus not known and the lag time between paracetamol administration to the mother and breast feeding also differed between individual infants. With varios assumptions on the amount of milk ingested and the time of breast feeding after paracetamol administration to the mother, it was estimated that on average an infant received only 1.1% of the weigt-adjusted maternal single dose. Under such restricted circumstances and assumptions, it was found that the percentage recovery of the sulphate conjugate in the infant's urine was lower than in adult volunteers. There was also increased excretion of the parent drug but there was no significant increase in the excretion of the cysteine and mercapturate metabolites. The authors made the conclusion that there is a deficiency of sulphate conjugation in infants, and that either the formation of the reactive metabolite or its detoxication may be incompletely developed. The interpretation of this study is hampered by the lack of knowledge of the dose, which was very small, received by each infants and the stringent assumptions.

The plasma paracetamol half-life has been noted to be prolonged in geriatric subjects when compared to young, healthy volunteers (Triggs, Nation, Long & Ashley, 1975; Briant, Dorrington, Cleal & Williams, 1976). Triggs *et al.* reported no significant difference in the plasma clearance or the apparent volume of distribution of paracetamol between geriatric and young subjects, whereas Briant *et al.* found the plasma clearance to be lower in geriatric subjects. In a more recent study where fit young subjects were compared with fit elderly subjects and frail elderly subjects, it was found that the elimination half-life was not significantly different between the fit young and fit elderly group but was prolonged in the frail elderly subjects (Wynne, Cope, Herd, Rawlins, James & Wood-house, 1990). Individual liver volume was estimated by ultrasound and paracetamol clearance expressed per unit volume of liver again showed no difference between the fit young and fit elderly subjects but a that of frail elderly subjects was significantly reduced. This study indicates that age-associated changes in paracetamol clearance are attributable to both changes in liver volume and in general health. The total paracetamol clearance per unit volume of liver was found to be similar in the fit young and elderly subjects but was significantly diminished in the frail elderly patients. Since the partial metabolic clearance to the glucuronide metabolite per unit volume of liver was significantly reduced, impairment of glucuronidation was suggested as another explanation of the diminished plasma clearance. An *in vitro* study using liver fractions from subjects of a wide age range (40–89) did not show a fall in glucuronidation and sulphation of paracetamol with increasing age and there was no significant correlation with age for the activity of these enzyme pathways (Herd, Wynne, Wright, James & Woodhouse, 1991). The authors concluded that age *per se* does not have a major effect on the activities of hepatic drug metabolising enzymes and that any age-related decrease in paracetamol clearance, observed in *in vivo* studies, is more likely to reflect reduced liver volume and liver blood flow.

Paracetamol clearance has been shown to be greater in males than females. In one investigation on 8 healthy males and 8 healthy females, paracetamol clearance was 22% greater in males (Miners *et al.*, 1983). In another study of 43 males and 71 females, the clearance in the males was 14% greater (Mucklow *et al.*, 1980). The elimination half-life was not found to be different between the sexes in either study. The difference was found to be entirely due to increased activity of the glucuronidation pathway in males. Sex differences in sulphation or oxidative metabolism have not been found (Miners *et al.*, 1983). Pregnant women seem to have enhanced glucuronidation and oxidation activities (Miners *et al.*, 1986). The apparent oral clearance was found to be 50% higher and the elimination half-life was 28% lower in a group of pregnant women, compared to a group of non-pregnant women of similar age. The metabolic clearances of the glucuronide and oxidative metabolites were 75% and 88% higher respectively in the pregnant group. This may be related to the effect of hormonal control on glucuronidation as similar findings were also noted in females who were oral contraceptive steroid users (Mucklow *et al.*, 1980; Miners *et al.*, 1983). In these women, paracetamol clearance was 49% greater than the control females, with an increase of 78% and 36% in the metabolic clearances of the glucuronide and oxidative metabolites respectively. Although in both the pregnant women study and the oral contraceptive steroid users study, neither metabolic clearance of the sulphate metabolite nor unchanged paracetamol was different from the control females, there is evidence from a study by Critchley *et al.* that there is evidence of increased glucuronide conjugation at the expense of sulphate conjugation, possibly due to competition for sulphation in women taking oral contraceptives (Critchley, Nimmo, Woolhouse & Prescott, 1983a). The authors from the pregnant women study and the oral contraceptive steroid users study concluded that these two groups of females may be under increased risks of developing paracetamol-induced hepatotoxicity and the dosage requirements for effective analgesia may need to be re-evaluated, but whether these findings are of real clinical significance is questionable. At the same time, paracetamol was found to cause an increase in plasma concentrations of ethinyloestradiol, as a result of a reduction in the sulphation of the steroid (Rogers, D.J., Stevenson, Grimmer & Orme, 1987b). Women on oral contraceptive steroids who also regularly take paracetamol, as suggested by the authors, may have higher than required plasma concentrations of the steroid, but again, the clinical significance of this is not known.

Since paracetamol is metabolised to a large extent by hepatic microsomal enzymes, drugs and other environmental factors, which alter the activity of these enzymes will affect paracetamol metabolism. Patients with enzyme induction due to treatment with anticonvulsants and rifampicin have lower plasma paracetamol concentrations, shorter paracetamol half-lives and higher plasma glucuronide concentrations compared to healthy controls (Prescott, Critchley, Balali-Mood & Pentland, 1981). These changes are mirrored in the pattern of urinary metabolite excretion. There are correspondingly lower percentages of unchanged paracetamol and its sulphate conjugate and a higher percentage of the glucuronide conjugate in 24 hour urine collections, but there is no difference in the urinary excretion of the cysteine and mercapturate conjugates. Shorter half-life values have been found in patients on long term antiepileptic treatment (Perucca & Richens, 1979; Prescott *et al.*, 1981; Miners, Attwood & Birkett, 1984). In one study, subjects were pre-treated with phenobarbitone for 5 days and a difference in the half-life value was not observed (Mitchell, Thorgeirsson, Potter, Jollow & Keiser, 1974). As oxidative metabolism has not been shown to be enhanced in patients on antiepileptic treatment, they do not seem to be at higher risk of developing hepatotoxicity from therapeutic doses of paracetamol, though laboratory animals pre-treated with enzyme-inducing agents such as phenobarbitone, 3-methylcholanthrene and ethanol are more susceptible to paracetamol hepatotoxicity (Mitchell *et al.*, 1973a; Jollow, Thorgeirsson, Potter, Hashimoto & Mitchell, 1974; Strubelt, Obermeier & Siegers, 1978; Teschke, Stutz & Strohmeyer, 1979).

The activation of paracetamol by specific cytochrome P450 has not been studied until quite recently except that the oxidative metabolic pathway can be induced or suppressed by pre-treatment with certain drugs. Raucy *et al.* studied the metabolic activation of paracetamol to the reactive intermediate by human liver microsomes. It was found that oxidation by cytochrome P450 CYP2E1 accounts for 52% (range 30–78%) of the metabolic activation of paracetamol and the other major cytochrome P450 enzymes that possesses extensive paracetamol-oxidising capacity is CYP1A2 (Raucy, Lasker, Lieber & Black, 1989).

Pre-treatment with cimetidine, a liver enzyme inhibitor, does not affect the clearance or the individual metabolic pathways of paracetamol (Critchley, Dyson, Scott, Jarvie & Prescott, 1983; Critchley, Scott, Jarvie, Dyson & Prescott, 1983b; Miners *et al.*, 1984), whereas sulphinpyrazone and propranolol pre-treatment increased and decreased paracetamol clearance, respectively (Miners *et al.*, 1984; Baraka, Truman, Ford & Roberts, 1990). Cigarette smoking was found to increase paracetamol clearance in a group of London factory and office workers (Mucklow *et al.*, 1980) but this was not confirmed by Miners *et al.* (Miners *et al.*, 1984). Cigarette smoke contains polycyclic hydrocarbons which are powerful enzyme inducers and paracetamol clearance may be increased due to enhanced glucuronidation activity (Mucklow *et al.*, 1980).

The concomitant use of alcohol can affect the metabolism of paracetamol. In animal studies, chronic administration of ethanol has been shown to increase paracetamol hepatotoxicity due to enhanced microsomal production of the reactive metabolite, whereas acute administration seems to provide some protection against hepatic injury, resulting from its competition for mixed function oxidase (Sato, Matsuda & Lieber, 1981; Maddrey, 1987). Acute administration of ethanol in human subjects also result in reduced urinary recovery of the oxidative metabolites following an oral dose of paracetamol (Critchley *et al.*, 1983; Critchley *et al.*, 1983b). There have been reports of severe liver damage in alcoholic patients who have taken paracetamol in therapeutic doses or doses which are not usually associated with severe hepatotoxicity (Goldfinger, Ahmed, Pitchumoni & Weseley, 1978; Seeff, Cuccherini, Hyman, Zimmerman, Adler & Benjamin, 1986; Florén, Thesleff & Nilsson, 1987). The increased paracetamol hepatotoxicity in people with chronic ethanol consumption may result from both an induced cytochrome P450 mixed function oxidase system and as a depletion of the hepatic GSH store. The latter is also reflected by the common increase of serum gamma glutamyl transferase, an enzyme also responsible for the degradation of GSH, in the alcoholics (Lauterburg & Velez, 1988).

Paracetamol metabolism is not altered in patients with chronic renal diseases. The volume of distribution and elimination half-life values are not significantly different in these patients when compared to healthy volunteers. But the more polar metabolites, the glucuronide and the sulphate, accumulated in the plasma and the apparent volumes of distribution of these metabolites were lower . This also indicates that the kidneys do not contribute significantly to the metabolism of paracetamol (Lowenthal *et al.*, 1976; Prescott, Speirs, Critchley, Temple & Winney, 1989; Martin, Temple, Winney & Prescott, 1991).

In patients with chronic liver disease but normal plasma albumin concentrations and prothrombin time ratio, the plasma paracetamol half-life and clearance is similar to that seen in healthy subjects. But in those patients with cirrhosis who have low plasma albumin and an increased prothrombin time ratio, the elimination of paracetamol is grossly abnormal. The plasma half-life was found to be 4.25 ± 1.15 hours compared with 2.43 ± 0.19 hours in the healthy controls (Forrest, Adriaenssens, Finlayson & Prescott, 1979). A good correlation was demonstrated between the plasma half-life or clearance and the serum albumin concentration (Forrest, Finlayson, Adjepon-Yamoah & Prescott, 1977; Forrest *et al.*, 1979; Forrest *et al.*, 1982). The 24-hour urinary excretion of paracetamol and its glucuronide, sulphate, cysteine and mercapturate conjugates were not reported to be significantly different among healthy subjects, patients with mild liver disease and patients with severe liver disease (Forrest *et al.*, 1979). There seemed to be no evidence that patients with impaired liver function are at increased risk of hepatotoxicity when given a single therapeutic dose of paracetamol (Forrest *et al.*, 1979).

Patients with non-insulin dependent diabetes mellitus show no significant difference in paracetamol clearance, half-life or partial clearance to the glucuronide conjugate, when compared to healthy control subjects, though drug conjugation has been shown to be impaired in rats with experimentally induced diabetes (Kamali, Thomas & Ferner, 1993). The partial clearance to the sulphate conjugate in diabetic patients is significantly reduced and the renal clearance is increased. The exact mechanism of these changes is uncertain.

Shively *et al.* found a temporal variation in the terminal elimination half-life of paracetamol, it being significantly longer in normal volunteers when the dose was given at 6:00am rather than at 2:00pm (Shively & Vesell, 1975). This was explained by a drop of 13% in the apparent volume of distribution value. This finding was not confirmed by a later study (Malan, Moncrieff & Bosch, 1985).

Greater inter-individual variation in paracetamol metabolism has been observed compared to intra-individual variation (Caldwell, Davies & Smith, 1980; Clements *et al.*, 1984). The range of inter-individual variation in the urinary recovery of the glucuronide and sulphate conjugates is only

3-fold but that of the oxidative metabolites is 60-fold (Critchley, Nimmo, Gregson, Woolhouse & Prescott, 1986). The contribution to inter-individual variation by the cysteine and mercapturate pathway is thus much greater than that of glucuronide and sulphate conjugation. In a study of paracetamol metabolism in twins, intra-twin variations in the rate of formation of the glucuronide and sulphate conjugates was found to be as large within monozygotic twins as within dizygotic twins. Also, the intra-twin correlation coefficients of these parameters in those living together were found to be almost twice those of twins living apart. These findings suggest that environmental factors are more predominant than genetic factors in the variations of paracetamol metabolism (Nash *et al.*, 1984).

Ethnic differences in the metabolism of paracetamol are well recognised. Mucklow *et al.* found that the plasma half-life was significantly longer and the plasma clearance was significantly slower in Asians working in London when compared with Caucasian subjects (Mucklow *et al.*, 1980). In another study, the fractional recovery of the cysteine and mercapturate conjugates of paracetamol in the urine was significantly lower in Ghanaians and Kenyans compared to Caucasians from Scotland –5.2% and 4.4% compared to 9.3% (Critchley *et al.*, 1986). This seems to indicate markedly reduced metabolic activation of paracetamol in Africans. Similarly, a lower fractional recovery of the oxidative metabolites has been found in Chinese and Indians living in Singapore (6% and 5.9% respectively) (Lee, Ti, Koh & Prescott, 1992), but the value in Chinese was not confirmed in another study done in Australia (Osborne, Tonkin & Miners, 1991). In this Australian study, the fractional recovery of the GSH derived conjugates in Chinese and Caucasian subjects was found to be 9.2% and 10.0% respectively and they were not significantly different. These ethnic differences in paracetamol metabolism may be related to genetic or environmental factors, including differences in diet and protein intake (Nash *et al.*, 1984; Critchley *et al.*, 1986).

Increased oxidative metabolism of a therapeutic dose of paracetamol has been found in certain groups of cancer patients. Mercapturate conjugate excretion was higher in patients with bladder carcinoma compared to healthy volunteers and it was suggested that increased formation of reactive metabolites might predispose an individual to bladder cancer (Dolara, Lodovici, Salvadori, Saltutti, Delle Rose, Selli & Kriebel, 1988). Similarly, Leung and Critchley found a higher proportion of oxidative metabolites in urine from patients with hepatocellular carcinoma. A few of their patients with chronic hepatitis B infection also excreted much higher than normal proportions of oxidative metabolites which again indicated increased microsomal cytochrome P450 activity (Leung & Critchley, 1991).

2.1.3.4 Excretion

Both paracetamol and its metabolites are excreted rapidly in man. As paracetamol is a moderately lipid-soluble weak acid (pKa 9.5) and plasma protein binding is minimal in therapeutic concentrations (Gazzard *et al.*, 1973; Lowenthal *et al.*, 1976; Morris & Levy, 1984), it undergoes considerable glomerular filtration with subsequent passive tubular reabsorption. Its renal clearance is independent of urine pH, but there is a significant correlation with flow rate (Prescott & Wright, 1973; Miners, Osborne, A.L. & Birkett, 1992). In healthy subjects given a dose of 20 mg/kg, the mean renal clearance of paracetamol was 13 ml/minute. The highly polar glucuronide and sulphate conjugates are both filtered at the glomerulus and actively secreted by the tubules. Their renal clearances are 130 ml/minute and 166 ml/minute, respectively (Prescott, 1980). Accumulation of these metabolites occur in chronic renal disease (Lowenthal *et al.*, 1976; Prescott *et al.*, 1989).

Biliary excretion and enterohepatic circulation of paracetamol has been shown both in rats and in man (Siegers, Rozman & Klaassen, 1983; Siegers, Loeser, Gieselmann & Oltmanns, 1984). In rats, within 8 hours after an intravenous administration of 100 mg/kg, 28.4% of the dose was excreted into bile (Siegers *et al.*, 1983). In man, after an oral dose of 1g, the percentage was 2.6% (Siegers *et al.*, 1984). The glucuronide, sulphate, cysteine, mercapturate metabolites of paracetamol, as well as the glutathione conjugate, were all found excreted in bile in the rat but the mercapturate and glutathione conjugates were not detected in bile in man. It was suggested that the glutathione conjugate is rapidly metabolised to the cysteine derivative before or during passage through the intestinal wall in the rat. The presence of high quantities of γ-glutamyl transpeptidase, the enzyme responsible for the degradation of reduced glutathione in human bile may be an explanation for its absence in human bile. However, these human subjects were patients with cholestasis and bile duct surgery and therefore might not have reflected the correct data in normal healthy subjects. In another study, bile was shown to be an important route of elimination for the cysteine conjugate in man and it accounts for 19.4% of the total excretion of the metabolite (Jayasinghe, Roberts & Read, 1986). One interesting observation from these studies is that, in man, the ratio of the uriniary recoveries of the cysteine and mercapturate conjugates of paracetamol is almost always unity but the mercapturate conjugate has never been detected in human bile. A survey of existing literature did not reveal where the N-acetylation of paracetamol cysteine takes place. Since the plasma levels of the mercapturate conjugate seems to be always lower than those of the cysteine conjugate following oral doses of paracetamol (see results, section 2.3.6.1), it may be speculated that at least some of the conversion of the cysteine conjugate to the mercapturate conjugate take place in the renal tubules prior to excretion .

2.1.4   Toxicity and Overdosage

Paracetamol is a drug with a long history, however, proper preclinical toxicity studies were not carried out before its marketing. It was not until it gained popularity that its hepatotoxicity with very high doses was recognised. Hepatic necrosis was first reported in cats and rats given large doses (Eder, 1964; Boyd & Bereczky, 1966) and these reports were soon followed by those of severe and fatal liver damage in man following paracetamol overdosage (Davidson & Eastham, 1966; Thomson & Prescott, 1966).

The clinical symptoms of paracetamol overdosage can be divided into three stages. There are non-specific symptoms including nausea, vomiting and malaise within the first 24 hours. During the second stage, between 24–48 hours after the overdose, these symptoms usually become less severe. Right upper quadrant and abdominal pain may develop, together with hepatic tenderness and mild jaundice. Maximum derangement of liver function tests does not occur until at least the third day. Renal damage, though not as common, may also occur as indicated by decreased urine output and back pain during the first 48 hours. Recovery at this stage is usually rapid and complete. Phase 3 only occurs as a result of fulminant hepatic failure after 3 to 5 days. There are dramatic increases in the liver enzymes in plasma, aspartate and alanine aminotransferases (AST and ALT) to over 10,000 iu/L, reflecting the release of these enzymes from acutely damaged hepatocytes. Deepening jaundice, hypoglycaemia, coagulation defects and coma may occur in severely poisoned patients. If death does not occur, normal liver function returns over a few weeks (Prescott, 1983; Prescott & Critchley, 1983; Clissold, 1986).

Other complications resulting from paracetamol poisoning include renal failure, pancreatitis, cardiotoxicity (Armour & Slater, 1993) and haematological abnormalities secondary to liver damage. Before specific antidotes were available, treatment was mainly supportive only. Severe liver damage following paracetamol overdose occurs in approximately 8% of patients and about 1% die from hepatic failure (Prescott, 1983).

Since clinical symptoms and biochemical changes are not seen in patients with paracetamol poisoning until 2–3 days after ingestion, it is difficult to assess the severity of poisoning apart from predictions based on plasma paracetamol concentrations. Prolongation of paracetamol elimination half-life is normally seen following liver damage (Prescott, Wright, Roscoe & Brown, 1971) but this cannot be used practically to for assessment of possible liver damage at an early stage. In practical clinical settings, assessment of paracetamol overdose is determined by the plasma concentration, usually a single measurement, in relation to the time after ingestion. A 'treatment line' is plotted by joining a 200 μg/ml paracetamol plasma concentration at 4 hours after ingestion with 30 μg/ml at 15 hours on a semilogarithmic graph of the paracetamol plasma concentrations against time after ingestion (Fig. 2.3). This is used to predict the possiblity of severe liver damage (Prescott *et al.*, 1971; James, Lesna, Roberts, Pulman, Douglas, Smith & Watson, 1975; Prescott, 1983). Patients with plasma concentrations above the treatment line on this graph are likely to develop some degree of liver damage. Concentrations above the parallel line joining 300 μg/ml at 4 hours and 45 μg/ml at 15 hours indicate a 90% chance of developing severe liver damage. The assessment of plasma paracetamol concentrations before 4 hours following ingestion is unreliable as absorption from the gastrointestinal tract may not be complete.

Other early markers of liver damage caused by paracetamol poisoning have been sought. Plasma glutathione S-transferase (GST) has found to be raised (> 100 times normal values) early after paracetamol overdose as a result of cellular damage (Beckett, Chapman, Dyson & Hayes, 1985). A change in the GST level can be seen 4 hours after taking paracetamol in overdose and in patients who are successfully treated with the antidote N-acetylcysteine, peak GST levels are much lower than those found in patients with severe liver damage. Two distinct peaks in the plasma GST level are seen, the first one occurring around 12–40 hours after overdose and the other one around 40–50 hours, suggesting two distinct phases of hepatotoxicity. Prescott *et al.* also suggested the possibility of early liver damage if the plasma half-life of paracetamol is prolonged from the outset (Prescott *et al.*, 1971). It has been postulated that the early release of GST

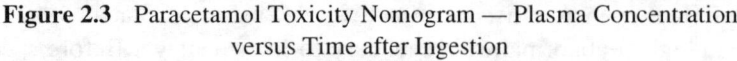

Figure 2.3 Paracetamol Toxicity Nomogram — Plasma Concentration versus Time after Ingestion

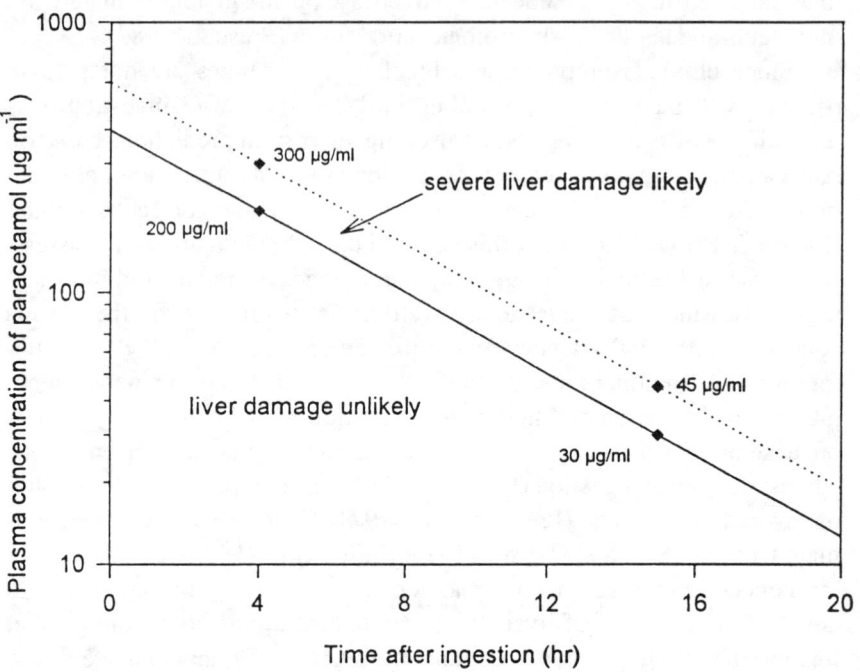

may be due to mild diffuse hepatocelluar damage or that a certain population of the liver cells are more vulnerable (Beckett *et al.*, 1985).The mechanism of paracetamol hepatotoxicity was elucidated by Mitchell and colleagues at the National Institutes of Health, Bethesda, U.S.A.. A difference in the degree of severity of hepatic damage was found in laboratory animals including rats and mice pre-treated with agents which altered the rate of metabolism of paracetamol. Phenobarbitone, a liver enzyme inducing agent, enhanced the clearance of paracetamol but at the same time, also markedly potentiated the degree of hepatic necrosis. In contrast, piperonyl butoxide pre-treatment inhibited paracetamol metabolism and was able to confer protection against hepatic necrosis. It was concluded that a toxic metabolite rather than paracetamol itself was the cause of hepatocellular damage (Mitchell *et al.*, 1973a). Further studies using [^{3}H]-paracetamol showed that large amounts of radiolabelled material were covalently bound to mouse liver protein *in vivo* when these animals were given an overdose. Both covalent binding and hepatic necrosis were shown to be dose dependent and the development of hepatic necrosis was always preceded by the occurrence of the peak level of radiolabel binding. The degree of binding in individual mice was also shown to be directly proportional to the severity of hepatic necrosis. These findings support the theory that paracetamol-induced hepatic necrosis is mediated through the covalent binding of a chemically reactive metabolite to vital hepatic macromolecules (Jollow *et al.*, 1973). *In vitro* studies confirmed that a metabolite generated by cytochrome P450-dependent mixed function oxidase covalently binds to microsomal proteins. The extent of *in vitro* binding is affected by treatments that alter hepatic necrosis and *in vivo* binding. Pretreatment of animals with cobaltous chloride, an inhibitor of cytochrome P-450 synthesis, lowered the extent of covalent binding which showed that it did not occur directly but was dependent on the conversion of paracetamol to an active metabolite formed in hepatic microsomes by a cytochrome-P450 mixed function oxidase (Potter *et al.*, 1973). It was also postulated that the reactive intermediate was formed through N-hydroxylation, since this same reaction took place to a much greater extent, with another substance of a similar structure to paracetamol (2-acetylaminofluorene), in species susceptible to paracetamol-induced hepatic injury (Davis, Potter, Jollow & Mitchell, 1974). More recently, the binding of the reactive intermediate of paracetamol to hepatocyte intracellular structure was demonstrated by immunohistochemical detection in rats using rabbit antiserum specific against the paracetamol-protein adduct (Roberts, Bucci, Benson, Warbritton, McRae, Pumford & Hinson, 1991).

The role played by GSH in conferring protection against paracetamol induced hepatic necrosis was demonstrated by Mitchell *et al.*. Diethyl maleate, an agent that depletes hepatic GSH, was shown to potentiate hepatotoxicity when given to mice before paracetamol treatment, whereas treatment with cysteine, a GSH precursor, was able to protect the animals from hepatic injury secondary to hepatotoxic doses of paracetamol. The administration of paracetamol caused dose dependent depletion of hepatic GSH up to a maximum of about 75% depletion. Significant covalent binding of radio-labelled paracetamol to liver proteins was evident only when the dose of paracetamol caused a 70% or more depletion of hepatic

GSH. Furthermore, pretreatments that alter hepatic GSH concentrations were shown to affect the extent of the covalent binding of the paracetamol metabolite to liver macromolecules. Diethyl maleate and cysteine increased and decreased the extent of binding to liver, respectively. No significant binding of paracetamol to skeletal or cardiac tissues was observed (Mitchell *et al.*, 1973b). Inter-species differences in the susceptibility to paracetamol hepatotoxicity correlated with the rate of paracetamol activation by hepatic microsomal enzymes to the potent reactive intermediate and also to the rate of hepatic GSH depletion (Davis *et al.*, 1974; Jollow *et al.*, 1974; Potter, Thorgeirsson, Jollow & Michell, 1974). These studies further support the theory that the reactive intermediate of paracetamol formed in vivo is preferentially detoxified by conjugation with GSH and that covalent binding to vital hepatic macromolecules only occurs when GSH availability is exceeded. The most susceptible animal, the hamster, produced the highest fraction of the mercapturate metabolite and the amount of this metabolite excreted in the urine was proportional to the dose administered until a hepatotoxic dose was reached. The fraction excreted as the mercapturate metabolite then decreased markedly, commensurated with the known depletion of hepatic GSH.

The protective role of GSH against injury by the reactive intermediate of paracetamol has also been studied in man. The urinary recovery of the mercapturate metabolite, derived from the GSH-conjugated intermediate, is proportional to the dose of paracetamol given, ranging from 900-1800 mg. Thus the availability of GSH was not rate-limiting for conjugation after these doses (Mitchell *et al.*, 1974). Extrapolating from animal studies that liver necrosis only occurs when more than 70% of hepatic GSH was depleted (Mitchell *et al.*, 1973b; Potter *et al.*, 1974), it was estimated that a dose of over 15 g would be hepatotoxic in normal human subjects. This was found to agree with clinical observations. Pre-treatment with phenobarbitone, an enzyme-inducing agents, was shown to increase the production of the mercapturate metabolite in human subjects (Mitchell *et al.*, 1974). It was estimated that patients with induced drug-metabolising enzymes may be susceptible to as low as 10 grams of paracetamol. On the other hand, Prescott *et al.* did not find any difference in the production of the mercapturate conjugate after oral doses of paracetamol between healthy subjects and patients on long term antiepileptic drugs, including phenobarbitone and carbamazepine, and rifampicin, which are all known enzyme-inducing agents (Prescott *et al.*, 1981). But the glucuronide conjugation was much enhanced in these epileptic patients and it was thought that the recovery of the mercapturate and cysteine conjugates much have been reduced, as has the recovery of unchanged drug and the sulphate conjugate. The author concluded that some induction of the oxidative metabolism was likely but might not have been clinically significant.

The highly reactive alkylating metabolite is most probably N-acetyl-p-benzoquinoneimine (NAPQI) (Miners & Kissinger, 1979; Dahlin *et al.*, 1984). The synthetic form of this reactive metabolite has been found to react, *in vitro*, with GSH, acetaminophen and reduced nicotinamide adenine dinucleotide phosphate (NADPH) (Potter & Hinson, 1986). NAPQI has been found to be severely cytotoxic, but not mutagenic, to *Salmonella typhimurium* and it has caused extensive DNA single-strand breaks in genotoxicity studies. This data seems to show that paracetamol can cause DNA interaction leading to damage at levels which are cytotoxic (Dybing, Holme, Gordon, Søderlund, Dahlin & Nelson, 1984).

Accompanying depletion of hepatic GSH, high molecular weight protein aggregates were found when the liver homogenates and microsomes of rats given hepatotoxic doses of paracetamol were separated by gel electrophoresis (Minamide, Horie & Awazu, 1992). This altered distribution pattern of proteins in the *in vivo* paracetamol-induced hepatotoxicity was the same as seen in *in vitro* lipid perioxidation in rat liver microsomes. Thus, lipid peroxidation was suggested as a contributing factor to paracetamol-induced hepatotoxicity.

The elucidation of the underlying pathogenesis of the hepatic injury caused by paracetamol overdosage provided indications to its management. Since the hepatic GSH stores must be depleted before hepatic injury by the reactive intermediate can take place, it follows that if the GSH store can be replenished in time, hepatic injury may be minimised.

Parenterally administered GSH, a natural and non-toxic substance, was not able to produce a direct increase of intracellular levels of GSH in liver cells as it does not penetrate hepatocytes (Hahn, Wendel & Flohé, 1978). However, Viña *et al.* did find an increase in hepatic GSH levels in mice treated with high doses of paracetamol after oral adminstration of GSH (Viña, Perez, Furukawa, Palacin & Viña, 1989). It was explained that oral GSH is converted to its constituent amino acids by intestinal enzymes and the increase in hepatic GSH requires active GSH synthesis in the liver from its constituents. It was found that the rate limiting factor of GSH synthesis is the availability of L-cysteine and so attempts to increase the hepatic levels of GSH have focused on the administration of sulphydryl compounds, including cysteamine, L-methionine, L-cysteine and N-acetyl-cysteine, which are all precursors of GSH. Another study on patients taking paracetamol daily in therapeutic doses showed that paracetamol caused a significant decrease in the concentration of reduced glutathione in plasma. This loss was more conspicuous in patients who had shown signs of microsomal enzyme induction, probably due to enhanced metabolic activation. It was suggested that these findings reflect the hepatic intracellular glutathione status (Trenti, Bertolotti, Castellana, Ferrari, Pini & Sternieri, 1992). In this study, intravenous injection of GSH resulted in a considerable increase in free plasma GSH but was cleared from the circulation with a half-life of about 12 minutes, in agreement with results published by Lauterburg (Lauterburg & Velez, 1988). It seemed that exogenous GSH could not raise itse hepatic level directly but could only serve as a precursor in replenishing intracellular GSH stores.

Of the possible precursors of glutathione that could be used in the treatment of acute paracetamol poisoning, cysteamine was the first sulphydryl compound used. Protection against paracetamol-induced hepatic injury was first shown in animal studies and later in man (Mitchell *et al.*, 1974; Prescott, Newton, Swainson, Wright, Forrest & Matthew, 1974; James *et al.*, 1975; Prescott, Park & Proudfoot, 1976). Although shown to be effective if given within 10–12 hours of poisoning, cysteamine was never made available as a pharmaceutical preparation. Due to its unpleasant gastrointestinal and central nervous system side effects, safer and more convenient alternatives were looked for.

Methionine can only be given orally and it was used with some enthusiasm in the past (Crome, Vale, Volan, Widdop & Goulding, 1976; Vale, Meredith & Goulding, 1981). However, it appears to be less effective than intravenous cysteamine and N-acetylcysteine, probably due to unreliable absorption, as nausea and vomiting are commonly associated with paracetamol overdosage. Methionine must also be given within 10–12 hours of paracetamol poisoning as late administration or delayed absorption may aggravate or precipitate hepatic encephalopathy (Canalese, Gimson, Davis & William, 1981). It has been suggested that addition of methionine to paracetamol tablets might protect against hepatotoxicity and nephrotoxicity and a formulation combining paracetamol and methionine is available in the U.K. ('Pameton') (Janes & Routledge, 1992).

N-acetylcysteine has been used with much success in the treatment of paracetamol poisoning in man and is now considered to be a very effective antidote preventing liver damage, renal failure and death (Prescott,

Ballantyne, Park, Adriaenssens & Proudfoot, 1977; Prescott, Illingworth, Critchley, Stewart, Adam & Proudfoot, 1979; BNF, 1993). Although previous guidelines recommended that N-acetylcysteine be given within 10 hours of a paracetamol overdose where virtually complete protection can be achieved, more studies are now showing that some benefits are seen with late administration of the antidote, up to and beyond 24 hours after an overdose episode (Smilkstein, Knapp, Kulig & Rumack, 1988; Keays, Gove, Forbes, Alexander & Williams, 1989; Harrison, Keays, Bray, Alexander & Williams, 1990). The intravenous route is preferred to the oral route to avoid unreliable absorption, though the latter is more prevalent in the United States (Prescott, 1983; Janes & Routledge, 1992). It is usually administered as a total intravenous dose of 300 mg/kg over 20 hours (BNF, 1993).

The protection offered by sulphydryl-containing compounds against paracetamol hepatotoxicity is presumed to be via the provision of GSH precursors but some direct combination with the reactive metabolite is possible. The exact mechanisms of protection are uncertain. They have all been found to reduce or prevent the covalent binding of the reactive intermediate of paracetamol, NAPQI, to vital cell structures. In addition, N-acetylcysteine stimulates the GSH conjugation of paracetamol in isolated rat hepatocytes and it is also capable of reacting with NAPQI itself (Huggett & Blair, 1983), whereas methionine does not react with NAPQI to any great extent. In overdose patients treated with N-acetylcysteine, the urinary excretion of the cysteine and mercapturate metabolites is increased (Prescott, 1980).

Since some beneficial effects were seen even with late administration of N-acetylcysteine when liver damage was evident, it was suggested that this antidote might have additional effects. Another postulated mechanism of paracetamol hepatotoxicity is that NAPQI oxidises thiol groups in key enzymes within the hepatocyte, in particular Ca^{2+}-translocases, leading to elevation of cytosolic calcium ions and eventual cell death. N-acetylcysteine may have an additional protective action through the reduction of these previously NAPQI-reduced thiol groups, permitting re-establishment of calcium homeostasis and thus preventing cell death (Janes & Routledge, 1992).

Further postulated mechanisms for the action of N-acetylcysteine in the protection against paracetamol hepatotoxicity were recently reviewed by Janes and Routledge (Janes & Routledge, 1992). These include the action of N-acetylcysteine as an antioxidant to prevent inflammatory responses initiated by oxidative damage; preventing microvascular plugging which extend ischaemia around the zone of injury in the liver; and improving the microcirculation in hepatic failure by restoring normal vascular responsiveness to endothelial derived relaxant factor (EDRF). It was suggested that, whatever the mechanism, the increase in oxygen delivery to injured tisuues may be important in any late response to N-acetylcysteine in paracetamol induced hepatotoxicity.

2.2 Estimation of paracetamol and its metabolites in plasma and urine by high performance liquid chromatography

2.2.1 Introduction

Paracetamol is an over-the-counter-sales antipyretic analgesic. Despite being extremely safe when used in normal therapeutic doses, it can lead to hepatotoxicity and possibly fatal hepatic necrosis following acute overdosage. The antidote N-acetylcysteine must be given early to prevent fulminant hepatic failure. Since the clinical symptoms of hepatic failure are not evident until 2–3 days after the ingestion of a paracetamol overdose, estimation of the plasma concentrations remains the only index of the likelihood of liver damage. A prediction nomogram was published by Prescott (Prescott *et al.*, 1971; Prescott, 1983) (see also Fig. 2.3) and a plethora of assays have been developed for the estimation of paracetamol concentrations for the purpose of aiding in diagnosis and management of overdose patients.

The methods available for the estimation of plasma paracetamol can be divided into 4 main groups:

(1) Colorimetry involving chemical derivatisation;
(2) Measurement of the absorbance of the unmodified compound by UV spectrophotometry;
(3) Chromatography including gas liquid chromatography and high performance liquid chromatography;
(4) Immunoassays

The earliest methods were based either on colorimetric techniques or the direct measurement of the ultraviolet absorbance of unmodified paracetamol following extraction from plasma. Colorimetric techniques involve several chemical derivatisations including hydrolysis of paracetamol to p-aminophenol, reaction with dyes and nitration. Both colorimetry and spectrophotometry, although they can be carried out relatively rapidly and easily, suffered from the disadvantage of non-specificity and interference from other compounds in the sample, in particular non-steroidal anti-inflammatory drugs (Spooner, Reavey & Mcintosh, 1976). Acid hydrolysis converts not only unchanged paracetamol, but also its inactive metabolites to p-aminophenol, leading to falsely high results (Stewart & Watson, 1987). A positive error of 40–100% was noted, when this technique was compared with a high performance liquid chromatographic reference method which measured only unchanged paracetamol (Stewart, Adriaenssens, Jarvie & Prescott, 1979). Despite the drawbacks with acid hydrolysis, further 'improved' versions of the colorimetric method were published due to its relative simplicity and the rapidity of performance (Glynn & Kendal, 1975; Chambers & Jones, 1976; Wiener, 1977; Wiener & Longlands, 1977; Archer & Richardson, 1980; Bailey, 1982). These improved methods offered improved sensitivity and specificity whereby paracetamol concentrations could be estimated in presence of its metabolites.

Further improvement in the specificity of the colorimetric method was achieved by an enzymic approach. A bacterial enzyme, acyl amidase (aryl acylamide amidohydrolase), specifically converts free paracetamol to p-aminophenol (Hammond & Scawen, 1981). This enzymic hydrolysis of paracetamol was coupled with the colorimetric chemical reaction, whereby the p-aminophenol formed was reacted with cresol to produce an indophenol dye. This method was evaluated and its sensitivity, linearity, precision and accuracy were found to be closely comparable to established HPLC methods (Brown, Campbell, Price, Rambohul, Widdop, Barbour, Roberts, Burnett, Atkinson, Scawen & Hammond, 1983; Price, Hammond & Scawen, 1983). This assay method was developed into a kit which has subsequently gained wide acceptance (Hallworth, 1983; Alkhayat, 1986).

Non-specificity remained a problem in using colorimetric and spectrophotometric methods for the estimation of paracetamol in biological fluids. For the purpose of research, the criteria for a method to be used for the estimation of paracetamol are different from those used for clinical purposes. Apart from being specific, accurate and relatively rapid, the method must also be able to measure therapeutic concentrations. For a study in the area of the metabolism of paracetamol, the method to be used must also be able to separate and measure the main metabolites. Chromatographic methods were sought to fulfil these requirements. Thin layer chromatography (Andrews *et al.*, 1976), ion-exchange chromatography (Mrochek, Katz, Christie & Dinsmore, 1974) and gas-liquid chromatography (Grove, 1971; Prescott, 1971; Stewart & Willis, 1975; Street, 1975; Dechtiaruk, Johnson & Solomon, 1976; Garland, Hsiao, Pantuck & Conney, 1977) have been used, but they suffer from various disadvantages including lengthy procedures, the need to use volatile solvents and to perform derivatisation.

The development of high performance liquid chromatography (HPLC) has brought about significant progress in the analysis of paracetamol and its metabolites in biological fluids due to its speed, accuracy, precision, selectivity and high sensitivity. The experimental procedures could be much simplified with minimal sample preparation and complete separation of the metabolites was possible. Knox and Jurand achieved separation of paracetamol and its major metabolites (but not quantification) by reversed-phase HPLC, which utilises a polar mobile phase with a non-polar support (Knox & Jurand, 1977). Since the conjugated metabolites of paracetamol are more polar than the unchanged drug, they are eluted first as their affinity for the eluent is greater. Chromatograms could be run with aqueous eluents and direct application of biological fluids without preliminary extraction was possible. They further modified this HPLC system to incorporate ion-pair systems to control the retention of the various metabolites (Knox & Jurand, 1978). A large number of HPLC methods for the estimation of paracetamol in biological fluids were published. Most of these only measured the unchanged drug but both therapeutic and overdose concentrations could be measured (Blair & Rumack, 1977; Gotelli, Kabra & Marton, 1977; Horvitz & Jatlow, 1977; Fletterick, Grove & Hohnadel, 1979; Korduba & Petruzzi, 1984). Estimation of paracetamol and its 4 major metabolites — glucuronide, sulphate, cysteine and mercapturate, in urine and plasma was successfully performed by both Howie *et al.* and Adriaenssens and Prescott, respectively (Howie, Adriaenssens & Prescott, 1977; Adriaenssens & Prescott, 1978). As more metabolites of paracetamol were discovered in very small quantities after overdosage, there were more attempts to completely separate these metabolites by HPLC, using gradient solvent systems (Aguilar, Hart & Calder, 1988).

Immunoassays for the estimation of paracetamol have been available since 1983. Comparison of enzyme multiplied immunoassay technique (EMIT) with HPLC showed comparable precision and accuracy (Hepler, Weber, Sutheimer & Sunshine, 1984). A fluorescence polarisation immunoassay (FPIA) was widely used in the U.S.A. despite its high cost as it was found to be extremely simple, requiring minimal skilled operator assistance (Keegan, Smith, Ungemach & Simpson, 1984). EMIT and FPIA are used by about 75% of all laboratories which participate in the quality control programme provided by the American Association for Clinical Chemistry (Stewart & Watson, 1987).

2.2.2   Analytical method

Although many analytical methods exist for the assay of paracetamol in biological fluids, they may not suit the requirements of a particular study. As the present study involves estimation of paracetamol *and* its main metabolites in both plasma and urine and that sample preparation is hoped to be minimised, a specific method needs to be developed. An HPLC method is favoured because of the specificity and sensitivity offered and semi-automation is possible. Following development of a specific assay, validations are required to ascertain its accuracy, sensitivity and recovery.

2.2.2.1 Materials

Paracetamol, paracetamol glucuronide, paracetamol sulphate, paracetamol cysteine and paracetamol mercapturate for reference standards were kindly donated by Sterling-Winthrop Research and Development Division, Alnwick, England. Potassium dihydrogen orthophosphate, propan-2-ol and 60% perchloric acid were obtained from E.Merck, acetic acid from BDH Chemical Ltd. The internal standard 2-acetamidophenol (AAP) was obtained from Sigma. Water was purified for HPLC by the Milli Q Water Purification System (Millipore, U.S.A.).

2.2.2.2 Instrumentation

The HPLC system consisted of a Waters 501 pump which delivered the mobile phase, degassed by sonification, via a filter to the system. The mobile phase then passed to a Waters Intelligent Sample Processor 712 (WISP), an automatic sample injection module.

Prior to passing through the analytical column, the solvent was passed through a Waters Guard-PAK precolumn containing the same packing material as the column. The column used was an 8 mm × 10 cm Waters Radial-PAK Cartridge. Packing material was Nova-Pak C_{18}, particle size

5 m. The cartridge was housed in a Waters Radial compression Module (RCM 8 × 10).

From the column, the eluate then passed through an ultraviolet (U.V.) absorbance detector (Waters 440 absorbance detector). The U.V. detector output was connected to a Waters 745B Data Module to produce the chromatograms and peak areas. A schematic presentation of the HPLC system is shown in Fig. 2.4.

2.2.2.3 Collection and storage of samples

Prior to analysis, all samples were stored at –20°C. Blood samples were collected into 10 ml heparinised tubes, centrifuged for 10 minutes at 1400 xg and the plasma separated for storage.

Urine volumes were recorded and a 20 ml aliquot stored. Paracetamol and paracetamol conjugates are stable under these conditions for a period of years (Adriaenssens, 1980).

2.2.2.4 Chromatographic conditions

For the estimation of paracetamol, paracetamol glucuronide, paracetamol sulphate, paracetamol cysteine and paracetamol mercapturate in urine and plasma, the following chromatographic conditions were used:

Mobile phase: 0.1 M potassium dihydrogen orthophosphate
                        containing 0.1% acetic acid and 0.75% propan-2-ol
Flow rate: 1.5 ml min^{-1}
Pressure: 1000 psi
Detector wavelength: 254 nm

2.2.3   Urine assay

2.2.3.1 Preparation of standards and test samples for urine assay

For estimating paracetamol and its metabolites in urine, standard solutions of paracetamol in blank urine with the internal standard AAP were prepared.

Paracetamol standards: 25, 250, 1250 and 2500 µg ml^{-1}
AAP (aq. solution):   250 µg ml^{-1}

The paracetamol standards and samples were prepared in the following way for analysis. To 500 µl of standard or sample, 1000 µl of water

Figure 2.4 A Schematic Presentation of the HPLC System Used

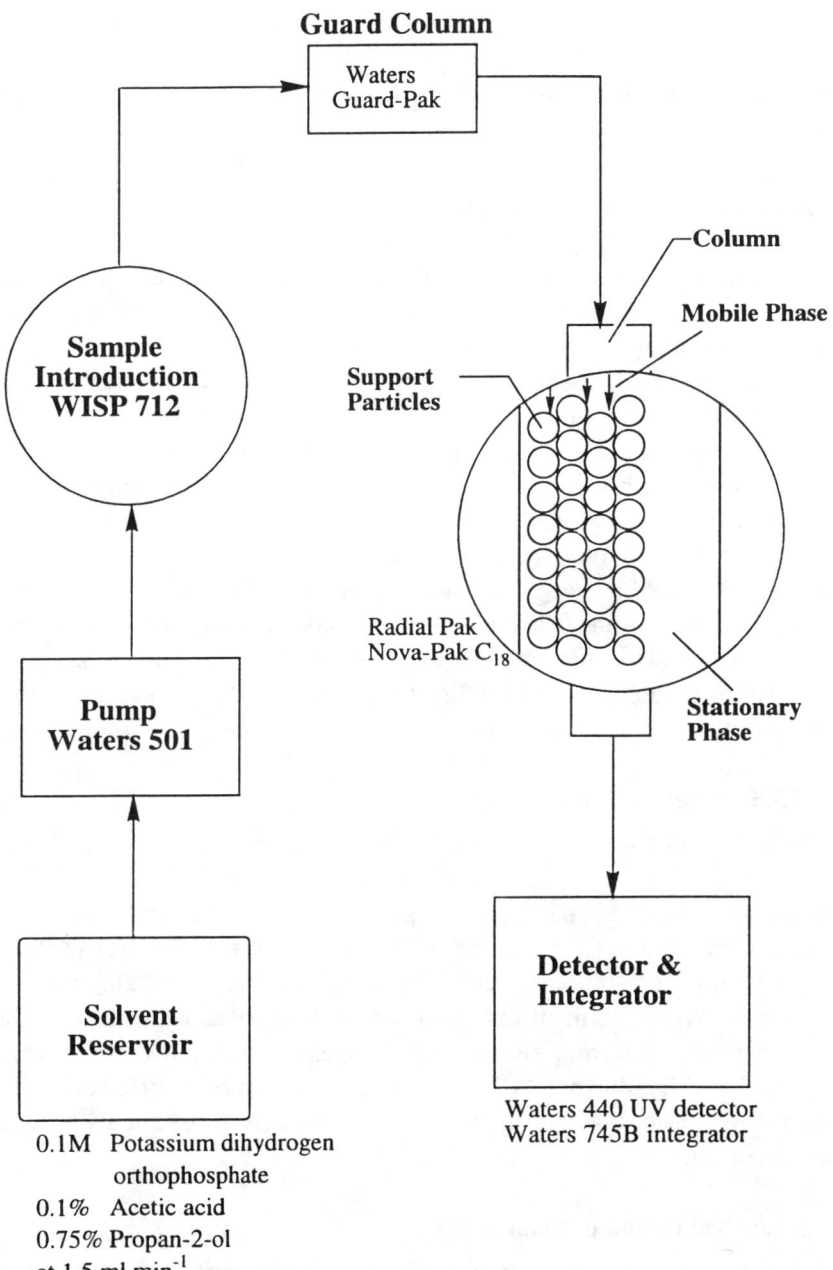

Waters 440 UV detector
Waters 745B integrator

0.1M Potassium dihydrogen
orthophosphate
0.1% Acetic acid
0.75% Propan-2-ol
at 1.5 ml min^{-1}

and 1000 µl of AAP solution were added. Effectively, the standards or samples were diluted 5-fold. The injection volume was 3 µl. Calibration standards were run with each batch of samples for calculation.

2.2.3.2 Calculation of results for urine assay

The concentrations of paracetamol and its metabolites in the samples were calculated in paracetamol equivalents from the peak area ratio of paracetamol and paracetamol conjugates to the internal standard AAP. The peak area alone instead of the peak area ratio was also used (see discussion). Standard curves were calculated by the least-squares regression analysis of the peak area ratio (or peak area) *versus* drug concentration. The reciprocal of the slope of the regression line is the factor by which the peak area ratios (or peak areas) are multiplied to give the paracetamol concentrations in µg ml^{-1}.

As only enough authentic paracetamol was available to be run as standards for each batch of samples, values obtained were only accurate for paracetamol. The absorbance of the glucuronide and sulphate conjugates of paracetamol are not the same as paracetamol and correction factors of 0.909 for the glucuronide conjugate and 0.945 for the sulphate conjugates at 254 nm must be applied. No correction factor was used for the cysteine and the mercapturate conjugates (Adriaenssens, 1980).

The area counts were used directly to calculate the percentage of each metabolite excreted in the 24 hour urine.

2.2.3.3 Results of urine assay

Chromatograms obtained from drug free urine and from urine collected following a therapeutic dose of paracetamol are shown in Fig. 2.5. The retention times of paracetamol glucuronide, paracetamol sulphate, paracetamol cysteine, unchanged paracetamol, internal standard AAP and paracetamol mercapturates were 3.7, 9.1, 9.9, 11.8, 23.0 and 28.7 minutes respectively. The limit of detection for the assay was dependent on the presence of interferring peaks from endogenous material present in the urine. Generally, down to 1–2 ng of paracetamol can be detected distinctly as a single peak, but this small amount is unlikely to be encountered in urine collections.

2.2.3.4 Validation of urine assay

A stock solution of paracetamol in blank urine was serially diluted to give

Figure 2.5 HPLC Chromatogram of Paracetamol and Its Glucuronide, Sulphate, Cysteine and Mercapturate Metabolites in Urine

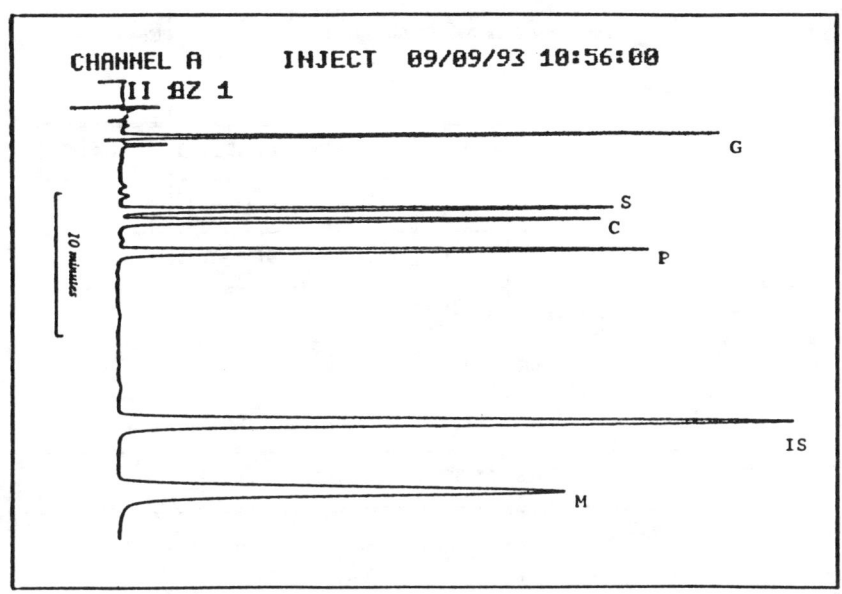

G	Paracetamol glucuronide
S	Paracetamol sulphate
C	Paracetamol cysteine
P	Paracetamol
IS	Internal standard
M	Paracetamol mercapturate

concentrations ranging from 5–500 μg ml^{-1}. Samples were assayed as described and analysed 4 times over a period of a few days.

The results are shown in Table 2.1. The coefficient of variation was 0.2%–1.7% using the peak area for calculation and 0.3–1.5% using the peak area ratio. The plot of mean peak area and mean peak area ratio against concentration was linear and passed through the origin. There was excellent agreement between the results obtained by the two methods of calculation (Fig. 2.6).

The precision and linearity of the urine assay for the metabolites were

Table 2.1a   Precision of HPLC Urine Paracetamol Assay (5–500 $\mu g\ ml^{-1}$)
Using Peak Area

Paracetamol Conc. ($\mu g\ ml^{-1}$)	Paracetamol Peak Area Ratio				Mean ± SD	Coefficient of Variation (%)
	Run 1	Run 2	Run 3	Run 4		
5	64082	64795	63167	65227	64318±901	1.4
25	296259	288685	290217	287074	290559±4011	1.4
50	627488	611196	624379	619946	620752±7083	1.1
100	1168293	1161967	1175135	1155627	1165256±8374	0.7
250	2817072	2796801	2801888	2900918	2829170±48601	1.7
350	3905591	3902292	3917460	3908555	3908475±6514	0.2
500	5579973	5533888	5548605	5558074	5555135±19319	0.3

Table 2.1b   Precision of HPLC Urine Paracetamol Assay (5–500 $\mu g\ ml^{-1}$)
Using Peak Area Ratio

Paracetamol Conc. ($\mu g\ ml^{-1}$)	Peak Area Ratio (Paracetamol/Internal Standard)				Mean ± SD	Coefficient of Variation (%)
	Run 1	Run 2	Run 3	Run 4		
5	0.189	0.197	0.188	0.194	0.191±0.003	1.5
25	0.872	0.865	0.856	0.848	0.860±0.011	1.2
50	1.860	1.831	1.838	1.834	1.841±0.013	0.7
100	3.468	3.485	3.462	3.458	3.468±0.012	0.3
250	8.348	8.156	8.393	8.410	8.327±0.117	1.4
350	11.550	11.453	11.549	11.400	11.488±0.074	0.6
500	16.354	16.277	16.610	16.097	16.335±0.213	1.3

Figure 2.6 Linearity of HPLC Urine Assay of Paracetamol Using
Area Counts and Area Ratios

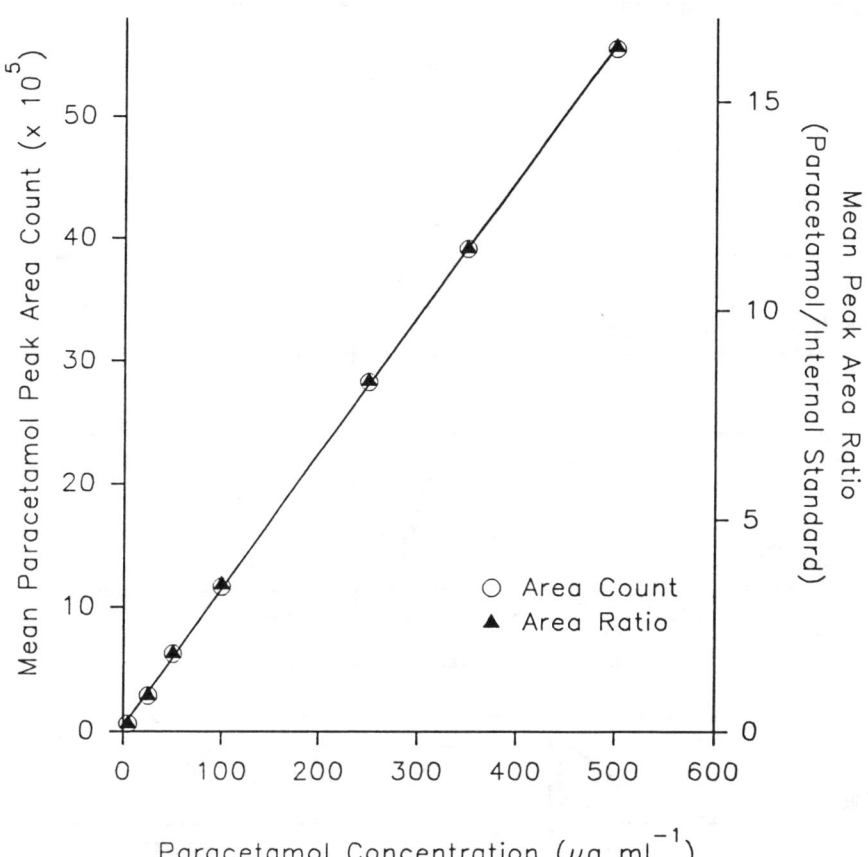

also established. Serial dilutions of stock solutions of the glucuronide, sulphate, cysteine and mercapturate metabolites were made and each sample was analysed 5 times. The results are shown in Tables 2.2 to 2.5. The highest coefficients of variation obtained were 1.2%, 2.1%, 2.4% and

Table 2.2   Precision of HPLC Urine Paracetamol Metabolite
Assay — Glucuronide

Paracetamol Glucuronide Conc. (μg ml^{-1})	Paracetamol Glucuronide Area Counts					Mean ± SD	Coefficient of Variation (%)
	Run 1	Run 2	Run 3	Run 4	Run 5		
5.70	107006	103769	104106	105005	105048	104897 ±1259	1.2
11.39	207403	205034	204577	205689	206605	205862 ±1150	0.6
22.79	416881	414821	413995	414028	411584	414262 ±1902	0.5
45.57	826647	818805	821548	820336	819825	821432 ±3078	0.4
91.15	1664764	1638337	1637783	1639303	1647478	1645733 ±11500	0.7
182.29	3283791	3282156	3326439	3309692	3310430	3302502 ±19050	0.6
364.58	6445926	6443917	6446038	6448985	6456356	6448244 ±4881	0.1
729.17	12815758	12778500	12823056	12844220	12815254	12815358 ±23722	0.2
1458.33	25525297	25633235	25645628	25610978	25664876	25616003 ±54350	0.2

Table 2.3 Precision of HPLC Urine Paracetamol Metabolite
Assay — Sulphate

Paracetamol Sulphate Conc. (μg ml^{-1})	Paracetamol Sulphate Area Counts					Mean ± SD	Coefficient of Variation (%)
	Run 1	Run 2	Run 3	Run 4	Run 5		
7.32	73189	72429	72569	72218	71927	72466 ±471	0.7
14.65	147790	147183	144811	146541	145739	146413 ±1175	0.8
29.30	298562	300676	295991	294772	292834	296567 ±3096	1.0
58.59	587567	580032	582675	588666	580884	583965 ±3927	0.7
117.19	1242396	1196237	1205563	1185318	1178841	1201671 ±24959	2.1
234.38	2458523	2503400	2468020	2495488	2475759	2480238 ±18774	0.8
468.75	4906596	4933380	4953472	4931486	4934060	4931799 ±16678	0.3
937.50	9864999	10020934	9914212	9931312	9930866	9932465 ±56381	0.6
1875.00	19834040	19826703	19767731	19847811	20004320	19856121 ±88314	0.4
3750.00	39296241	39266952	39273448	39356659	39735638	39395787 ±198749	0.5

16.3% for the glucuronide, sulphate, cysteine and mercapturate conjugates, respectively. The peak areas all showed excellent linearity over the range of concentration studied (Fig. 2.7).

Table 2.4   Precision of HPLC Urine Paracetamol Metabolite
Assay — Cysteine

Paracetamol Cysteine Conc. (μg ml^{-1})	Paracetamol Cysteine Area Counts					Mean ± SD	Coefficient of Variation (%)
	Run 1	Run 2	Run 3	Run 4	Run 5		
3.05	33428	31637	32805	33404	33505	32956 ±789	2.4
6.10	67825	66805	68513	67909	67403	67691 ±634	0.9
12.21	138332	135424	135537	134959	135138	135878 ±1391	1.0
24.41	268057	275919	277748	275497	274659	274376 ±3709	1.4
48.83	546273	546694	551185	550641	554254	549809 ±3337	0.6
97.66	1119533	1115887	1117896	1114787	1118304	1117281 ±1914	0.2
195.31	2308590	2299574	2306469	2327945	2317761	2312068 ±11000	0.5
390.62	4625395	4627355	4674038	4636319	4657658	4644153 ±21041	0.5
781.25	9269628	9282387	9256645	9395146	9237146	9288190 ±62085	0.7
1562.50	18665814	18635154	18555954	18577464	18640388	18614955 ±46174	0.3
3125.00	36988957	37526174	37267842	37645617	37397623	37365243 ±253296	0.7

Table 2.5   Precision of HPLC Urine Paracetamol Metabolite
Assay — Mercapturate

Paracetamol Mercapturate Conc. (μg ml⁻¹)	Paracetamol Mercapturate Area Counts					Mean ± SD	Coefficient of Variation (%)
	Run 1	Run 2	Run 3	Run 4	Run 5		
5.86	19683	13031	19414	15659	17119	16981 ±2765	16.3
11.72	42112	40854	36883	36379	41520	39550 ±2707	6.8
23.44	89460	82531	79051	77000	76383	80885 ±5361	6.6
46.88	148118	165088	155663	161066	155324	157052 ±6431	4.1
93.75	346258	334247	329887	324404	330005	332960 ±8214	2.5
187.50	691835	662512	677728	668098	672214	674477 ±11190	1.7
375.00	1362617	1340908	1352183	1366533	1377396	1351927 ±12848	1.0

2.2.4   *Plasma assay*

2.2.4.1   Preparation of standards and test samples for plasma assay

For estimating therapeutic concentrations of paracetamol and its metabolites, spiked plasma standards containing 5, 15 and 25 μg ml⁻¹ of
paracetamol were prepared. These were run in between every 4 samples.
An internal standard was not used in the plasma assay (see under validation). The calibration standards and samples were prepared in the

Figure 2.7   Linearity of HPLC Urine Assay of Paracetamol Metabolities

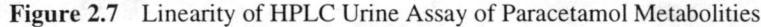

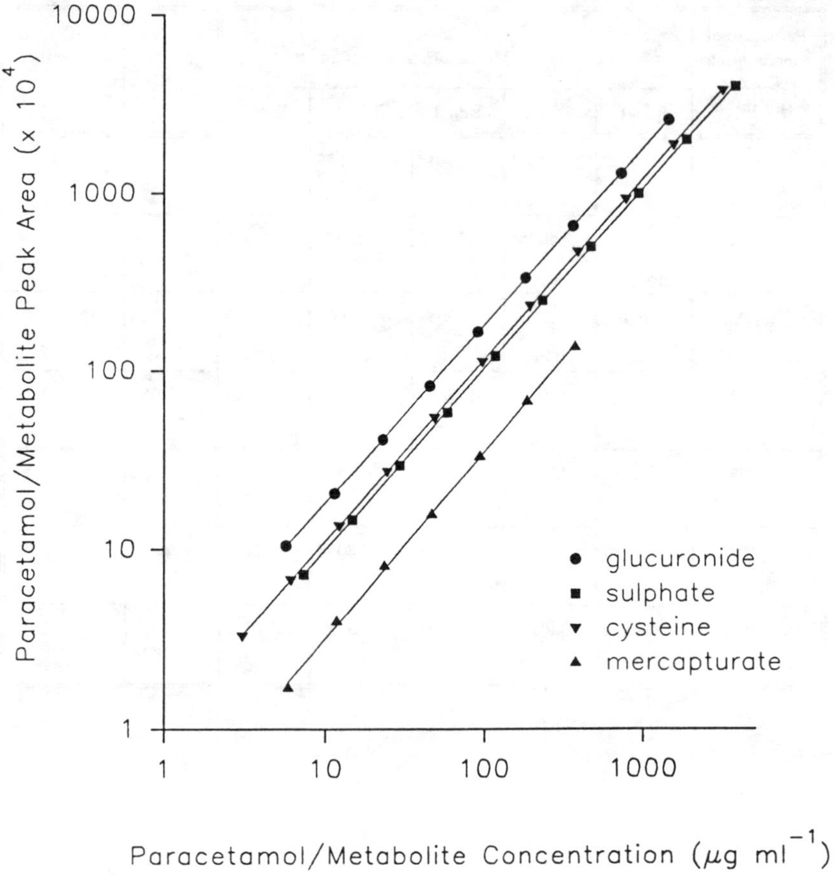

Paracetamol/Metabolite Concentration (μg ml^{-1})

following way for analysis. To 500 µl of plasma in a 1.5 ml eppendorf tube, 50 1 of 30% w/v aqueous perchloric acid was added with continuous mixing (Auto Vortex Mixer MT19, Chiltern Scientific) to precipitate the plasma proteins. The tubes were centrifuged for 10 minutes at 1400 x*g* and up to 30 µl of the clear supernatant was injected directly into the HPLC system.

2.2.4.2 Calculation of results for plasma assay

Concentrations of paracetamol and its metabolites in plasma were calculated in paracetamol equivalents from the peak area values. Standard curves were calculated by the least-squares regression analysis of peak area versus drug concentration. The reciprocal of the slope of the regression line is the factor by which the peak area are multiplied to give the paracetamol concentrations in $\mu g\ ml^{-1}$.

As only enough authentic paracetamol was available to be run as standards for each batch of samples, values obtained were only accurate for paracetamol. The absorbance of glucuronide and sulphate conjugates of paracetamol are not the same as paracetamol and correction factors of 0.835 for the glucuronide conjugate and 1.027 for the sulphate conjugates at 254 nm must be applied. No correction factor was used for the cysteine and the mercapturate conjugates (Adriaenssens & Prescott, 1978).

2.2.4.3 Results of plasma assay

Chromatograms for a plasma sample spiked with paracetamol and its metabolites is shown in Fig. 2.8. The retention times of paracetamol glucuronide, paracetamol sulphate, paracetamol cysteine, unchanged paracetamol and paracetamol mercapturate were essentially the same as in the urine assay as the chromatographic conditions were almost identical. They were 3.7, 9.1, 9.9, 11.8 and 28.7, respectively. Paracetamol cysteine and paracetamol mercapturate could be detected by this HPLC system but they exist only in very low concentrations following therapeutic doses. The paracetamol cysteine peak could be seen in some of the plasma samples following a therapeutic dose in our study subjects but the paracetamol mercapturate peak was not seen in any of the plasma samples. The absence of the mercapturate conjugate in the plasma samples of our study subjects is most likely due to the extremely low concentrations. Most previous studies could only detect the glucuronide and sulphate conjugates of paracetamol in the plasma following therapeutic doses. In the present study, the plasma assay developed could detect the cysteine conjugate in some of the plasma samples. The non-detection of the mercapturate metabolite in *all* plasma samples under study indicate that it can only exist in minute quantity.

The detection limit of paracetamol was about 1–2 ng and there was no interference from commonly used medications.

Figure 2.8　HPLC Chromatogram of Paracetamol and Its Glucuronide, Sulphate, Cysteina dn mercapturate Metabolites in Plasma

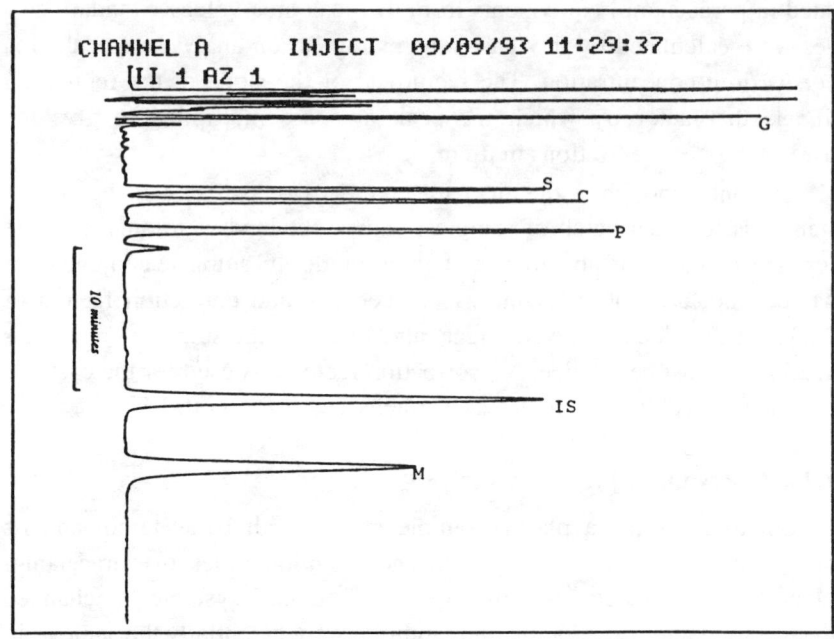

G	Paracetamol glucuronide
S	Paracetamol sulphate
C	Paracetamol cysteine
P	Paracetamol
IS	Internal standard
M	Paracetamol mercapturate

2.2.4.4　Validation of plasma assay

1. *Precision & linearity.* The linearity and the precision for the plasma assay was determined by repeated analysis of plasma paracetamol standards, with concentrations ranging from 5–25 1 ml^{-1}. Samples were assayed as described and analysed 5 times over a period of 2 days. The results are shown in Table 2.6a. The coefficients of variation ranged from 0.1–3.3% using the peak area counts forcalculation, while the calibration plots were linear and passed through the origin (Fig. 2.9).

Table 2.6a Precision of HPLC Plasma Paracetamol Assay Using
Peak Area Counts

Conc. (μg ml⁻¹)	Paracetamol Peak Area Counts						Mean ± SD	Coefficient of Variation (%)
	Run 1	Run 2	Run 3	Run 4	Run 5	Run 6		
5	558775	504427	549119	550004	550602	542721	542608 ±17702	3.3
10	1205727	1208426	1208321	1214228	1211151	1208136	1209332 ±2694	0.2
15	1793812	1813156	1810012	1806486	1800857	1800821	1804191 ±6451	0.4
20	2401440	2406252	2406346	2407065	2406207	2409202	2406085 ±2322	0.1
25	3059761	3061039	3057895	3065258	3051001	3041512	3056078 ±7786	0.3

Table 2.6b Precision of HPLC Plasma Paracetamol Assay Using
Peak Area Ratio

Paracetamol Conc. (μg ml⁻¹)	Paracetamol Peak Area Ratio (Paracetamol/Internal Standard)					Mean ± SD	Coefficient of Variation (%)
	Run 1	Run 2	Run 3	Run 4	Run 5		
5	0.536	0.492	0.486	0.503	0.467	0.497 ±0.025	5.1
10	0.951	0.971	1.008	0.992	0.929	0.970 ±0.032	3.3
15	1.416	1.403	1.466	1.464	1.354	1.421 ±0.046	3.3
20	1.909	1.887	1.943	1.860	1.829	1.885 ±0.044	2.3
25	2.359	2.294	2.268	2.572	2.311	2.361 ±0.123	5.2

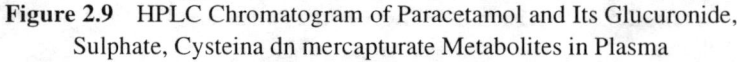

Figure 2.9   HPLC Chromatogram of Paracetamol and Its Glucuronide, Sulphate, Cysteina dn mercapturate Metabolites in Plasma

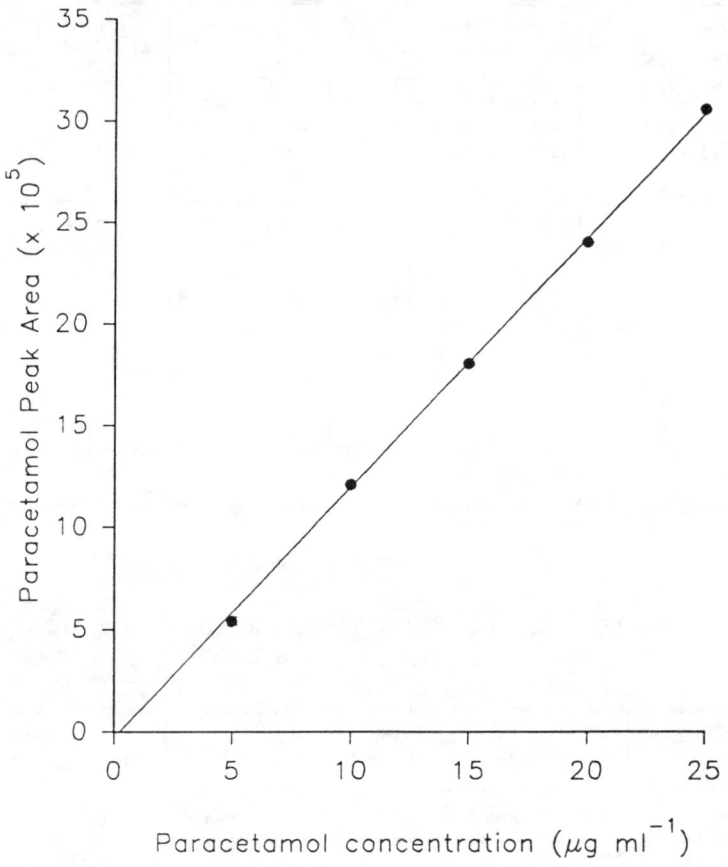

In comparison with another set of precision tests using the peak area ratios (paracetamol peak area to internal standard peak area) for calculations, the variation in the peak areas of the internal standard has a larger percentage of error. The coefficient of variation in this case varied from 2.3–5.1%. The coefficient of variation of the peak area counts of the internal standard was 3.8% (Table 2.6b). Although the standard of accuracy and precision of modern laboratory pipette are extremely good, the introduction of another variable, the dispensing of the internal standard in this case, is still liable to produce a slight increase in the coefficient of variation in the calculated result.

2. *Recovery.* Using the method of standard addition, the percentage of recovery was found to be consistently high, being very close to 100% (Table 2.7).

Table 2.7 Recovery of HPLC Plasma Paracetamol Assay Using Method of Standard Addition

	Paracetamol Area Counts	Calculated Paracetamol Concentration (μg ml^{-1})	Expected Paracetamol Concentration (μg ml^{-1})	Recovery (%)
Baseline (B)	1357881	13.58	13.64	99.6
500 μl of 15 μg ml^{-1}	1347283	13.47		98.8
+	1343479	13.44		98.5
50 μl blank plasma	1332395	13.33		97.7
B +	1593451	15.91	15.91	100.0
1.25 μg/ 50 μl	1580693	15.79		99.2
	1570506	15.68		98.6
	1561082	15.59		98.0
B +	1823175	18.18	18.18	100.0
2.5 μg/ 50 μl	1809284	18.05		99.3
	1795566	17.91		98.5
	1783409	17.79		97.9
B +	2262295	22.53	22.73	99.1
5.0 μg/ 50 μl	2244680	22.36		98.4
	2235913	22.27		98.0
	2230630	22.22		97.8

Sample preparation: To 500 μl of a paracetamol plasma sample (15 μg ml^{-1}), 50 μl of plasma containing different amounts of paracetamol standard was added. 50 μl of blank plasma was added to the baseline sample. Sample volume was effectively increased to 550 μl. Plasma protein precipitation was carried out in the normal manner.

Another set of recovery tests was done using commercially available plasma paracetamol standards for an ELISA method for the estimation of paracetamol concentrations, routinely employed by the Chemical Pathology Department of the Prince of Wales Hospital, Hong Kong. The concentrations of these standards estimated by the HPLC method were very close to their nominal value, as used in the ELISA assays, giving recoveries ranging from 94.9–96.3% over a range of 10–200 μg ml^{-1} (Table 2.8).

Table 2.8   Recovery of HPLC Plasma Paracetamol Assay Using
Commercial Available Paracetamol Standards

Sample	Peak Area of Paracetamol	Calculated Paracetamol Concentration (μg ml^{-1})	Nominal Paracetamol Concentration (μg ml^{-1})	Recovery (%)
A	0	0	0	-
A	0	0	0	-
A	0	0	0	-
B	964167	9.49	10.00	94.9
B	969433	9.54	10.00	95.4
B	962742	9.48	10.00	94.8
C	1948185	19.18	20.00	95.9
C	1946623	19.16	20.00	95.8
C	1936329	19.06	20.00	95.3
D	4908800	48.32	50.00	96.6
D	4859982	47.84	50.00	95.7
D	4864914	47.89	50.00	95.8
E	9774972	96.22	100.00	96.2
E	9825479	96.72	100.00	96.7
E	9783287	96.30	100.00	93.3
F	19638342	193.31	200.00	96.7
F	19402915	191.00	200.00	95.5
F	19388033	190.85	200.00	95.4

It was deemed satisfactory to use the area counts for all calculations instead of the area ratio. The coefficient of variation of the area ratio (2.3%–5.2%, median 3.3%) was found to be higher than the coefficient of variation of the area counts (0.1%–3.3%, median 0.3%). As precision, linearity and recovery were all above the required standard, it was decided not to use the internal standard. Thus standard curves calculated by the least-squares regression analysis of the peak area count *versus* drug concentration were used.

The linearity of the plasma assay for the metabolites was also established up to about 25 μg ml^{-1}, greater concentrations are unlikely to be reached after a therapeutic dose of paracetamol. The coefficients of correlations are shown in Table 2.9. The linearity of all the metabolites and of paracetamol was found to be excellent (Fig. 2.10).

The peak area counts obtained from paracetamol spiked in plasma and in water were found to be different when they were subjected to identical sample treatment. Peak area counts from paracetamol standards spiked in plasma were consistently lower than those spiked in water (Table 2.9). However, all reference standards to be run with plasma samples were prepared in the same matrix.

2.2.5 Summary

Many analytical methods are available for the estimation of paracetamol concentrations in biological fluids. HPLC assays are sensitive and accurate and they can be employed to measure both therapeutic and overdose concentrations of paracetamol, but only methods where the major metabolites of paracetamol, the glucuronide, sulphate, cysteine and mercapturate conjugates can also be co-chromatographed in the same assay can fulfil the requirements of a study involving its *in vivo* metabolism.

An HPLC method with excellent performance in precision, accuracy and linearity for the estimation of paracetamol and its metabolites is described. The same assay can be used to analyse both plasma samples and urine samples. The method described above required minimal sample preparation with a relatively short run time. Validation tests showed that this assay method for plasma and urine samples is reliable. This assay was used throughout for the study on the metabolism of paracetamol in healthy subjects and in patients with liver diseases and hepatocellular carcinoma.

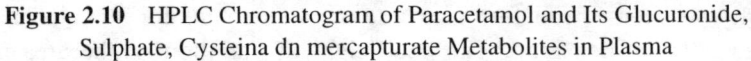

Figure 2.10   HPLC Chromatogram of Paracetamol and Its Glucuronide, Sulphate, Cysteina dn mercapturate Metabolites in Plasma

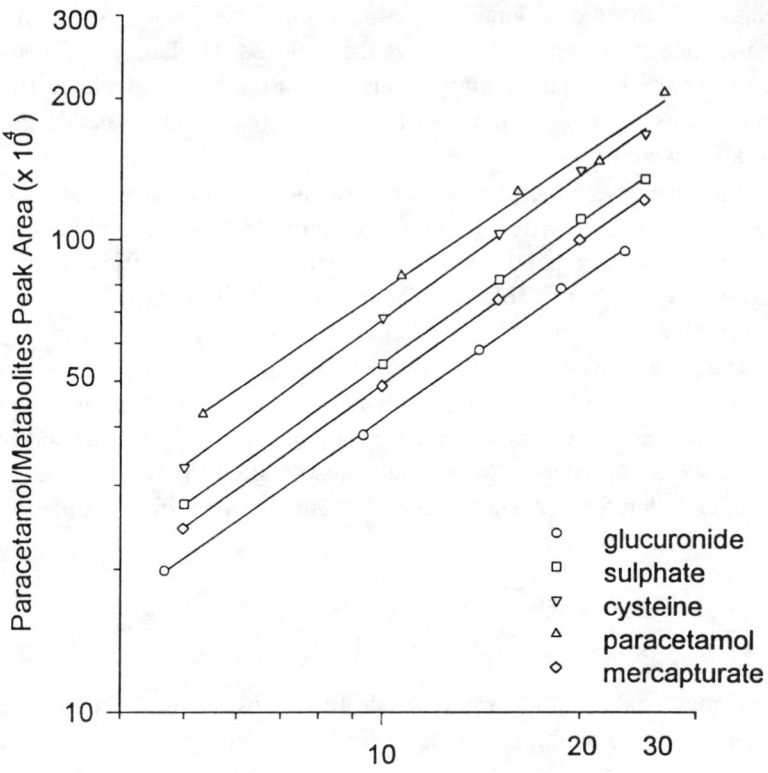

2.3   The pharmacokinetics of paracetamol in healthy subjects

2.3.1   *Introduction*

Although many studies on paracetamol metabolism in healthy subjects have been previously reported, it is unclear as to the most suitable duration of plasma sampling in such studies. In some studies, plasma samples were taken up to 8 hours after a dose of paracetamol while in others, blood

Table 2.9 Linearity of HPLC Plasma Paracetamol Metabolite Assay Using Peak Area Counts and Peak Area Ratio, in Aqueous and in Plasma

a. glucuronide

Conc. (µg ml⁻¹)	Aqueous		Plasma	
	Peak Area	Peak Area Ratio	Peak Area	Peak Area Ratio
4.67	168254	0.29	198178	0.36
9.33	331258	0.58	383919	0.71
14.00	494995	0.88	580447	1.07
18.67	663463	1.16	784790	1.42
23.33	822570	1.50	943690	1.75
r	1.000	1.000	0.999	1.000

b. sulphate

Conc. (µg ml⁻¹)	Aqueous		Plasma	
	Peak Area	Peak Area Ratio	Peak Area	Peak Area Ratio
5.00	313497	0.55	273492	0.50
10.00	624936	1.10	542358	1.00
15.00	930965	1.66	820081	1.51
20.00	1260614	2.21	1106928	2.00
25.00	1582384	2.88	1347861	2.49
r	1.000	0.999	1.000	1.000

c. cysteine

Conc. (µg ml⁻¹)	Aqueous		Plasma	
	Peak Area	Peak Area Ratio	Peak Area	Peak Area Ratio
5.00	318787	0.57	328297	0.60
10.00	653574	1.15	679938	1.26
15.00	963274	1.71	1028195	1.90
20.00	1314422	2.31	1405652	2.54
25.00	1613774	2.94	1683046	3.11
r	1.000	1.000	0.999	1.000

d. paracetamol

Conc. (µg ml⁻¹)	Aqueous		Plasma	
	Peak Area	Peak Area Ratio	Peak Area	Peak Area Ratio
5.33	441434	0.77	425203	0.77
10.67	868628	1.53	835922	1.54
16.00	1291443	2.30	1264082	2.33
21.33	1617669	2.84	1472114	2.66
26.67	2158753	3.93	2061368	3.81
r	0.998	0.995	0.992	0.988

e. mercapturate

Conc. (µg ml⁻¹)	Aqueous		Plasma	
	Peak Area	Peak Area Ratio	Peak Area	Peak Area Ratio
4.98	258140	0.45	243736	0.44
9.97	507636	0.89	488191	0.90
14.95	755035	1.34	745155	1.37
19.93	1001379	1.76	1000066	1.80
24.92	1288737	2.35	1216869	2.25
r	1.000	0.998	1.000	1.000

samples were taken up to 24 hours after the dose. In some of the published studies, a terminal elimination half-life value was quoted, but it was not clear which period of time this value referred to.

As a forerunner for the main pharmacokinetic study, a study was carried out on healthy control subjects to evaluate the differences in the pharmacokinetic parameters calculated using different sampling regimens. This would help in choosing the most appropriate sampling regimen for the study which followed.

2.3.2   Study protocol

All studies were carried out in the Clinical Pharmacology Studies Unit, Department of Clinical Pharmacology, The Chinese University of Hong Kong, at the Prince of Wales Hospital, Shatin, Hong Kong.

2.3.3   Methods

2.3.3.1 Subjects

Subjects for the healthy control study were volunteers responding to recruitment appeal posters for clinical research posted around the Hospital. Fourteen healthy Chinese males with a mean age of 29.4 ± 11.6 years, mean body weight 57.9 ± 8.3 kg and mean height 164 ± 8 cm were entered into the study. Each was given a physical examination and screening tests for plasma biochemistry and haematology were performed, together with urinalysis. The results in all subjects were normal.

Details of the age, body weight and height of the subjects are shown in Table 2.10 and the plasma biochemistry and haematology screen data are shown in Tables 2.11 and 2.12. None of the subjects was on any medication and none smoked or consumed alcohol regularly. Informed consent was given by each subject and the study was approved by the Hospital Ethics Committee.

2.3.3.2 Drug administration and sampling

The subjects attended the Clinical Pharmacology Studies Unit in the Department of Clinical Pharmacology in the morning after an overnight fast. An in-dwelling cannula (Angiocath 20G 2 inch, Becton Dickson) was inserted into a forearm vein. The cannula stayed *in situ* until after the 12 hour sample was drawn. The 24 hour blood sample was taken at a different site by venepuncture. Paracetamol was administered as the syrup (Panadol

Table 2.10   Details of 14 Chinese Healthy Subjects

Subject Number	Sex	Age	Body Weight (kg)	Height (cm)
1	M	21	69.4	175
2	F	32	46.1	155
3	M	26	56.3	160
4	F	26	47.4	161
5	F	22	48.9	156
6	F	23	48.1	154
8	M	23	70.5	178
10	F	23	60.1	157
11	F	23	52.8	161
14	M	22	61.2	175
15	M	22	60.8	169
23	M	42	68.2	163
24	F	54	63.0	162
25	M	53	57.6	167
Mean	7M/7F	29.4	57.9	163.8
S.D.		11.6	8.3	7.9

Table 2.11 Plasma Biochemistry Screen in 14 Chinese Healthy Subjects

	Mean	Range	Normal Range*
Total Protein (g l⁻¹)	76.2	70 - 84	66 - 81
Albumin (g l⁻¹)	46.0	42 - 50	36 - 48
Total Bilirubin (μmol l⁻¹)	10.2	6 - 16	0 - 15
Alkaline Phosphatase (IU l⁻¹)	60.8	35 - 81	40 - 136
ALT (IU l⁻¹)	14.1	2 - 56	0 - 58
Gamma GT (U l⁻¹)	11.0	4 - 21	0 - 84(F) 0 - 100(M)
Fasting Glucose (mmol l⁻¹)	4.9	4.2 - 5.8	3.5 - 6.0
Sodium (mmol l⁻¹)	139.6	137 - 142	134 - 145
Potassium (mmol l⁻¹)	3.9	3.4 - 4.8	3.5 - 5.1
Urea (mmol l⁻¹)	5.2	3.2 - 7.4	3.4 - 8.9
Creatinine (μmol l⁻¹)	78.8	64 - 96	44 - 107(F) 57 - 126(M)
Calcium (mmol l⁻¹)	2.31	2.17 - 2.46	2.13 - 2.51

* From the Department of Chemical Pathology, Prince of Wales Hospital, Shatin

Syrup 160 mg ml^{-1}, Sterling Drug (Malaya) Sdn., Bhd., Kuala Lumpur for Winthrop Product Inc., New York, U.S.A.) at a dose of 20 mg/kg body weight, together with 150 ml of water. Food and beverages were withheld for at least 3 hours after drug administration which and only water was allowed. Lunch was available at 4 hours and after that fluid and food intake

Table 2.12 Haemotology Screen in 14 Chinese Healthy Subjects

	Mean	Range	Normal Range*
Haemoglobin (g dl^{-1})	14.6	12.0 - 17.5	11.5 - 14.3(F) 13.2 - 16.7(M)
Haematocrit	0.441	0.357 - 0.533	0.32 - 0.43(F) 0.39 - 0.50(M)
RBC (x 10^{12} l^{-1})	5.25	4.12 - 7.04	3.7 - 4.9(F) 4.2 - 5.7(M)
MCHC (g dl^{-1})	33.1	30.9 - 34.2	32 - 35
MCH (pg)	28.1	20.6 - 31.5	27 - 33
MCV (fl)	85	67 - 93	81 - 97
Platelets (x 10^9 l^{-1})	213	153 - 275	140 - 380
WBC (x 10^9 l^{-1})	5.6	3.2 - 7.9	4.0 - 10.8
Neutrophils (%)	62.9	49 - 82	40 - 60
Lymphocytes (%)	28.8	13 - 43	20 - 40
Monocytes (%)	4.9	4 - 6	4 - 8
Eosinophils (%)	1.8	1 - 5	1 - 4
Basophils (%)	1.1	1 - 2	~ 1

* From the Department of Chemical Pathology, Prince of Wales Hospital, Shatin

were unrestricted. 5 ml venous blood samples were drawn into heparinised tubes at 0, 0.5, 1, 1.5, 2, 3, 4, 5, 6, 7, 8, 9, 10, 11, 12 and 24 hours after dosing. Blood samples were centrifuged at 1400 xg for 10 minutes and the plasma separated for storage at –20°C prior to analysis. Urine was collected for the time period 0–4, 4–8, 8–12 and 12–24 hours after dosing. The volume of urine excreted at each time period was noted and a 20 ml aliquot was taken from each collection and stored at $-20°C$ until analysis.

2.3.3.3 Drug analysis

The concentrations of paracetamol, the glucuronide, sulphate, cysteine and mercapturate metabolites in plasma and in urine were measured by the HPLC assay described in this chapter, section 2.2.2. Metabolite concentrations were expressed as paracetamol equivalents.

2.3.3.4 Calculations

Plasma concentrations of paracetamol and the glucuronide, sulphate and cysteine metabolites of individual subjects were calculated from the respective peak area counts and the paracetamol standards according to section 2.2.4.2. The recovery of paracetamol and its metabolites in the urine was calculated according to section 2.2.3.2. The individual peak plasma concentrations (C_{max}) and time to reach peak plasma concentrations (t_{max}) were noted.

The metabolic clearance was calculated according to the method of Miners *et al.* (Miners *et al.*, 1983; Miners *et al.*, 1986). This calculation assumes that the clearance of paracetamol (Cl) is the sum of the individual clearances involved in paracetamol elimination. i.e.

$$Cl = Cl_P + Cl_G + Cl_S + Cl_C + Cl_M$$

where Cl is the overall clearance of paracetamol and Cl_P, Cl_G, Cl_S, Cl_C, and Cl_M are the metabolic clearances to unchanged paracetamol, the glucuronide, sulphate, cysteine and mercapturate conjugates, respectively. The metabolic clearance to each metabolite Cl_M was calculated as:

$$Cl_M = f_m \, Cl$$

where f_m is the fractional recovery of the respective metabolite in the urine.

2.3.4 Pharmacokinetic analysis

Pharmacokinetic analysis was done using the pharmacokinetic modelling programme SIPHAR/base, Version 4.0 (1991, SIMED, Créteil, Cedex, France). Pharmacokinetic modelling and estimation of the pharmacokinetic parameters for individual plasma data were done as follows.

The semilogarithmic plot of plasma concentrations against time was displayed on the screen. After visual inspection of the plot, the number of exponentials suitable to describe the data and the number of observations belonging to each exponential phase were decided. After having chosen these criteria, the goodness of fit of this model was verified by a visual analysis of the theoretical curve superimposed on the experimental data points. This was done by the programme using the method of residuals, also known as *peeling* or *feathering* (SIMED, 1991; Shargel & Yu, 1993). The parameters of each phase computed were then displayed and were used as the initial parameters for the next iterative procedure in the data modelling. In the second stage of parameters estimation, the extended least squares method was used, and the minimization algorithm employed was that of Powell. Using the extended least squares method, both the structural model and the error model parameters were estimated simultaneously by minimizing the log-likelihood function L:

$$L = \sum_{i}^{N} \frac{(Y_i - M_i)^2}{V_i} + \log V_i$$

where N is the number of experimental points, Y_i is the i-th observation, M_i is the i-th predicted value and V_i is the error variance of the i-th observation. The error model utilised in the iteration was

$$V = a\, M_i^b$$

where a and b are the two error model parameters. This model generalizes the usual weighting scheme applied to standard weighted regression analysis.

Very often different equations can be used to fit the same data set. For each set of data and a chosen model, a number of fitted curves can be generated with slightly differing pharmacokinetic parameters. A plot of the residual *versus* time and/or the computed values are provided by SIPHAR for the assessment of the adequacy of the structural model. The residuals should be randomly distributed. Apart from the residual plot, the programme also computes firstly the correlation coefficient between the observed and theoretical values and secondly the coefficient of variation (CV) of each parameter. The value of the CV gives an indication of the accuracy of the estimate.

SIPHAR also provides three values for the assessment of the appropriateness of the model — the Akaike value, the Schwartz value and the Leonard value. The calculation of the Schwartz value takes into account the number of data points and was chosen as one of the criteria to decide the best-fit model. The Schwartz value is defined as

$$S = -Log\ likelihood + \tfrac{1}{2} \log N$$

where N is the number of data points.

The equations used to describe a 2 phase model and a 3 phase model are:

2 phase model $Y = -Ae^{-at} + Be^{-bt}$

3 phase model $Y = -Ce^{-ct} + Ae^{-at} + Be^{-bt}$ $(C = A+B)$

A, B and C are the coefficients and a, b and c are the exponentials of the respective phases. Both equations describe curves which are forced through the origin.

The following parameters are provided by the programme following data modelling:

AUCT$_{ex}$ Total area under the curve extrapolated to infinity, calculated by the trapezoidal rule (model independent)

AUC   Total area under the curve of the fitted model

$t_{1/2}$ Half-life, calculated as $t_{1/2} = 0.693/k$, where k is the exponential of the phase to which the half-life refers

Cl   Clearance, calculated as $Cl = Dose/AUCT_{ex}$ (assuming complete absorption)

V_d Volume of distribution of the terminal elimination phase (ß phase), calculated as $V_d = Cl/beta$ where beta is the terminal slope

MRT   Mean residence time is defined as the average time that all the drug molecules reside in the body. It is a measure of the mean transit time of the drug molecules. The model independent MRT is calculated normally calculated as MRT = AUMC/AUC, where AUMC is the area under the first moment versus time curve from t = 0 to infinity and AUC is also known as the zero moment curve. In this pharmacokinetic modelling programme, the MRT of the fitted model is calculated as $MRT = \Sigma\ Coef_i / Exp_i^2$, where $Coef_i$ and Exp_i are the coefficient and exponential of the ith phase, respectively

To determine if there was any difference in data modelling when the sampling times were different, 5 different models using different sampling times were compared. The parameters obtained from these 5 different curve fittings were analysed for any statistically significant difference. The sampling times used in these models were as follows:

Model	Sampling times (hour)	No. of phases
1	0, 0.5, 1, 1.5, 2, 3, 4, 5, 6, 7, 8, 9, 10, 11, 12, 24	3
2	0, 0.5, 1, 1.5, 2, 3, 4, 5, 6, 7, 8, 9, 10, 11, 12	3
3	0, 0.5, 1, 1.5, 2, 3, 4, 5, 6, 7, 8, 24	3
4	0, 0.5, 1, 1.5, 2, 3, 4, 5, 6, 7, 8, 9, 10, 11, 12	2
5	0, 0.5, 1, 1.5, 2, 3, 4, 5, 6, 7, 8	2

In particular, a comparison between model 1 and model 2 was used to demonstrate the importance of the plasma level at 24 hour in influencing the pharmacokinetic parameters of a 3-phase model, whereas a comparison between model 1 and model 3 was used to show the importance of extra sampling times at 9, 10, 11 and 12 hours.

Model 2 and model 4 used the same sampling times and the former was fitted to a 3-phase model with an initial elimination phase between about 2 to 8 hours and a terminal elimination phase following that. Model 4 was fitted using a 2-phase model with only 1 terminal elimination phase. A comparison between model 2 and model 4 was used to demonstrate the difference in the pharmacokinetic parameters when the same sampling points were force-fitted to two different models.

Sampling time was only taken up to 8 hours in model 5. A comparison between model 4 and model 5 was used to demonstrate if the extra sampling times at 9, 10, 11 and 12 hours had any influence on the estimated pharmacokinetic parameters when the two models were both used to fit a 2-phase model.

Therefore, the pharmacokinetic parameters estimated from these different models were compared together by analysis of variance but the following comparisons were also made in particular:

model 1 *vs* model 2
model 1 *vs* model 3
model 2 *vs* model 4
model 4 *vs* model 5

2.3.5 Statistical analysis

Mean values with the standard deviation (SD) are presented. All statistical analyses were carried out using the computer statistics package SPSS for

Windows (Version 5, 1992, SPSS Inc., Chicago, U.S.A.), supplemented by SigmaStat (Version 1.01, 1993, Jandel Scientific, San Rafael, California, U.S.A.) when the desired tests were not available on SPSS. Geigy Scientific Tables (Geigy Scientific Tables, 1982) was also consulted when the coefficient of correlation was tested for statistical significance.

Bland-Altman plots (Bland & Altman, 1986) were done using a modification of the original authors' method (see results and discussion, sections 2.3.6.4 and 2.3.7). The calculations for the intraclass correlation coefficient of reliability was based on the method given in Chapter 1 (p. 11) of *The Design and Analysis of Clinical Experiments* (Fleiss, 1986).

2.3.6   Results

2.3.6.1 Plasma Results

Mean plasma concentrations of paracetamol and its metabolites following oral administration of a 20 mg kg^{-1} body weight dose to 14 healthy subjects are shown in Table 2.13. and Fig. 2.11. The mercapturate conjugate was not detected in any of the plasma samples, probably due to very low concentrations. Plasma concentrations for each subject are shown in Appendices 2.2–2.5. Individual values for peak concentration (C_{max}) and time to reach peak concentration (t_{max}) are shown in Table 2.14.

The absorption of paracetamol was rapid with a mean C_{max} of 22.5 ± 5.81 µg ml^{-1} (range 16.53–33.83), occurring at a mean t_{max} of 0.89 ± 0.40 hr (range 0.5–1.5). A semilogarithmic plot of paracetamol concentrations against time showed a linear decline up to around 8–12 hr post dose. Beyond this period, the decline in paracetamol concentration seemed to be much slower as the plasma concentration at 24 hr did not seem to fit with a single elimination phase.

The mean plasma concentration of paracetamol glucuronide rose steadily and peaked at 3.07 ± 0.73 hr (range 2.0–4.0 hr). The C_{max} ranged from 5.65–15.10 µg ml^{-1} (mean 9.62 ± 2.64 g ml^{-1}). After paracetamol glucuronide t_{max}, the plasma concentration of the glucuronide conjugate was always higher than the parent drug. In contrast, the mean plasma concentration of paracetamol sulphate was always lower than paracetamol, with mean C_{max} 5.14 ± 1.30 µg ml^{-1} (range 2.85–7.15). The time to peak concentration was reached early, mean t_{max} was at 1.50 ± 0.28 hr (range 1.0–2.0).

Only very low concentrations of the cysteine conjugate were detected in the plasma samples (see Appendix 2.5).

Table 2.13   Mean Plasma Concentrations of Paracetamol and the Glucuronide, Sulphate and Cysteine Conjugates in 14 Healthy Subjects Following Ingestion of a 20 mg kg^{-1} Body Weight Dose

Time After Dosing (hr)	Plasma Concentration (μg ml^{-1})			
	Paracetamol	Glucuronide	Sulphate	Cysteine
	Mean $\pm$ SD	Mean $\pm$ SD	Mean $\pm$ SD	Mean $\pm$ SD
0	0	0	0	0
0.5	20.99 $\pm$ 7.20	2.05 $\pm$ 1.00	2.90 $\pm$ 1.12	0.01 $\pm$ 0.02
1	19.21 $\pm$ 4.02	5.60 $\pm$ 1.48	4.66 $\pm$ 1.35	0.04 $\pm$ 0.05
1.5	16.58 $\pm$ 3.31	7.63 $\pm$ 2.23	5.08 $\pm$ 1.37	0.08 $\pm$ 0.06
2	14.23 $\pm$ 2.79	8.78 $\pm$ 2.57	5.03 $\pm$ 1.30	0.10 $\pm$ 0.05
3	11.21 $\pm$ 2.37	9.47 $\pm$ 2.60	4.71 $\pm$ 1.28	0.14 $\pm$ 0.07
4	8.54 $\pm$ 1.86	9.31 $\pm$ 2.57	4.07 $\pm$ 1.19	0.19 $\pm$ 0.07
5	6.36 $\pm$ 1.35	8.18 $\pm$ 2.06	3.47 $\pm$ 1.04	0.19 $\pm$ 0.06
6	4.84 $\pm$ 1.17	6.93 $\pm$ 1.80	2.96 $\pm$ 1.01	0.16 $\pm$ 0.05
7	3.80 $\pm$ 0.94	5.58 $\pm$ 1.53	2.45 $\pm$ 0.84	0.13 $\pm$ 0.08
8	2.96 $\pm$ 0.79	4.53 $\pm$ 1.41	1.98 $\pm$ 0.72	0.12 $\pm$ 0.07
9	2.19 $\pm$ 0.61	3.62 $\pm$ 1.07	1.56 $\pm$ 0.60	0.11 $\pm$ 0.08
10	1.90 $\pm$ 0.57	3.58 $\pm$ 1.96	1.62 $\pm$ 1.21	0.11 $\pm$ 0.07
11	1.40 $\pm$ 0.44	2.44 $\pm$ 0.84	1.02 $\pm$ 0.37	0.08 $\pm$ 0.06
12	1.13 $\pm$ 0.36	1.96 $\pm$ 0.71	0.86 $\pm$ 0.32	0.07 $\pm$ 0.05
24	0.24 $\pm$ 0.07	0.32 $\pm$ 0.12	0.17 $\pm$ 0.08	0.01 $\pm$ 0.02

Figure 2.11   Mean Plasma Concentrations of Paracetamol, Paracetamol
Glucuronide and Paracetamol Sulphate in 14 Healthy Subjects
Following Ingestion of a 20 mg kg^{-1} Body Weight Dose

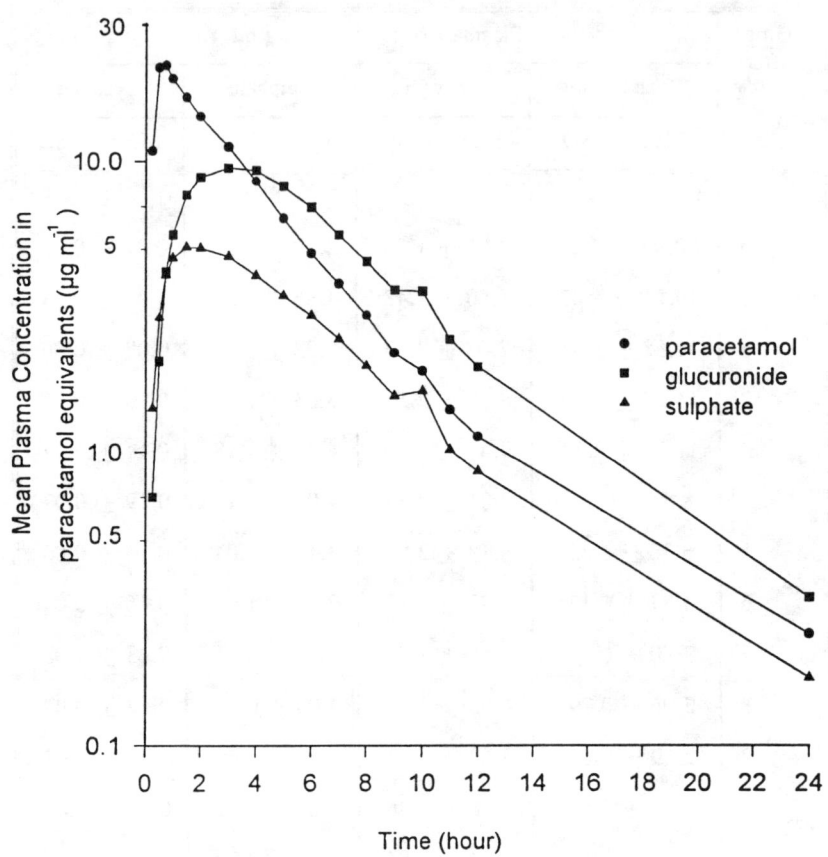

2.3.6.2   Urine Results

Table 2.15 shows the overall recovery and fractional recovery of
paracetamol and its four major metabolites in the 24 hour urine collections
of the 14 healthy subjects. The mean total recovery of paracetamol and all
metabolites in the 24 hour urine collection was 94.2 ± 15.4% of the
administered dose. The mean fractional recovery in the 24 hr urine collection was 54.8 ± 8.9%, 33.7 ± 8.0%, 3.3 ± 1.2%, 2.5 ± 0.9% and 5.6 ± 1.6%

Table 2.14   Peak Plasma Concentration (C_{max}) and Time to Reach Peak Plasma Concentrations (T_{max}) of Paracetamol and Its Glucuronide and Sulphate Metabolites in 14 Healthy Subjects Following a 20 mg kg^{-1} Dose

Subject	Paracetamol		Glucuronide		Sulphate	
	Cmax	Tmax	Cmax	Tmax	Cmax	Tmax
	(μg ml-1)	(hr)	(μg ml-1)	(hr)	(μg ml-1)	(hr)
CWH	21.16	0.50	11.79	3.00	4.43	1.50
WR	17.66	1.00	6.30	4.00	2.85	1.00
WKKW	16.53	0.50	12.23	2.00	3.88	1.50
KWSC	17.55	1.50	8.25	3.00	4.25	1.50
CSYC	23.55	0.50	7.45	2.00	6.22	1.50
LHY	19.44	1.00	5.65	3.00	5.35	1.50
CWSD	19.75	1.00	12.57	4.00	3.12	2.00
NPSD	28.88	0.50	8.89	2.00	5.49	1.00
LCKY	28.81	1.00	8.76	4.00	7.15	1.50
WP	18.59	1.00	10.63	4.00	6.10	1.50
WH	31.23	0.50	9.40	3.00	5.78	1.50
YAS	16.77	1.50	7.56	3.00	5.20	1.50
SPY	21.18	1.50	15.10	3.00	5.28	2.00
KKH	33.83	0.50	10.15	3.00	6.89	1.50
Mean	22.50	0.89	9.62	3.07	5.14	1.50
SD	5.81	0.40	2.64	0.73	1.30	0.28
Min	16.53	0.50	5.65	2.00	2.85	1.00
Max	33.83	1.50	15.10	4.00	7.15	2.00

for the glucuronide, sulphate, cysteine, mercapturate conjugate and unchanged paracetamol, respectively. For unchanged paracetamol and the glucuronide and sulphate conjugates, more than 70% of the recovered amount was excreted within 8 hours of the ingestion of paracetamol. More than 50% of the oxidative metabolites was also excreted within 8 hours and the proportion of the excreted cysteine conjugate and mercapturate conjugate was almost parallel at all stages. The mean cumulative recovery

　　　　　　　Metabolic Activation of Drugs and Other Xenobiotics

Table 2.15　Urinary Recovery of Paracetamol and Its Glucuronide, Sulphate, Cysteine and Mercapturate Metabolites in 24 h Following Ingestion of a 20 mg kg^{-1} Dose in 14 Healthy Subjects

Subject	Percentage of Total Amount Recovered in Urine Over 24 hours						Total Recovery as % of Dose
	G	S	C	P	M	M+C	
CWH	63.9	24.1	3.6	5.2	3.2	6.7	69.0
WR	56.2	30.3	5.0	5.4	3.2	8.1	63.6
WKKW	67.1	24.9	2.5	3.1	2.4	4.9	96.8
KWSC	56.5	30.0	5.0	6.1	2.4	7.4	94.2
CSYC	44.2	46.4	2.2	5.4	1.8	4.0	81.3
LHY	40.7	43.7	4.2	9.0	2.3	6.5	79.9
CWSD	68.6	22.3	2.1	5.0	2.0	4.1	113.7
NPSD	55.0	36.7	2.0	4.8	1.6	3.6	99.6
LCKY	45.5	45.9	2.5	4.2	2.0	4.5	112.9
WP	52.5	37.5	3.5	4.1	2.5	6.0	104.5
WH	55.7	34.3	2.4	6.5	1.0	3.5	107.2
YAS	49.3	35.3	4.4	6.5	4.5	8.9	95.4
SPY	65.0	25.3	1.7	5.5	2.6	4.2	103.0
KKH	47.5	35.7	4.7	8.1	4.1	8.7	98.2
Mean	54.8	33.7	3.3	5.6	2.5	5.8	94.2
SD	8.9	8.0	1.2	1.6	0.9	1.9	15.4

G = paracetamol glucuronide
S = paracetamol sulphate
C = paracetamol cysteine
P = paracetamol
M = paracetamol mercapturate

of paracetamol and its metabolites in the urine was shown in Table 2.16 and Fig. 2.12. Individual urinary excretion data are shown in Appendices 2.6–2.10.

Table 2.16 Mean Cumulative Percentage Recovery of Paracetamol and Its Metabolites in 14 Healthy Subjects Following Ingestion of a 20 mg kg–1 Body Weight Dose

Time After Ingestion (hr)	Mean Cumulative Percentage Recovery											
	Glucuronide		Sulphate		Cysteine		Paracetamol		Mercapturate		M + C	
	Mean	SD	Mean	SD	Mean	SD	Mean	SD	Mean	SD	Mean	SD
Predose	0	0	0	0	0	0	0	0	0	0	0	0
4	20.4	6.5	14.6	3.9	0.7	0.2	3.1	0.9	0.6	0.2	1.2	0.4
8	40.1	7.9	25.4	6.1	1.7	0.6	4.4	1.1	1.4	0.4	3.1	0.8
12	49.1	8.0	30.4	7.4	2.5	0.9	5.1	1.4	2.0	0.6	4.5	1.3
24	54.8	8.9	33.7	8.0	3.3	1.2	5.6	1.6	2.5	0.9	5.8	1.9

Figure 2.12   Mean Culumative Percentage Recovery of Paracetamol and
Its Metabolites in 14 Healthy Subjects Following Ingestion of
a 20 mg kg^{-1} Body Weight Dose

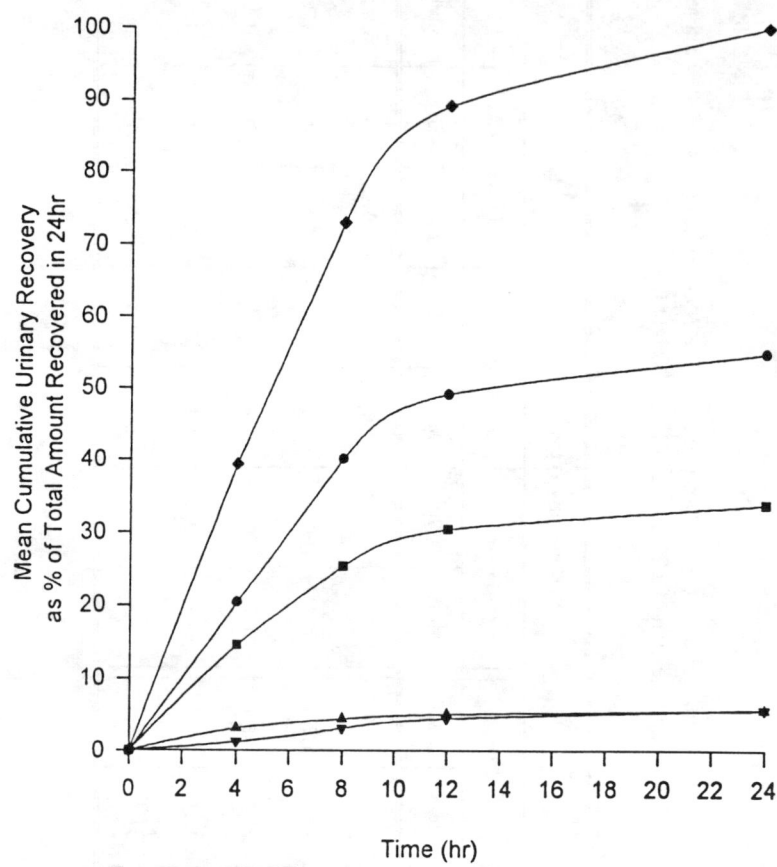

•   glucuronide
■   sulphate
▲   paracetamol
▼   mercapturate & cysteine
◆   total recovery

The mean percentages of total drug excreted as paracetamol and its
metabolites in divided urine collections are shown in Table 2.17 and Fig.
2.13. At all times the greatest proportion was excreted as the glucuronide

Table 2.17 Mean Percentage Recovery of Paracetamol and Its Metabolites in Divided Urine Collection in 14 Healthy Subjects Following Ingestion of a 20 mg kg−1 Body Weight Dose

Time After Ingestion (hr)	Mean Percentage Recovery											
	Glucuronide		Sulphate		Cysteine		Paracetamol		Mercapturate		M + C	
	Mean	SD	Mean	SD	Mean	SD	Mean	SD	Mean	SD	Mean	SD
0-4	51.2	9.5	37.5	8.2	1.7	0.5	8.2	3.0	1.4	0.5	3.1	0.8
4-8	58.7	9.1	32.0	8.2	3.2	1.1	3.8	1.1	2.4	0.8	5.5	1.8
8-12	56.6	9.3	31.1	9.1	4.8	2.0	4.0	1.6	3.5	1.1	8.3	2.7
12-24	51.7	9.7	31.7	9.3	6.6	2.7	5.1	1.7	4.9	2.2	11.5	4.4
0-24	54.8	8.9	33.7	8.0	3.3	1.2	5.6	1.6	2.5	0.9	5.8	1.9

Figure 2.13   Mean Percentage Recovery of Paracetamol and Its Metabolites in Divided Urine Collections in 14 Healthy Subjects Following Ingestion of a 20 mg kg^{-1} Body Weight Dose

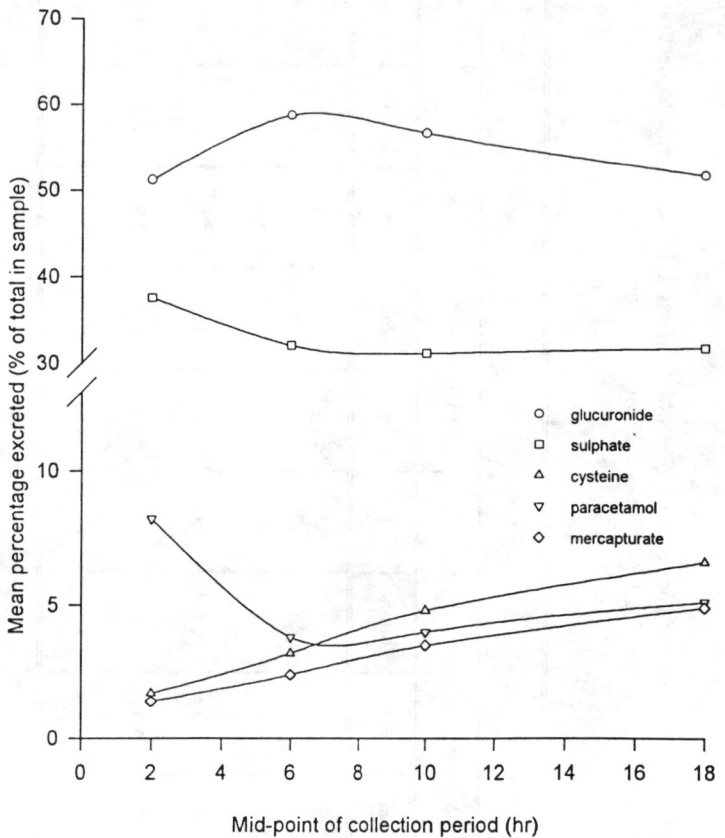

conjugate, the percentage being between 50–60%. There was a slight increase in the percentage recovery of glucuronide during the period between 4 to 8 hours, thereafter, it decreased again. This change in the percentage recovery was mirrored in the opposite pattern by that of the sulphate conjugate.

The percentage recovery of unchanged paracetamol during the first urine collection period between 4–8 hours was high at 8.2% and then decreased rapidly to 3–4%. The excretion patterns of the cysteine and mercapturate conjugates were very similar. The initial percentage recovery of these two metabolites was low, at below 2%, but increasing steadily to about 5–6%.

2.3.6.3 Pharmacokinetic Results

The pharmacokinetic parameters calculated for the different models are shown in Table 2.18 to Table 2.22, including AUC, Cl, terminal $t_{1/2}$, MRT and Vd.

Table 2.18   Area Under Curve (AUC) of the Plasma Concentration-Time Curves of Paracetamol of 5 Fitted Models in 14 Healthy Subjects Following Ingestion of a 20 mg kg^{-1} Body Weight Dose

Subject	Area Under Curve of Fitted Model (μg ml^{-1} hr)				
	Fitted Model				
	1	2	3	4	5
CWH	92.1	88.3	100.2	86.5	85.0
WR	84.9	80.3	98.0	79.9	82.7
WKKW	48.4	46.4	51.3	46.0	45.1
KWSC	85.9	81.2	95.5	80.7	81.4
CSYC	84.9	81.1	92.2	77.7	75.6
LHY	95.5	94.9	104.5	88.2	87.1
CWSD	94.3	91.8	103.7	89.8	88.6
NPSD	90.0	86.6	98.4	85.2	74.0
LCKY	118.8	112.3	130.1	110.7	110.4
WP	86.8	82.1	96.0	81.7	81.1
WH	75.4	70.9	84.3	69.7	80.8
YAS	94.9	89.8	105.4	88.9	87.0
SPY	112.7	106.0	126.5	105.7	106.0
KKH	123.4	117.9	136.2	115.5	115.4
Mean	92.0	87.8	101.6	86.2	85.7
SD	18.6	17.7	20.9	17.4	17.3

As the AUC is that of the fitted model and also extrapolated to infinity, the values obtained from different models were quite different. The mean values for the 5 models were 92 ± 18.6, 87.8 ± 17.7, 101.6 ± 20.9, 86.2 ± 17.4 and 85.7 ± 17.3 g ml^{-1} hr, respectively (Table 2.18). The highest value was obtained in Model 3. The mean AUC values of Model 4 and Model 5 were very close, as well as the standard deviation. The only difference between these two models was that the sampling time was up to 12 hours in Model 4 and only up to 8 hours in Model 5.

Clearance values for individual subjects in different fitted models are shown in Table 2.19. The mean values for the 5 models were 3.80 ± 1.01,

Table 2.19 Clearance (Cl) of Paracetamol in 5 Fitted Models in 14 Healthy Subjects Following Ingestion of a 20 mg kg^{-1} Body Weight Dose

Subject	Clearance of Paracetamol in Fitted Model (ml min^{-1} kg^{-1})				
	Fitted Model				
	1	2	3	4	5
CWH	3.62	3.77	3.33	3.85	3.92
WR	3.93	4.15	3.40	4.17	4.03
WKKW	6.89	7.18	6.49	7.25	7.39
KWSC	3.88	4.11	3.49	4.13	4.09
CSYC	3.93	4.11	3.62	4.29	4.41
LHY	3.49	3.51	3.19	3.78	3.83
CWSD	3.54	3.63	3.21	3.71	3.76
NPSD	3.71	3.85	3.39	3.91	4.51
LCKY	2.81	2.97	2.56	3.01	3.02
WP	3.84	4.06	3.47	4.08	4.11
WH	4.42	4.70	3.95	4.78	4.13
YAS	3.51	3.71	3.16	3.75	3.83
SPY	2.96	3.14	2.64	3.15	3.15
KKH	2.70	2.83	2.45	2.89	2.89
Mean	3.80	3.98	3.45	4.05	4.08
SD	1.01	1.05	0.97	1.05	1.07

3.98 ± 1.05, 3.45 ± 0.97, 4.05 ± 1.05 and 4.08 ± 1.07, respectively. Again, the mean values between Model 4 and Model 5 were very close with similar standard deviations. As Cl and AUC have an inverse relationship (Cl = Dose/AUC), it was as expected that the mean Cl value was found to be lowest in Model 3.

The terminal $t_{1/2}$ values tabulated in Table 2.20 refer to different time periods in the various models. In Models 1 to 3, where a 3-phase model was fitted, the terminal elimination $t_{1/2}$ refers to the time period around 7 to 8 hr to the last sampling time. For Models 1 and Model 3, this was 24 hr and for Model 2, the last sampling time was 12 hr. The terminal elimination $t_{1/2}$ for Model 4 refers to the time about 2 to 12 hr and for Model 5, about 2 to 8 hr. As a result, the terminal $t_{1/2}$ values of a particular subject in these different fitted models were very different. The mean terminal $t_{1/2}$ estimated by these models were 5.4 ± 1.1, 3.5 ± 0.9, 4.3 ± 0.4, 2.6 ± 0.3 and 2.6 ± 0.4 hr, respectively (Table 2.20).

The mean $t_{1/2}$ estimated by Model 1 was the longest, followed by Model 3. In these two models, the last sampling time used was 24 hr. The plasma concentration at this terminal point seemed to contribute to the estimation of a longer $t_{1/2}$ value. The difference between the mean estimated $t_{1/2}$ value in Model 4 and Model 5 was very small. It seemed that the sampling points at 9 to 12 hr, the extra sampling times used in Model 4, fitted very well into the elimination phase between 2 and 8 hr, the time period for the estimation of terminal $t_{1/2}$ in Model 5. The mean $t_{1/2}$ in these two models were much lower than those estimated in Model 1 and Model 3.

Model 2 used sampling time up to 12 hr and was fitted to a 3-phase model. The mean $t_{1/2}$ was between the longer values of Model 1 and 3, and the shorter value of Model 4 and 5.

The mean residence time (MRT), defined as the average time for all the drug molecules to reside in the body, is a measure of the mean transit time of the drug molecules. It takes into account all the different phases and not just the terminal elimination phase. The mean MRT values estimated in the different models were 5.0 ± 0.5, 4.4 ± 0.6, 4.9 ± 0.4, 4.1 ± 0.5 and 4.0 ± 0.5, respectively (Table 2.21). When comparing the mean MRT in the different models, it was seen that the values estimated in Model 1 and Model 3 were close with comparable standard deviations and the mean at around 5 hr. Similar findings were seen with Model 4 and Model 5, with mean MRT at around 4 hr. The mean MRT value in Model 2, like the mean $t_{1/2}$ again, lay midway between the values of the other models.

Table 2.20   Terminal Elimination Half-life of Paracetamol in 5 Fitted Models in 14 Healthy Subjects Following Ingestion of a 20 mg kg^{-1} Body Weight Dose

Subject	Terminal Elimination Half-Life of Paracetamol (hr)				
	Fitted Model				
	1	2	3	4	5
CWH	4.4	3.6	4.6	2.6	2.6
WR	4.5	3.1	4.1	2.9	3.1
WKKW	5.8	2.7	4.9	1.9	1.8
KWSC	5.3	2.8	4.2	2.5	2.6
CSYC	6.9	4.6	4.9	2.2	2.1
LHY	5.3	5.9	4.6	2.9	2.8
CWSD	3.8	3.8	3.8	2.8	2.7
NPSD	3.9	4.0	3.6	2.5	2.6
LCKY	7.5	3.4	4.6	2.2	2.2
WP	5.1	2.9	4.1	2.6	2.5
WH	6.9	3.3	4.5	2.3	2.3
YAS	4.8	3.5	4.3	3.0	2.7
SPY	5.6	2.8	4.4	2.6	2.6
KKH	5.2	3.1	4.5	3.0	3.0
Mean	5.4	3.5	4.3	2.6	2.6
SD	1.1	0.9	0.4	0.3	0.4

The volume (V_d) of distribution of the terminal phase was calculated by dividing the clearance by the slope of the terminal phase. The mean values for V_d in the different models were 1.77 ± 0.64, 1.20 ± 0.33, 1.31 ± 0.45, 0.88 ± 0.15 and 0.88 ± 0.15 l kg^{-1}, respectively (Table 2.22). Model 4 and Model 5, had the shortest $t_{1/2}$ (and thus the largest terminal slope value), the mean V_d in these two models were the biggest. The mean values were actually identical in these two models. Since the mean $t_{1/2}$ estimated in Model 1 was longest, it was as expected that the mean V_d was also largest

Table 2.21   Mean Residence Time of Paracetamol in 5 Fitted Models in 14 Healthy Subjects Following Ingestion of a 20 mg kg^{-1} Body Weight Dose

Subject	Mean Residence Time of Paracetamol (hr)				
	Fitted Model				
	1	2	3	4	5
CWH	4.9	4.5	4.8	4.1	4.0
WR	5.3	4.6	5.3	4.6	4.9
WKKW	3.9	3.2	3.9	3.0	2.9
KWSC	4.8	4.0	4.8	3.9	4.0
CSYC	5.3	4.5	5.0	3.8	3.5
LHY	5.6	6.0	5.3	4.5	4.4
CWSD	4.8	4.8	4.7	4.4	4.3
NPSD	4.5	4.6	4.4	4.0	4.4
LCKY	4.9	3.8	4.6	3.5	3.5
WP	4.9	4.1	4.8	4.0	3.9
WH	5.3	4.2	5.1	3.9	3.4
YAS	5.6	5.0	5.4	4.9	4.6
SPY	5.1	4.2	5.0	4.2	4.2
KKH	5.2	4.3	5.0	4.3	4.3
Mean	5.0	4.4	4.9	4.1	4.0
SD	0.5	0.6	0.4	0.5	0.5

among the 5 models. The V_d values in Model 2 and Model 3 were in between.

The metabolic clearances to the various metabolites of paracetamol estimated in the different models are governed by the plasma clearance of paracetamol; therefore, the comparisons of these metabolic clearance values in the different models were similar to the comparisons of the plasma clearance. The mean values are shown in Table 2.23. The metabolic clearance to all the metabolites in the different models followed a

Table 2.22   Volume of Distribution of Terminal Elimination Phase of Paracetamol in 5 Fitted Models in 14 Healthy Subjects Following Ingestion of a 20 mg kg^{-1} Body Weight Dose

Subject	Volume of Distribution of the Terminal Elimination Phase of Paracetamol (l kg-1)				
	Fitted Model				
	1	2	3	4	5
CWH	1.38	1.18	1.32	0.87	0.90
WR	1.53	1.12	1.20	1.04	1.10
WKKW	3.43	1.71	2.74	1.17	1.17
KWSC	1.80	1.01	1.26	0.88	0.93
CSYC	2.34	1.63	1.52	0.82	0.79
LHY	1.59	1.80	1.26	0.95	0.94
CWSD	1.15	1.21	1.06	0.89	0.88
NPSD	1.27	1.32	1.04	0.85	1.01
LCKY	1.83	0.87	1.02	0.58	0.58
WP	1.71	1.01	1.23	0.91	0.87
WH	2.65	1.36	1.54	0.95	0.81
YAS	1.47	1.11	1.17	0.99	0.91
SPY	1.44	0.75	1.00	0.71	0.70
KKH	1.22	0.76	0.95	0.74	0.75
Mean	1.77	1.20	1.31	0.88	0.88
SD	0.64	0.33	0.45	0.15	0.15

similar pattern. The values between Model 4 and Model 5 were very close and so were the values between Model 2 and Model 4. The individual metabolic clearance values are shown in Appendices 2.11–2.15.

2.3.6.4 Statistical Results

Each of the pharmacokinetic parameters from the 5 different models was first compared by a global analysis using the one-way repeated measures analysis of variance (RM ANOVA) for a parametric comparison and a

Table 2.23 Mean Metabolic Clearance of Paracetamol and Its Glucuronide, Sulphate, Cysteine and Mercapturate Conjugates in 14 Healthy Subjects Following Ingestion of a 20 mg kg^{-1} Body Weight Dose

	Mean Metabolic Clearance of Paracetamol and Metabolites ± SD (ml min^{-1} kg^{-1})				
	Fitted Model				
	1	2	3	4	5
T	3.80 ± 1.01	3.98 ± 1.05	3.45 ± 0.97	4.05 ± 1.05	4.08 ± 1.07
G	2.12 ± 0.82	2.22 ± 0.86	1.93 ± 0.78	2.26 ± 0.86	2.27 ± 0.87
S	1.26 ± 0.33	1.32 ± 0.35	1.14 ± 0.31	1.35 ± 0.36	1.35 ± 0.37
C	0.12 ± 0.05	0.13 ± 0.05	0.11 ± 0.04	0.13 ± 0.05	0.13 ± 0.05
P	0.21 ± 0.05	0.22 ± 0.05	0.19 ± 0.05	0.22 ± 0.06	0.22 ± 0.05
M	0.09 ± 0.04	0.10 ± 0.04	0.09 ± 0.03	0.10 ± 0.04	0.10 ± 0.04
M+C	0.22 ± 0.08	0.23 ± 0.08	0.20 ± 0.07	0.23 ± 0.08	0.23 ± 0.08

T = Total clearance
S = Metabolic clearance to the sulphate conjugate
P = Metabolic clearance to unchanged paracetamol
M+C = Sum of the metabolic clearances
　　　to the cysteine and mercapturate conjugate

G = Metabolic clearance to the glucuronide conjugate
C = Metabolic clearance to the cysteine conjugate
M = Metabolic clearance to the mercapturate conjugate

Friedman repeated measures analysis of variance (FRM ANOVA) for a non-parametric comparison. Multiple comparisons of paired models were done by the Student-Newman-Keuls (SNK) test. The results are shown in Table 2.24 and Table 2.25.

In all the global analyses, the means of the various models were significantly different ($p < 0.001$). This is the same for both the parametric and non-parametric ANOVAs. Following the global analyses, multiple comparisons by the SNK test revealed that the various pharmacokinetic parameters were not significantly different between all the paired models. For all the parameters including AUC, Cl, $t_{1/2}$, MRT, V_d and the metabolic clearance to various metabolites, there was no statistically significant difference between Model 4 and Model 5 by either the parametric or non-parametric comparison. Any difference in the estimated parameters between these two models seemed to be attributable to random variation.

A statistically significant difference was found only in the terminal $t_{1/2}$, MRT and Vd in the comparisons between Model 2 and Model 4 ($p < 0.05$), with both the parametric and non-parametric SNK tests.

With the comparisons between Model 1 and Model 3, using parametric SNK test, it was found that all the pharmacokinetic parameters were significantly different except the MRT. But these statistically significant differences seemed to be borderline only as they became non-significant when the comparisons were done by the non-parametric SNK test using ranks only. i.e. the AUC, Cl, $t_{1/2}$, V_d and the metabolic clearances, which were significantly different between Model 1 and Model 3 by the parametric SNK test, were all found not to be so by the non-parametric SNK test.

Parametric SNK tests showed that all of the pharmacokinetic parameters were significantly different between Model 1 and Model 2. Again, some of these statistically significant differences might be borderline only as by non-parametric SNK tests, the AUC, Cl, $t_{1/2}$, V_d and the metabolic clearances to glucuronide and sulphate were no longer significantly different.

The *intraclass correlation coefficient of reliability (R)* is a single quantity that can usefully express the magnitude of the two components of the variability among a series of measurements on different subjects — variability among their steady-state values and the variability of the random errors; or the between subject variation and the within subject variation. *R* is distinguished from the traditional product-moment correlation coefficient. It is directly interpretable as a proportion of variance. It is the

Table 2.24 Statistical Analysis — One Way Repeated Measures Analysis of Variance (RM ANOVA)

Parameter	RM ANOVA p Value	Multiple Comparisons Between Models: Student-Newman-Keuls Test p Value			
		1 vs 2	1 vs 3	4 vs 5	2 vs 4
AUC	< 0.001	< 0.05	< 0.05	> 0.05	> 0.05
Cl	< 0.001	< 0.05	< 0.05	> 0.05	> 0.05
$t_{\frac{1}{2}}$ (terminal phase)	< 0.001	< 0.05	< 0.05	> 0.05	< 0.05
MRT	< 0.001	< 0.05	> 0.05	> 0.05	< 0.05
Vd (terminal phase)	< 0.001	< 0.05	< 0.05	> 0.05	< 0.05
Met.Cl. glucuronide	< 0.001	< 0.05	< 0.05	> 0.05	> 0.05
Met.Cl. sulphate	< 0.001	< 0.05	< 0.05	> 0.05	> 0.05
Met.Cl. cysteine	< 0.001	< 0.05	< 0.05	> 0.05	> 0.05
Met.Cl. paracetamol	< 0.001	< 0.05	< 0.05	> 0.05	> 0.05
Met.Cl. mercapturate	< 0.001	< 0.05	< 0.05	> 0.05	> 0.05
Met.Cl. cysteine+mercapturate	< 0.001	< 0.05	< 0.05	> 0.05	> 0.05

Shaded cells indicate p values > 0.05, difference not statistically significant

Table 2.25 Statistical Analysis — Friedman Repeated Measures Analysis of Variance on Ranks (FRM ANOVA)

Parameter	FRM ANOVA p Value	Multiple Comparisons Between Models: Student-Newman-Keuls Test p Value			
		1 vs 2	1 vs 3	4 vs 5	2 vs 4
AUC	< 0.001	> 0.05	> 0.05	> 0.05	> 0.05
Cl	< 0.001	> 0.05	> 0.05	> 0.05	> 0.05
t½ (terminal phase)	< 0.001	> 0.05	> 0.05	> 0.05	< 0.05
MRT	< 0.001	< 0.05	> 0.05	> 0.05	< 0.05
Vd (terminal phase)	< 0.001	> 0.05	> 0.05	> 0.05	< 0.05
Met.Cl. glucuronide	< 0.001	> 0.05	> 0.05	> 0.05	> 0.05
Met.Cl. sulphate	< 0.001	> 0.05	> 0.05	> 0.05	> 0.05
Met.Cl. cysteine	< 0.001	< 0.05	> 0.05	> 0.05	> 0.05
Met.Cl. paracetamol	< 0.001	< 0.05	> 0.05	> 0.05	> 0.05
Met.Cl. mercapturate	< 0.001	< 0.05	> 0.05	> 0.05	> 0.05
Met.Cl. cysteine + mercapturate	< 0.001	< 0.05	> 0.05	> 0.05	> 0.05

Shaded cells indicate p values > 0.05, difference not statistically significant

proportion of the variance of an observation due to subject-to-subject variability in error-free scores. Therefore, R approaches the maximum value of unity when variations due to random error decrease and the reliability of the measurement increases. R is calculated as:

$$R = \frac{(BMS - WMS)}{BMS + (K_o - 1)\ WMS}$$

where
WMS = within subject mean squares
BMS = between subject mean squares
ss = sum of squares
ms = mean squares
K_o = number of comparisons (measurements)

The R values calculated for the comparisons between Model 1 and Model 2, Model 1 and Model 3, Model 4 and Model 5, and Model 2 and Model 4 for Cl, terminal $t_{1/2}$ and AUC are tabulated in Table 2.26. For the clearance of paracetamol, the best R value was found in the comparison between Model 2 and Model 4 at 0.99, followed by the comparison between Model 1 and Model 2, then that between Model 4 and Model 5. Since unity is the best reliability value that could be obtained, the R values of these 3 comparisons were quite high. The lowest R was obtained from the comparison between Model 1 and Model 3 at 0.88.

The R values calculated for the different comparisons of AUC for Models 1 & 2, 2 & 4, and 4 & 5 were high at 0.94, 0.98 and 0.94, respectively, similar to those for Cl values. The lowest R again was obtained from the comparison between Model 1 and Model 3 at 0.77.

As mentioned before, the terminal $t_{1/2}$ in the different models referred to different time periods and there could be large differences in the mean values with different models. It was not unexpected that the reliability test showed that the $t_{1/2}$ values in one model did not quite agree with the $t_{1/2}$ values in another model. The R values in the comparison between Models 1 & 2, 1 & 3 and 2 & 4 were negative and indicated that the variation between the two values from the same subject in the two models was far in excess of the between subjects variation. The only reasonable R value was 0.85, obtained from the comparison between Model 4 and Model 5.

The Bland-Altman method is an assessment of the agreement between two sets of measurements on the same subjects. It is essentially a plot of the difference between the methods (models) against their mean. Instead of

Table 2.26 Statistical Analysis — Interclass Correlation
Coefficient of Reliability

1. Cl

Comparisons between models		4 vs 5	1 vs 2	1 vs 3	2 vs 4
WMS	ss	0.43	0.26	0.89	0.07
	df	14	14	14	14
	ms	0.031	0.018	0.063	0.005
BMS	ss	14.44	13.75	12.68	14.37
	df	13	13	13	13
	ms	1.111	1.058	0.975	1.105
R		0.95	0.97	0.88	0.99

2. $t_{\frac{1}{2}}$

Comparisons between models		4 vs 5	1 vs 2	1 vs 3	2 vs 4
WMS	ss	0.13	36.66	12.63	11.37
	df	14	14	14	14
	ms	0.009	2.619	0.902	0.812
BMS	ss	1.51	6.32	6.46	3.15
	df	13	13	13	13
	ms	0.116	0.486	0.497	0.242
R		0.85	-0.69	-0.29	-0.54

3. AUC

Comparisons between models		4 vs 5	1 vs 2	1 vs 3	2 vs 4
WMS	ss	135.58	140.07	694.10	38.25
	df	14	14	14	14
	ms	9.685	10.005	49.579	2.732
BMS	ss	3827.49	4289.52	5059.55	3991.86
	df	13	13	13	13
	ms	294.422	329.963	389.196	307.066
R		0.94	0.94	0.77	0.98

WMS = *within subject mean squares*   BMS = *between subject mean squares*
ss = *sum of squares*   df = *degrees of freedom*   ms = *mean squares*
R = *intraclass correlation coefficient of reliability, calculated as*

$$R = \frac{(BMS - WMS)}{BMS + (K_o - 1)\,WMS}$$

K_o = *number of comparisons*

the absolute values of the difference between the models, the difference, as a percentage of the mean, was plotted against the mean. These modified Bland-Altman plots are shown in Fig. 2.14 to Fig. 2.16. The Mean ±2SD lines gives the 95% confidence intervals of the percentage differences. The acceptability of the agreement between two models was assessed by the confidence limits. The ideal would be very a small percentage difference of the means. A summary of the percentage differences of the means for AUC, Cl and $t_{1/2}$ for the various comparisons between the models is shown in Table 2.27. The individual data are shown in Appendices 2.16 to 2.27.The percentage difference of the mean for the comparison between Model 4 and Model 5 was small for Cl, $t_{1/2}$ and AUC. The mean values were $3.3 \pm 4.7\%$, $3.9 \pm 3.1\%$ and $3.3 \pm 4.6\%$ respectively. For the other comparisons, the percentage difference of the mean were below 10% for Cl and AUC, but an agreement between the compared models for $t_{1/2}$ was not expected as the mean % were high at 42.7%, 20.1% and 30.0% for the comparisons of Models 1 & 2, Models 1 & 3 and Models 2 & 4 respectively.

From Fig. 2.14 to Fig. 2.16, it can be seen that the spread of the percentage differences for the different comparisons was not wide except for the comparison of $t_{1/2}$ for Models 1 & 2, Models 1 & 3 and Models 2 & 4. Except for these three comparisons, the 95% confidence interval lines

Table 2.27   Statistical Analysis — Modified Bland-Altman Method for the Assessment of Agreement Between two Models

	Mean value of individual percentage difference of the mean (± SD)			
	Comparisons between models			
	4 vs 5	1 vs 2	1 vs 3	2 vs 4
Cl	3.3 ± 4.7	4.6 ± 1.5	9.8 ± 1.9	1.9 ± 1.8
$t_{1/2}$	3.9 ± 3.1	42.7 ± 25.3	20.1 ± 13.5	30.0 ± 21.1
AUC	3.3 ± 4.6	4.6 ± 1.4	9.8 ± 1.9	1.9 ± 1.8

Figure 2.14 Modified Bland-Altman Plots of Comparisons of Clearance of Paracetamol between Regimens 1 & 2, Regimens 1 & 3, Regimens 2 & 4 and Regimens 4 & 5

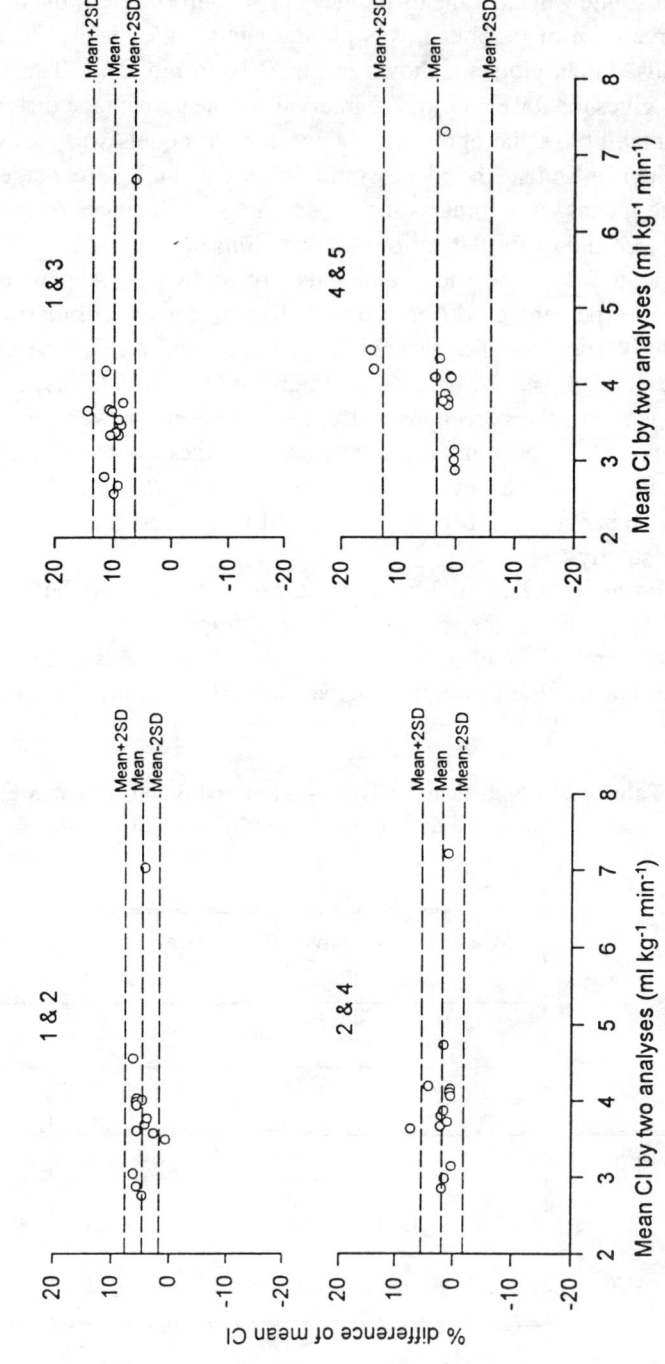

Figure 2.15 Modified Bland-Altman Plots of Comparisons of Elimination Half-life of Paracetamol between Regimens 1 & 2, Regimens 1 & 3, Regimens 2 & 4 and Regimens 4 & 5

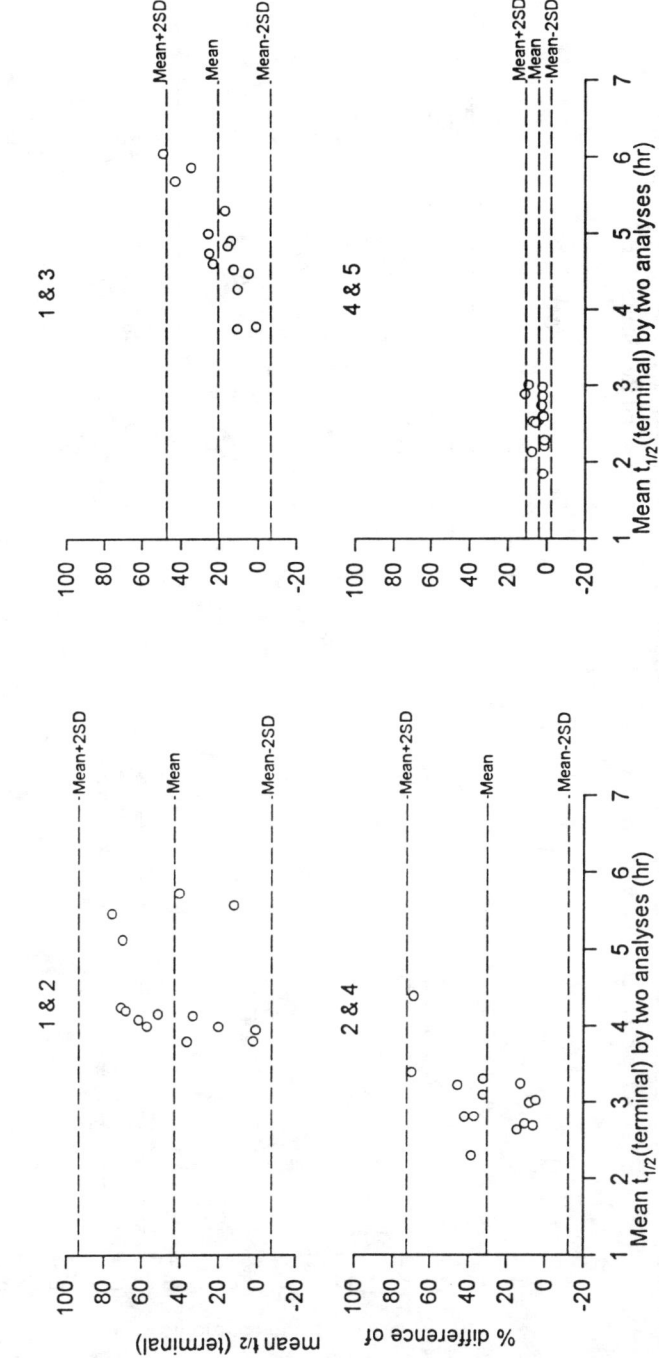

Figure 2.16 Modified Bland-Altman Plots of Comparisons of Area Under Curve of the Paracetamol Plasma Concentration-Time Curve between Regimens 1 & 2, Regimens 1 & 3, Regimens 2 & 4 and Regimens 4 & 5

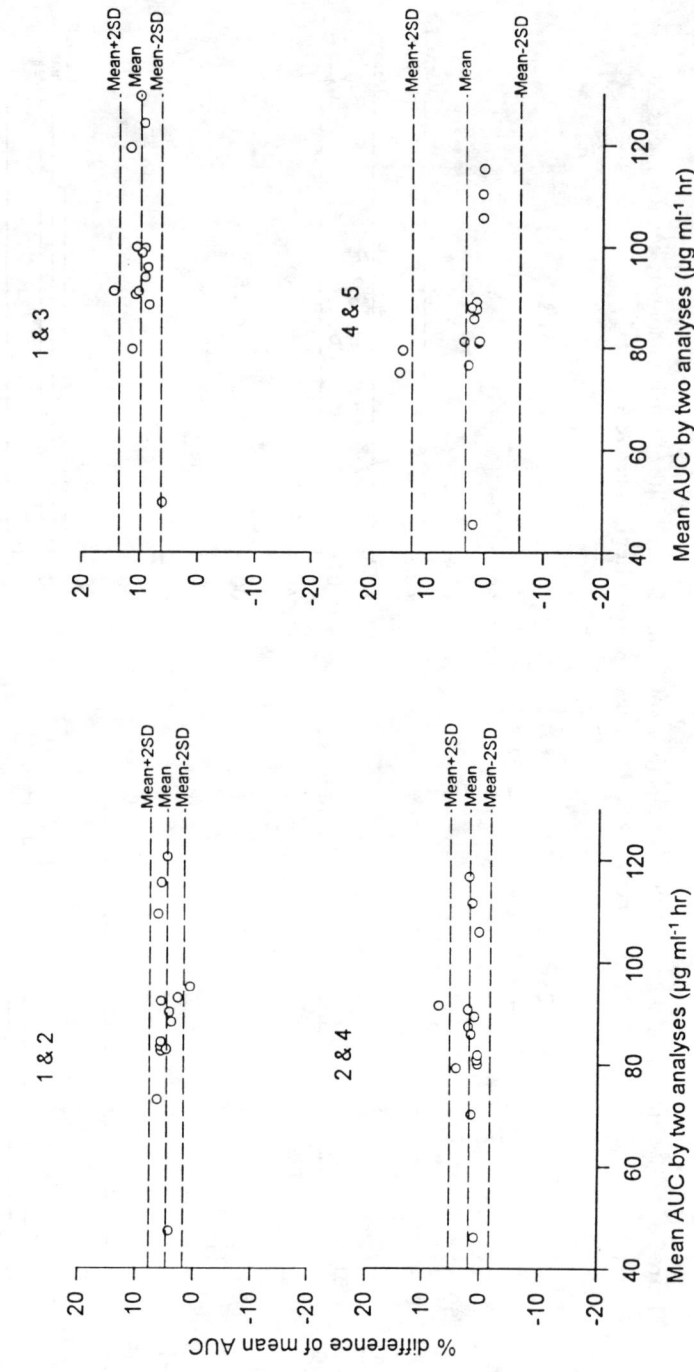

were close to the mean, showing quite good agreement between the two models

2.3.7   Discussion

The absorption of paracetamol in healthy volunteers in this study was rapid. The peak plasma concentration was reached early, mean t_{max} being 0.89 ± 0.40 hr. All subjects were fasted overnight for the study and paracetamol was administered as a solution, therefore factors that could affect the rate of absorption were minimised. Following absorption, there was a very brief distribution phase which could be missed very easily as elimination also takes place at the same time. The half-life of this distribution phase was found to be only around 3 to 19 minutes (Prescott, 1980) and thus is not always characterised in pharmacokinetic studies of paracetamol. The distribution phase is usually complete at approximately 1.5 hr when equilibrium is achieved between the tissues and the circulation. Paracetamol is distributed throughout most tissues but not fat.

Plasma paracetamol is removed mainly by hepatic metabolism and the decrease in plasma paracetamol concentrations follows first order kinetics. On a semilogarithmic graph, the plasma concentration of paracetamol declined in a linear fashion against time up to around 8–12 hr. Using this part of the slope for estimation, the mean $t_{1/2}$ of paracetamol was 2.6 ± 0.3 hr (range 1.9–3.0, Model 4). Beyond this period, the decline in paracetamol concentration seemed to be much slower as the plasma concentration at 24 hr did not seem to fit-in with a single elimination phase. The $t_{1/2}$ of this apparently slower elimination phase between 8–24 hr was estimated to be 5.4 ± 1.1 hr (range 3.8–7.5, Model 1), but this estimation is dominated by the 24 hr measurement.

Metabolism of paracetamol by the gastrointestinal tract is insignificant in man (Clements *et al.*, 1984), but following absorption, which is almost complete, it reaches the systemic circulation. First pass metabolism of paracetamol is extensive and the oral bioavailability is about 70–80% (Rawlins *et al.*, 1977; Perucca & Richens, 1979; Clements *et al.*, 1984). The extent of paracetamol metabolism was reflected in the finding that along with all metabolites excreted in the 24 hr urine collection (mean total recovery 94.2%), only 5.6% was recovered as unchanged paracetamol. The rate of metabolism was also high as over 40% of all metabolites was recovered within 4 hr in the urine and over 70% within 8 hr.

Forrest *et al.* that approximately 85–95% of a therapeutic dose of paracetamol is excreted in the urine within 24 hr (Forrest *et al.*, 1982). In the present study, the mean total recovery in the 24 hr urine collection was $94.2 \pm 15.4\%$ of the dose (63.6–113.7%). The mean value is comparable to published data. The between subject variation was likely due to inaccuracies or incomplete in the collection of urine samples.

The glucuronide and sulphate conjugates are the major metabolites of paracetamol. In this study, their sum represented a mean of 88.5% of all metabolites recovered in the 24 hr urine collection. The mean fractional recovery of the cysteine and mercapturate metabolites were 3.3% and 2.5%, respectively. The fractional recoveries of the various metabolites were comparable to published data in the Caucasians (Prescott, 1980) but with slightly lower values for the oxidative metabolites. The mean of the sum of the fractional recoveries of the cysteine and mercapturate metabolites in this study was found to be $5.8 \pm 1.9\%$, comparing to 9.3% among Caucasians in Scotland (Critchley *et al.*, 1986). This genetic difference in the fractional recoveries of the oxidative metabolites of paracetamol was also found in a study among Chinese living in Singapore. The value was at 6.0% (Lee *et al.*, 1992).

Inter-individual variation in paracetamol metabolism is well recognised (Caldwell *et al.*, 1980; Clements *et al.*,; Critchley *et al.*, 1986). In the present study, the fractional recovery of the glucuronide conjugate ranged from 40.7% to 68.6% and that of the sulphate conjugate was 22.3–46.4%. Those subjects with lower fractional recoveries of the glucuronide conjugate made up for it by producing more of the sulphate conjugate. Overall, the fractional recoveries of the cysteine conjugate, unchanged paracetamol and the mercapturate conjugate among the subjects varied by about 3 to 4 fold. Factors such as age and diet may influence the metabolism of paracetamol.

In the different models for analysis in this study, though the same plasma concentration data were used, there was much difference in the estimated pharmacokinetic parameters, as different sampling times were used. Global analyses by repeated measures ANOVA showed that the AUC, Cl, $t_{1/2}$, MRT and V_d estimated in these 5 models were significantly different, but paired comparison between models revealed that some of the individual comparisons were not significantly different.

The comparison between Model 1 and Model 2 was used to demonstrate the importance of the 24 hr point in influencing the pharmacokinetic parameters of a 3-phase model. All the pharmcokinetic parameters estimated were significantly different between these 2 models.

The AUC and V_d (terminal phase) were significantly larger and the terminal $t_{1/2}$ was significantly longer in Model 1. Cl was thus found to be lower. It was evident that the contribution of the 24 hr point to the characterisation of a 3-phase model is important and a terminal phase could not be adequately described for sampling times up to 12 hr only.

On the other hand, none of the pharmacokinetic parameters estimated was significantly different between Model 4 and Model 5. They were both describing a 2-phase model but the sampling time was up to 12 hr in Model 4 and for Model 5, only up to 8 hr. This seems to indicate that the extra sampling points at 9, 10, 11 and 12 hr did not affect the overall pharmacokinetic model at all when the model chosen was a 2-phase one. In comparison, the parameters obtained in a 2-phase model (Model 4 or 5) to those in Model 1, the AUC and V_d (terminal phase) were smaller, the terminal $t_{1/2}$ and MRT were shorter and the Cl was higher.

Combining the findings from these two comparisons, it seemed that up to 12 hr after oral administration, the pharmacokinetics of paracetamol could be adequately described by a 2-phase model. The sampling times from 9 to 12 hr did not fit very well in the terminal elimination phase of a 3-phase model, but extremely well in the elimination phase of a 2-phase model. The existence of a second, slower elimination phase seemed to hinge on the existence of a higher than expected plasma concentration at 24 hr. If the 24 hr plasma sample was not taken or if this sampling time was ignored, then a 2-phase model could be used to describe the pharmacokinetics of paracetamol adequately, regardless of whether the sampling time was up to 8 or 12 hr.

The comparison between Model 1 and Model 3 addressed the importance of extra sampling times between 9 to 12 hr in a 3-phase model. All pharmacokinetic parameters estimated, except MRT, were significantly different between the 2 models. This indicated that there was a significant difference between fitting the terminal elimination phase through the sampling points at 8, 9, 10, 11, 12 and 24 hours or just between the 8 and 24 hr points. In the comparison between Model 4 and Model 5, it has been demonstrated already that the sampling points from 9–12 hr fitted almost perfectly in the terminal elimination phase of a 2-phase model. With that in mind, it was not surprising to find that the pharmacokinetic parameters between Model 1 and Model 3 were significantly different.

The same sampling times were used in Model 2 and Model 4, the former fitted to a 3-phase model and the latter to a 2-phase model. A comparison between these 2 models was used to demonstrate the difference in the pharmacokinetic parameters when the same sampling points were force-fitted to 2 different models. The AUC and Cl were not significantly different between these 2 models but the terminal $t_{1/2}$, V_d and MRT were. The force-fitting of the sampling points between 8 to 12 hr put these points into a second elimination phase and thus the terminal $t_{1/2}$ in Model 2 and Model 4 were essentially describing a different time period. Nevertheless, this did not alter the AUC and Cl significantly enough to produce a difference.

The lack of difference between Model 4 and Model 5 was further demonstrated by the results of the intraclass correlation coefficient of reliability study. Among the 4 different between-models comparisons, only that between Model 4 and Model 5 scored a high R value with all 3 parameters studied — Cl, $t_{1/2}$ and AUC. This result indicated that Model 4 and Model 5 could quite reliably interchange with one another. It should also be noted that though R was a negative value in the comparison of $t_{1/2}$ between Model 2 and Model 4, the comparisons of Cl and AUC scored excellent R values. There were similar findings for the comparison between Model 1 and Model 2.

The Bland-Altman method was originally devised as a statistical method for the assessment of agreement between two methods of clinical measurement (Bland & Altman, 1986), e.g. a comparison of a new measurement technique with an established one. The use of the product-moment correlation coefficient between the results of the two measurement methods is inappropriate because it measures the strength of a relation between the two sets of variables, not the agreement between them. Bland and Altman thus devised this method which is essentially a plot of the difference between the two methods against their mean, with the 95% confidence interval lines as an aid in assessing the agreement. If the mean difference between the two sets of data in study is close to zero and the 95% confidence intervals are within tolerated limits, then the two methods show reasonable agreement and they are interchangeable.

In this study, this plot was altered slightly. Instead of the absolute value of the difference, the percentage difference was plotted against the mean. This modification was realised to be necessary and would improve the presentation of results. For a parameter whose normal value is high, then a difference arising from two measurements would be of a small percentage of the mean value. Take AUC in this study, the commonly reported values was around 100 g ml^{-1} hr. A difference of a magnitude of 10 or below between two measurements in comparison would constitute only a 10% difference. On the other hand, a difference of 2 to 3 between two measurements of $t_{1/2}$ whose commonly reported value was only about 4 hr would be an unaceptably high percentage of difference of the mean value. To be able to evaluate the comparisons of pharmacokinetic parameters between two modelling regimens in this study, which encompass parameters of varying magnitudes, it is necessary to find a common unit that would describe the differences of all parameters between the two regimens in compariosn. By expressing the difference as a percentage of the mean instead of the absolute value, this became possible. This principle also applies to a parameter whose value can span over a wide range. The mean value between two particular methods may be much smaller than that of another two. It would be misleading to compare the absolute value of the difference and by expressing the difference as a percentage of the mean, this problem can also be negated. Thus, in this study, all Bland-Altman plots were presented and results calculated as the percentage differences versus the mean values of two regimens in comparison. This has made a major improvement in the presentation of comparative results.

Like the intraclass correlation coefficient of reliability, the results of the Bland-Altman comparisons again showed that there was excellent agreement between Model 4 and Model 5. The mean percentage difference for Cl, $t_{1/2}$ and AUC were all below 4%. For the comparison between Model 2 and Model 4, there was excellent agreement in Cl and AUC with the mean percentage difference at below 2%, but that for $t_{1/2}$ stood out as high at 30%. This observation also applies to the comparisons of Model 1 & 2, and Model 1 & 3.

In summary, the results of this study indicate that up to 12 hr after oral administration, the pharmacokinetics of paracetamol could be adequately described by a 2-phase model. The sampling times from 9 to 12 hr did not fit very well in the terminal elimination phase of a 3-phase model, but extremely well in the elimination phase of a 2-phase model. The existence of a second, slower elimination phase seemed to hinge on the existence of a higher than expected plasma concentration at 24 hr. If the 24 hr plasma sample was not taken or if this sampling time was ignored, then a 2-phase model could be used to describe the pharmacokinetics of paracetamol adequately, regardless of whether the sampling time was up to 8 or 12 hr. The intraclass correlation coefficient of reliability and the Bland-Altman plots showed excellent agreement between Model 4 and Model 5 for Cl, $t_{1/2}$ and AUC, but not for other between-model comparisons. Model 5 is thus an adequate model for the study of the pharmacokinetics of paracetamol.

In this study of 14 healthy Chinese subjects, the mean Cl of paracetamol after an oral dose of 20 mg kg^{-1}, estimated by Model 5 was 4.08 ± 1.07 ml min^{-1} kg^{-1} and mean terminal $t_{1/2}$ was 2.6 ± 0.4 hr. The mean V_d of this terminal phase was found to be 0.88 l kg^{-1} and the mean MRT was 4.0 ± 0.5 hr.

A prolonged second elimination phase in the pharmacokinetics of paracetamol has seldom been reported. The well published elimination $t_{1/2}$ usually refers to the period between 2 to 8 hr after drug administration. The reason for the higher than expected plasma level at 24 hr in this study was not clear. One suggestion is that previously, the detection limit of paracetamol in plasma might be higher than what can be achieved now. This low level at 24 hr might not be detectable in previous studies. Another explanation for this higher than expected plasma level at 24 hr may be that this is not entirely due to a slower, second elimination phase, but due to some enterohepatic circulation. Biliary excretion and enterohepatic circulation of paracetamol has been shown both in the rat and in man (Siegers *et al.*, 1983; Siegers *et al.*, 1984). In man, 2.6% of an oral 1 g dose is excreted into bile within 8 hours. Bile has been shown to be an important route of elimination for the cysteine conjugate and it accounts for 19.4% of the total excretion of the metabolite (Jayasinghe *et al.*, 1986), but the extent of enterohepatic circulation is not known. It may be possible that some of the paracetamol and its metabolites excreted in bile is recirculated, thus contributing to a prolonged, higher plasma concentration.

2.4   The pharmacokinetics of paracetamol in healthy subjects, patients with liver disease and hepatocellular carcinoma

2.4.1   Introduction

Previous work in the Department of Clinical Pharmacology at The Chinese University of Hong Kong has shown that the percentage of urinary recovery of the oxidative metabolites of paracetamol in 24 hr urine collections was much greater in patients with hepatocellular carcinoma (Leung & Critchley, 1991). There were a few outliers in a group of patients with chronic hepatitis B infection who also excreted a much higher percentage as the oxidative metabolites than the rest of the group. This indicated increased microsomal cytochrome P450 activity. The patients with hepatocellular carcinoma had correspondingly reduced glucuronide conjugation but the proportions of the sulphate conjugate excreted were similar. These findings suggested that the increased production of oxidative metabolites was not a consequence of a primary impairment in glucuronidation because a corresponding increase in sulphate conjugation would be expected. Nevertheless, due to the limitations of this study, full interpretations could not be made as only 24 hr urine data was available. To make clearer interpretations of the finding of a much enhanced oxidative metabolism of paracetamol in patients with hepatocellular carcinoma, a full comparative study of the pharmacokinetics of paracetamol in healthy subjects and patients with liver disease or hepatocellular carcinoma is needed. Clearance and elimination half-lives calculated from the plasma data would provide more information about the mechanism of the altered metabolism.

In section 2.3, the differences in the estimated pharmacokinetic parameters in different models were assessed. Model 5 was chosen as a pharmacokinetic model that could be used to describe the pharmacokinetics of paracetamol adequately and this 2-phase model would be used in the following study.

2.4.2   Study protocol

All studies were carried out in the Clinical Pharmacology Studies Unit, Department of Clinical Pharmacology, The Chinese University of Hong Kong, at the Prince of Wales Hospital, Shatin.

2.4.3   Methods

2.4.3.1 Subjects

Subjects were recruited for 5 categories:

    Group A: Healthy controls
    Group B: Patients with alcoholic liver disease
    Group C: Patients with chronic hepatitis B infection/liver cirrhosis
    Group D: Patients with hepatocellular carcinoma
    Group E: Patients with renal impairment

The healthy subjects were volunteers responding to recruitment appeal posters for clinical research posted around the Hospital, or patients attending other clinics at the Prince of Wales Hospital, who were not on any medication or suffering from any disease affecting liver function or drug metabolism. Subjects in Group B and Group C were patients recruited from the Liver Clinic at the Li Ka Shing Specialist Clinic, Prince of Wales Hospital and those in Group D, from the Joint Hepatoma Clinic. These patients all had detailed patient records and previous laboratory tests to confirm diagnoses and were referred by their physicians-in-charge. Subjects with renal impairment were added on as a group for interest of comparison. They were diabetic patients attending the Metabolic Investigation Unit at the Prince of Wales Hospital. It was aimed to recruit 8 subjects for each study group. Every subject was given a physical examination and screening tests for plasma biochemistry were performed together with urinalysis. Group D, the group of patients with hepatocellular carcinoma was later split into two. The first 8 subjects recruited remained as Group D. A further 8 patients with hepatocellular carcinoma were recruited later and they formed Group D' (see Discussions p. 195).

A summary of the age, body weight and height of the subjects in each group is shown in Table 2.28 and the plasma biochemistry screen data are shown in Table 2.29. Informed consent was given by each subject and the study was approved by the Hospital Ethics Committee.

2.4.3.2 Drug administration and sampling

The procedures were essentially the same as in 2.3.3.2 with a slight modification in the sampling times. The subjects attended the Clinical Pharmacology Studies Unit in the Department of Clinical Pharmacology in the morning, after an overnight fast. An in-dwelling cannula (Angiocath 20G 2 inch, Becton Dickson) was inserted into a forearm vein. The cannula stayed *in situ* until after the 8 hr sample was drawn. The 24 hr blood sample was taken at a different site by venepuncture. Paracetamol was administered as the syrup (Panadol Syrup 160 mg ml^{-1}, Sterling Drug (Malaya) Sdn., Bhd., Kuala Lumpur for Winthrop Product Inc., New York, U.S.A.) at a dose of 20 mg/kg body weight. Food and beverage were withheld for at least 3 hours after drug administration and only water was allowed. Lunch was available at 4 hour and after that fluid and food intake were unrestricted.

5 ml venous blood samples were drawn into heparinised tubes at 0, 0.5, 1, 1.5, 2, 3, 4, 5, 6, 7, 8, and 24 hours after dosing. Blood samples were centrifuged at 1400 xg for 10 minutes and the plasma separated for storage

Table 2.28 Details of Subjects in Different Study Groups

Group		Group A Healthy Control	Group B Alcoholic	Group C Chronic Heaptitis B Infection	Group D Hepato- cellular Carcinoma	Group R Renal Impairment	Group D' Hepato- cellular Carcinoma
Sex	M	5	7	8	8	5	7
	F	2	1	1	0	2	1
Age	Mean	47.3	52.5	48.6	59.1	60.1	59.8
	SD	12.1	11.2	10.0	12.4	9.2	12.8
	Range	23 - 60	38 - 70	35 - 60	38 - 76	40 - 69	38 - 74
Weight (kg)	Mean	66.3	53.9	61.0	54.4	59.2	56.2
	SD	8.2	10.6	11.7	13.7	13.1	5.4
	Range	60.2 - 84.0	37.8 - 73.8	51.6 - 83.6	36.2 - 78.8	44.5 - 83.6	48.0 - 63.0
Height (cm)	Mean	161.5	165.5	166.0	166.3	155.9	162.1
	SD	7.9	3.1	5.8	3.8	11.5	4.1
	Range	150 - 168	162 - 169	162 - 178	163 - 170	141 - 174	154 - 168

Table 2.29   Plasma Biochemistry Screen of Subjects in Different Study Groups

		Group A	Group B	Group C	Group D	Group R	Group D'	Normal Range*
Na	Mean	140.9	135.4	138.4	137.1	139.1	137.0	137 - 142
(mmol l⁻¹)	SD	2.0	8.4	7.0	5.1	1.5	4.5	
	Range	138 - 144	115 - 141	122 - 144	127 - 142	138 - 142	128 - 143	
K	Mean	3.9	4.2	4.2	4.1	4.3	4.5	3.5 - 5.1
(mmol l⁻¹)	SD	0.4	0.7	0.8	0.4	0.4	0.5	
	Range	3.7 - 4.7	3.3 - 5.3	2.8 - 5.4	3.3 - 4.5	3.7 - 4.9	4.0 - 5.3	
Urea	Mean	5.6	4.2	6.2	8.3	20.1	8.3	3.4 - 8.9
(mmol l⁻¹)	SD	1.1	1.4	1.8	3.2	11.6	2.4	
	Range	4.2 - 7.5	1.9 - 6.6	3.9 - 9.1	5.1 - 13.5	9.0 - 44.6	5.0 - 11.3	
Creatinine	Mean	80.6	82.9	83.8	81.2	269.7	100.6	64 - 96
(μmol l⁻¹)	SD	9.8	7.4	8.2	9.0	159.2	10.4	
	Range	62 - 90	70 - 95	70 - 94	72 - 93	128 - 609	88 - 115	
Total Protein	Mean	81.1	82.6	79.1	78.4	71.4	80.0	66 - 81
(g l⁻¹)	SD	2.0	6.6	8.8	8.3	7.0	6.7	
	Range	77 - 83	72 - 93	65 - 91	67 - 92	64 - 82	72 - 90	
Albumin	Mean	45.6	39.5	38.3	36.0	34.3	37.2	35 - 48
(g l⁻¹)	SD	2.4	5.0	9.1	6.2	19.3	5.3	
	Range	42 - 49	29 - 44	22 - 50	29 - 47	5 - 64	29 - 45	
Total	Mean	9.7	52.8	18.9	91.1	13.2	109.9	0 - 15
Bilirubin	SD	3.6	57.3	17.8	185.6	17.9	229.9	
(μmol l⁻¹)	Range	5 - 16	7 - 165	4 - 52	14 - 550	3 - 45	6 - 630	
Alkaline	Mean	77.0	141.1	104.5	281.8	95.2	326.4	40 -136
Phosphatase	SD	20.1	46.9	45.6	306.3	38.2	261.3	
(IU l⁻¹)	Range	58 - 116	84 - 223	68 - 210	99 - 902	59 - 162	2.5 - 785	
ALT	Mean	34.0	39.5	88.8	81.0	10.2	99.4	0 - 58
(IU l⁻¹)	SD	25.2	33.7	110.8	69.3	6.1	48.8	
	Range	9 - 66	20 - 116	16 - 351	22 - 243	2 - 18	60 - 190	
Gamma GT	Mean	36.3	328.3	177.5	201.1			0 - 84 (F)
(U l⁻¹)	SD	23.5	239.1	297.2	155.5			0 - 100 (M)
	Range	11 - 68	53 - 739	18 - 778	52 - 466			
α-foetoprotein	Mean						156936.7	< 10
(IU ml⁻¹)	SD						228374.5	
	Range						10 - 563500	

* From the Department of Clinical Pathology, Prince of Wales Hospital, Shatin

at -20°C prior to analysis. Urine was collected for the time periods 0–4, 4–8 and 8–24 hours after dosing. The volume of urine excreted at each time period was noted and a 20 ml aliquot was take from each collection and stored at -20°C until analysis.

2.4.3.3 Drug analysis

The concentrations of paracetamol, the glucuronide, sulphate, cysteine and mercapturate metabolites in plasma and in the urine were measured by the HPLC assay as described in section 2.2.2 of this chapter. Metabolite concentrations were expressed as paracetamol equivalents.

2.4.3.4 Calculations

Plasma concentrations of paracetamol and the glucuronide, sulphate and cysteine metabolites for each subject were calculated from the respective peak area counts and the paracetamol standards according to section 2.2.4.2. The recovery of paracetamol and its metabolites in the urine was calculated according to section 2.2.3.2. The individual peak plasma concentrations (C_{max}) and time to reach peak plasma concentration (t_{max}) were noted.

The metabolic clearance was calculated according to the Method of Miners *et al.* (Miners *et al.*, 1983; Miners *et al.*, 1986), as described in section 2.3.3.4.

2.4.4 Pharmacokinetic analysis

Pharmacokinetic analysis was done using the pharmacokinetic modelling programme Siphar/base, Version 4.0 (1991, SIMED, Créteil, Cedex, France). Pharmacokinetic modelling and estimation of the pharmacokinetic parameters of individual plasma data was done as described in section 2.3.4. The following parameters were calculated for each study subject: AUC, Cl, $t_{1/2}$, V_d and MRT, as defined in section 2.3.4.

2.4.5 Statistical analysis

Mean values with the standard deviation (SD) are presented. All statistical analyses were carried out using the computer statistics package SPSS for Windows (Version 5, 1992, SPSS Inc., Chicago, U.S.A.), supplemented by SigmaStat (Version 1.01, 1993, Jandel Scientific, San Rafael, California, U.S.A.) when some of the tests were not available. The Geigy Scientific

Tables (Geigy Scientific Tables, 1982) was also consulted when the coefficient of correlation was tested for statistical significance.

2.4.6   Results

2.4.6.1   Plasma Results

Mean plasma concentrations of paracetamol and its metabolites following oral administration of a 20 mg kg^{-1} body weight dose in the different groups are shown in Table 2.30 to Table 2.33 and Fig. 2.17 to Fig. 2.20.

Figure 2.17   Mean Plasma Concentration of Paracetamol in Subjects in Different Study Groups Following Ingestion of a 20 mg kg^{-1} Body Weight Dose

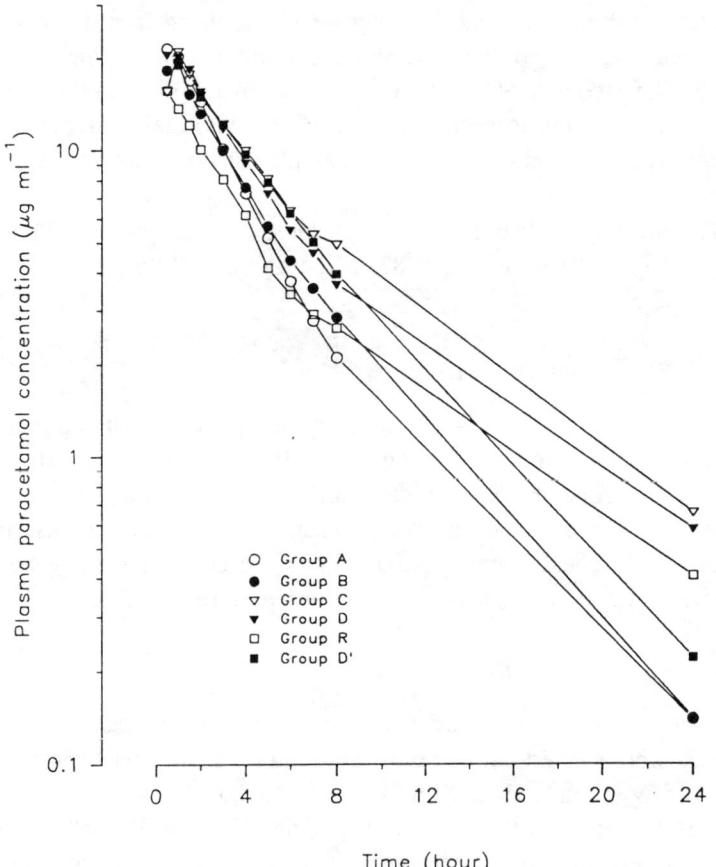

Table 2.30 Mean Plasma Concentration of Paracetamol in Different Study Groups Following Ingestion of a 20 mg kg^{-1} Body Weight Dose

Time (hr)	Paracetamol Plasma Concentration (μg ml^{-1}) Mean ± SD					
	Group A	Group B	Group C	Group D	Group R	Group D'
0	0	0	0	0	0	0
0.5	21.50 ± 3.91	18.27 ± 7.32	15.73 ± 5.40	20.66 ± 6.45	15.69 ± 10.03	18.32 ± 11.10
1	20.23 ± 5.22	19.49 ± 6.30	21.08 ± 4.03	20.33 ± 6.39	13.70 ± 3.99	19.07 ± 7.24
1.5	16.99 ± 4.33	15.28 ± 4.91	17.84 ± 4.55	18.53 ± 7.42	12.09 ± 4.77	
2	14.50 ± 2.64	13.18 ± 4.21	15.22 ± 4.06	15.63 ± 5.92	10.07 ± 4.48	14.97 ± 3.99
3	10.13 ± 1.88	10.01 ± 3.88	12.20 ± 5.12	11.84 ± 4.42	8.07 ± 3.96	12.14 ± 2.85
4	7.26 ± 1.74	7.59 ± 3.61	9.99 ± 4.64	9.14 ± 3.29	6.16 ± 3.14	9.72 ± 2.26
5	5.19 ± 1.26	5.68 ± 3.11	8.11 ± 4.99	7.27 ± 2.80	4.13 ± 2.50	7.88 ± 2.03
6	3.73 ± 1.05	4.38 ± 2.73	6.36 ± 3.98	5.53 ± 2.18	3.38 ± 2.01	6.25 ± 1.56
7	2.77 ± 0.84	3.55 ± 2.39	5.34 ± 3.66	4.65 ± 2.07	2.90 ± 1.62	5.04 ± 1.55
8	2.10 ± 0.75	2.85 ± 1.98	4.95 ± 3.78	3.66 ± 1.77	2.62 ± 1.45	3.94 ± 1.28
24	0.14 ± 0.03	0.14 ± 0.16	0.66 ± 1.02	0.58 ± 0.80	0.41 ± 0.56	0.22 ± 0.11

Table 2.31 Mean Plasma Concentration of Paracetamol Glucuronide in Different Study Groups Following Ingestion of a 20 mg kg^{-1} Body Weight Dose

Time (hr)	Paracetamol Glucuronide Plasma Concentration (μg ml^{-1}) Mean ± SD					
	Group A	Group B	Group C	Group D	Group R	Group D'
0	0	0	0	0	0	0
0.5	4.53 ± 1.78	3.94 ± 1.54	3.12 ± 2.38	3.45 ± 1.85	4.78 ± 2.13	2.88 ± 1.32
1	10.17 ± 4.05	9.94 ± 4.09	8.32 ± 4.83	7.60 ± 4.65	10.76 ± 4.14	6.23 ± 2.31
1.5	11.89 ± 2.46	15.59 ± 7.97	11.74 ± 7.10	9.43 ± 5.29	14.57 ± 3.70	
2	13.76 ± 3.69	14.98 ± 7.71	12.81 ± 7.82	11.03 ± 5.41	17.59 ± 3.98	9.57 ± 3.14
3	14.32 ± 2.68	14.82 ± 6.16	12.80 ± 7.23	11.53 ± 4.81	21.26 ± 3.95	10.10 ± 3.70
4	12.93 ± 2.30	13.12 ± 4.30	12.15 ± 6.16	10.95 ± 5.19	22.94 ± 4.53	9.91 ± 3.77
5	11.04 ± 2.26	10.70 ± 2.99	10.22 ± 4.43	10.39 ± 4.68	22.35 ± 6.19	9.35 ± 3.62
6	9.11 ± 2.20	8.59 ± 2.15	8.53 ± 3.45	9.09 ± 4.43	22.56 ± 6.47	8.26 ± 3.30
7	7.48 ± 2.13	7.11 ± 1.90	7.21 ± 2.64	8.40 ± 4.85	22.17 ± 6.39	7.56 ± 2.95
8	6.02 ± 2.00	5.63 ± 1.93	6.19 ± 2.08	7.39 ± 4.46	21.32 ± 6.54	6.65 ± 2.59
24	0.87 ± 0.41	0.35 ± 0.24	0.75 ± 0.60	2.53 ± 3.89	7.46 ± 6.21	0.78 ± 0.42

Table 2.32 Mean Plasma Concentration of Paracetamol Sulphate in Different Study Groups Following Ingestion of a 20 mg kg^{-1} Body Weight Dose

Time (hr)	Paracetamol Sulphate Plasma Concentration (μg ml^{-1}) Mean ± SD					
	Group A	Group B	Group C	Group D	Group R	Group D'
0	0	0	0	0	0	0
0.5	4.03 ± 0.72	2.84 ± 1.30	2.07 ± 1.54	2.75 ± 1.57	5.38 ± 2.07	2.37 ± 1.13
1	6.17 ± 0.94	4.95 ± 1.94	4.00 ± 1.83	4.15 ± 1.46	8.58 ± 2.69	4.17 ± 1.16
1.5	6.10 ± 1.17	5.13 ± 1.84	4.52 ± 1.81	4.56 ± 1.27	10.14 ± 3.01	
2	6.41 ± 1.23	5.32 ± 1.91	4.46 ± 1.64	4.79 ± 1.03	10.79 ± 3.60	5.45 ± 1.44
3	5.75 ± 1.30	4.80 ± 1.65	4.03 ± 0.95	4.65 ± 1.10	12.03 ± 4.57	5.68 ± 1.80
4	4.96 ± 1.49	4.13 ± 1.80	3.72 ± 0.64	4.36 ± 1.45	11.86 ± 5.30	5.57 ± 2.21
5	4.02 ± 1.31	3.38 ± 1.67	3.25 ± 0.56	3.90 ± 1.64	11.14 ± 7.53	5.06 ± 2.40
6	3.14 ± 1.15	2.62 ± 1.35	2.64 ± 0.60	3.33 ± 1.75	11.00 ± 7.99	4.42 ± 2.38
7	2.43 ± 0.99	2.11 ± 1.22	2.22 ± 0.64	2.97 ± 1.95	10.69 ± 8.31	3.85 ± 2.19
8	1.90 ± 0.89	1.67 ± 1.05	1.93 ± 0.65	2.43 ± 1.74	10.16 ± 8.06	2.88 ± 2.42
24	0.10 ± 0.08	0.09 ± 0.10	0.23 ± 0.31	0.85 ± 1.35	3.17 ± 5.91	0.30 ± 0.28

Table 2.33 Mean Plasma Concentration of Paracetamol Cysteine in Different Study Groups Following Ingestion of a 20 mg kg^{-1} Body Weight Dose

Time (hr)	Paracetamol Cysteine Plasma Concentration ($\mu g \cdot ml^{-1}$) Mean $\pm$ SD					
	Group A	Group B	Group C	Group D	Group R	Group D'
0	0	0	0	0	0	0
0.5	0.06 ± 0.04	0.09 ± 0.06	0.08 ± 0.09	0.11 ± 0.09	0.11 ± 0.08	0.12 ± 0.10
1	0.10 ± 0.09	0.16 ± 0.08	0.12 ± 0.10	0.16 ± 0.04	0.20 ± 0.09	0.28 ± 0.12
1.5	0.14 ± 0.08	0.18 ± 0.12	0.17 ± 0.08	0.22 ± 0.07	0.30 ± 0.20	
2	0.18 ± 0.12	0.24 ± 0.15	0.20 ± 0.07	0.27 ± 0.11	0.37 ± 0.18	0.51 ± 0.20
3	0.21 ± 0.13	0.33 ± 0.19	0.22 ± 0.06	0.34 ± 0.16	0.48 ± 0.32	0.71 ± 0.26
4	0.23 ± 0.11	0.35 ± 0.26	0.24 ± 0.07	0.36 ± 0.21	0.54 ± 0.34	0.82 ± 0.38
5	0.22 ± 0.11	0.36 ± 0.29	0.25 ± 0.13	0.37 ± 0.22	0.59 ± 0.48	0.83 ± 0.45
6	0.20 ± 0.14	0.28 ± 0.22	0.21 ± 0.09	0.32 ± 0.23	0.60 ± 0.54	0.81 ± 0.48
7	0.20 ± 0.09	0.19 ± 0.14	0.20 ± 0.07	0.31 ± 0.24	0.60 ± 0.58	0.79 ± 0.45
8	0.17 ± 0.09	0.16 ± 0.11	0.19 ± 0.08	0.29 ± 0.21	0.61 ± 0.58	0.72 ± 0.46
24	0.02 ± 0.04	0.01 ± 0.03	0.06 ± 0.09	0.11 ± 0.15	0.25 ± 0.41	0.09 ± 0.07

Figure 2.18   Mean Plasma Concentration of Paracetamol Glucuronide in
Subjects in Different Study Groups Following Ingestion of
a 20 mg kg^{-1} Body Weight Dose

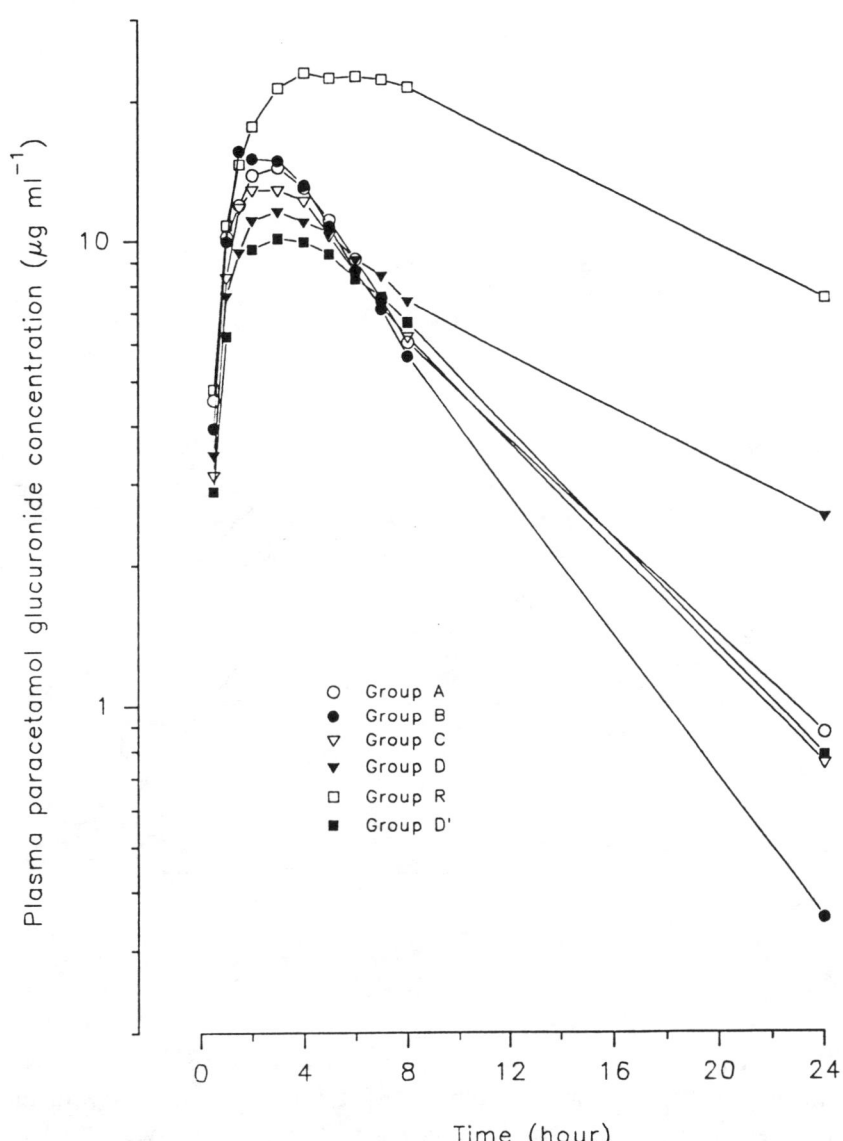

Figure 2.19   Mean Plasma Concentration of Paracetamol Sulphate in
Subjects in Different Study Groups Following Ingestion of
a 20 mg kg^{-1} Body Weight Dose of Paracetamol

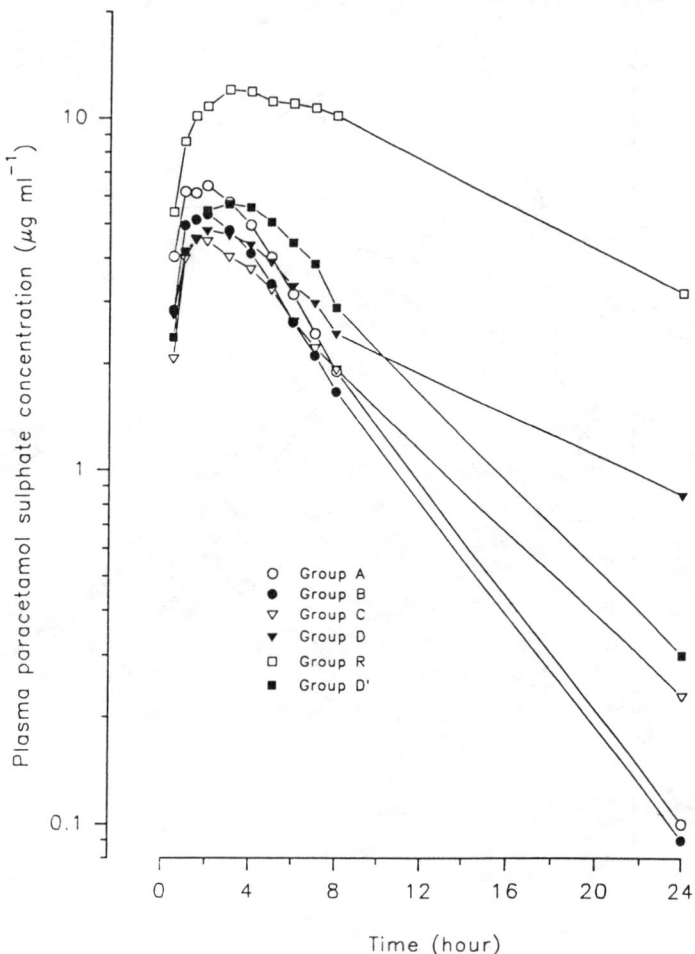

The mercapturate conjugate was not detected in any of the plasma samples probably due to very low concentrations. Plasma concentrations for individual subjects are shown in Appendices 2.28–2.51. Individual values for peak concentration (C_{max}) and time to reach peak concentration (t_{max}) for paracetamol, paracetamol glucuronide and paracetamol sulphate are

Figure 2.20   Mean Plasma Concentration of Paracetamol Cysteine in
Subjects in Different Study Groups Following Ingestion of
a 20 mg kg^{-1} Body Weight Dose of Paracetamol

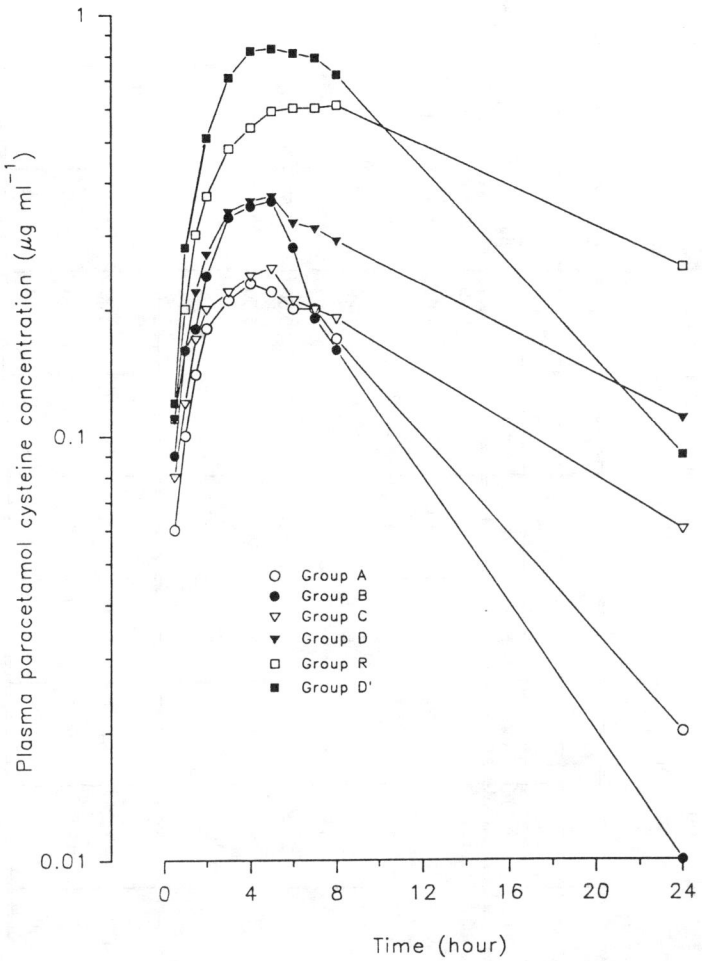

shown in Table 2.34 to Table 2.36. They are also shown as scattergraphs in
Fig. 2.21.

Mean C_{max} and t_{max} of paracetamol in Group A, the healthy controls,
were 22.91 ± 4.57 g ml^{-1} and 0.71 ± 0.27 hr. These values are comparable
to those of the 14 healthy volunteers studied in section 2.3. The mean C_{max}

Table 2.34 Peak Plasma Concentration (C_{max}) and Time to Reach Peak Plasma Concentrations (t_{max}) of Paracetamol in Different Study Groups Following a 20 mg kg^{-1} Dose

Subject	Group A		Group B		Group C		Group D		Group R		Group D'	
	C_{max} ($\mu g\ ml^{-1}$)	T_{max} (hr)	C_{max} ($\mu g\ ml^{-1}$)	T_{max} (hr)	C_{max} ($\mu g\ ml^{-1}$)	T_{max} (hr)	C_{max} ($\mu g\ ml^{-1}$)	T_{max} (hr)	C_{max} ($\mu g\ ml^{-1}$)	T_{max} (hr)	C_{max} ($\mu g\ ml^{-1}$)	t_{max} (hr)
1	15.52	0.50	12.57	0.50	21.88	1.00	22.49	0.50	20.74	1.50	17.13	2.00
2	19.72	0.50	26.92	0.50	29.15	1.00	19.73	1.00	9.82	1.00	20.12	1.00
3	21.23	1.00	15.39	0.50	22.93	1.00	20.23	0.50	17.85	0.50	19.45	1.00
4	23.59	0.50	31.38	1.00	21.59	0.50	31.05	1.50	18.52	0.50	30.83	1.00
5	29.21	1.00	30.24	0.50	15.59	1.00	30.81	1.00	11.35	0.50	8.78	3.00
6	24.26	1.00	24.39	1.00	27.15	1.50	23.89	0.50	11.67	1.00	31.63	0.50
7	26.87	0.50	19.53	1.00	23.51	1.00	16.29	1.50	33.51	0.50	15.90	1.00
8			14.69	1.00	21.31	0.50	25.04	0.50			30.30	0.50
9					17.73	1.00						
Mean	22.91	0.71	21.89	0.75	22.31	0.94	23.69	0.88	17.64	0.79	21.77	1.25
SD	4.57	0.27	7.35	0.27	4.18	0.30	5.22	0.44	8.15	0.39	8.32	0.85
Min	15.52	0.50	12.57	0.50	15.59	0.50	16.29	0.50	9.82	0.50	8.78	0.50
Max	29.21	1.00	31.38	1.00	29.15	1.50	31.05	1.50	33.51	1.50	31.63	3.00

Table 2.35 Peak Plasma Concentration (C_{max}) and Time to Reach Peak Plasma Concentrations (t_{max}) of Paracetamol Glucuronide in Different Study Groups Following a 20 mg kg^{-1} Dose

Subject	Group A C_{max} ($\mu g\ ml^{-1}$)	Group A T_{max} (hr)	Group B C_{max} ($\mu g\ ml^{-1}$)	Group B T_{max} (hr)	Group C C_{max} ($\mu g\ ml^{-1}$)	Group C T_{max} (hr)	Group D C_{max} ($\mu g\ ml^{-1}$)	Group D T_{max} (hr)	Group R C_{max} ($\mu g\ ml^{-1}$)	Group R T_{max} (hr)	Group D' C_{max} ($\mu g\ ml^{-1}$)	Group D' t_{max} (hr)
1	16.40	3.00	19.02	2.00	6.43	4.00	10.28	3.00	24.79	7.00	8.13	5.00
2	20.41	2.00	13.98	3.00	7.77	5.00	12.62	4.00	21.17	4.00	17.09	3.00
3	13.10	3.00	7.19	3.00	17.78	3.00	16.41	1.50	27.94	6.00	6.93	2.00
4	10.79	3.00	30.52	2.00	5.81	5.00	18.44	5.00	29.93	4.00	7.22	3.00
5	15.95	3.00	14.48	2.00	13.23	2.00	21.04	2.00	18.77	3.00	8.65	4.00
6	15.64	4.00	14.15	3.00	23.21	3.00	5.14	3.00	29.97	6.00	12.78	4.00
7	11.08	3.00	8.38	4.00	16.44	1.50	9.55	5.00	20.77	3.00	10.25	3.00
8			18.55	1.50	8.25	4.00	7.35	3.00			11.17	2.00
9					24.88	2.00						
Mean	14.77	3.00	15.78	2.56	13.76	3.28	12.60	3.31	24.76	4.71	10.28	3.25
SD	3.39	0.58	7.29	0.82	7.24	1.30	5.58	1.28	4.63	1.60	3.41	1.04
Min	10.79	2.00	7.19	1.50	5.81	1.50	5.14	1.50	18.77	3.00	6.93	2.00
Max	20.41	4.00	30.52	4.00	24.88	5.00	21.04	5.00	29.97	7.00	17.09	5.00

Table 2.36 Peak Plasma Concentration (C_{max}) and Time to Reach Peak Plasma Concentrations (t_{max}) of Paracetamol Sulphate in Different Study Groups Following a 20 mg kg^{-1} Dose

Subject	Group A		Group B		Group C		Group D		Group R		Group D'	
	C_{max} ($\mu g\ ml^{-1}$)	T_{max} (hr)	C_{max} ($\mu g\ ml^{-1}$)	T_{max} (hr)	C_{max} ($\mu g\ ml^{-1}$)	T_{max} (hr)	C_{max} ($\mu g\ ml^{-1}$)	T_{max} (hr)	C_{max} ($\mu g\ ml^{-1}$)	T_{max} (hr)	C_{max} ($\mu g\ ml^{-1}$)	t_{max} (hr)
1	5.33	1.00	6.06	1.00	4.32	4.00	5.95	1.50	28.33	7.00	9.99	4.00
2	7.25	1.00	4.05	3.00	4.17	5.00	4.31	2.00	13.25	3.00	5.21	3.00
3	7.64	2.00	2.72	2.00	5.57	1.50	4.89	1.00	13.58	3.00	4.65	2.00
4	6.48	1.50	7.57	1.50	3.71	5.00	7.52	7.00	13.29	3.00	4.75	2.00
5	8.33	2.00	6.22	1.50	5.92	1.50	5.57	2.00	5.87	1.00	4.92	4.00
6	5.54	1.50	6.76	2.00	7.24	1.00	6.31	1.50	9.49	4.00	6.68	3.00
7	5.26	1.50	8.33	2.00	6.59	1.50	3.63	4.00	13.27	1.50	4.72	3.00
8			3.59	1.50	3.05	4.00	4.11	1.50			7.37	2.00
9					7.17	2.00						
Mean	6.55	1.50	5.66	1.81	5.30	2.83	5.29	2.56	13.87	3.21	6.04	2.88
SD	1.23	0.41	2.00	0.59	1.55	1.64	1.30	2.01	6.99	1.95	1.89	0.83
Min	5.26	1.00	2.72	1.00	3.05	1.00	3.63	1.00	5.87	1.00	4.65	2.00
Max	8.33	2.00	8.33	3.00	7.24	5.00	7.52	7.00	28.33	7.00	9.99	4.00

Figure 2.21 Scattergraphs of Maximum Plasma Concentration (C_{max}) and Time to Reach C_{max} (t_{max}) of Paracetamol of Subjects in Different Study Groups Following Ingestion of a 20 mg kg^{-1} Body Weight Dose

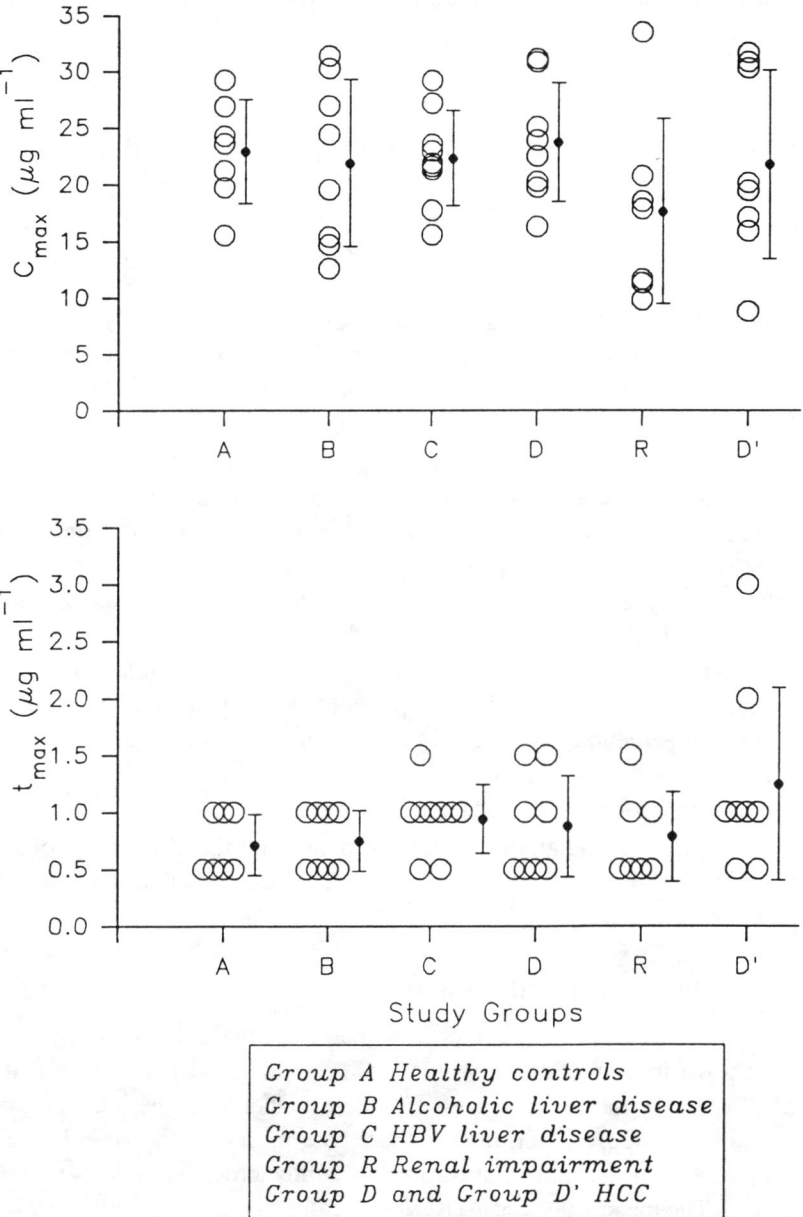

for the glucuronide and sulphate conjugates of Group A are 14.77 ± 3.39 g ml^{-1} and 6.55 ± 1.23 g ml^{-1}, and the mean t_{max} 3.00 ± 0.58 hr and 1.50 ± 0.41 hr, respectively. As expected, only very low concentrations of the cysteine conjugate was detected in the plasma samples (see Appendices 2.46–2.51).

2.4.6.2 Urine Results

Table 2.37 shows the overall recovery and fractional recovery of paracetamol and its 4 major metabolites in the 24 hour urine collection of the various study groups. The mean total recovery of paracetamol and all metabolites in the 24 hour urine collection were $89.8 \pm 10.7\%$, $94.4 \pm 18.8\%$, $85.9 \pm 20.8\%$, $99.7 \pm 28.6\%$, $62.5 \pm 24.1\%$ and $78.1 \pm 8.3\%$ for Groups A, B, C, D, R and D', respectively. The total recovery was much lower in the Group R, patients with renal impairment and this lower percentage of reocovery in the 24 hour urine collection is comparable to a previous study (Prescott *et al.*, 1989).

The percentage recovery as the glucuronide, sulphate conjugate and as unchanged paracetamol was comparable in the various groups. The mean percentage recovery as the glucuronide conjugate ranged from $42.9 \pm 10.86\%$ to $58.50 \pm 5.18\%$, from $31.22 \pm 11.58\%$ to $36.24 \pm 9.98\%$ as the sulphate conjugate and from $3.28 \pm 1.79\%$ to $4.95 \pm 1.62\%$ as unchanged paracetamol. There was no significant difference in these mean values but the mean percentage as the cysteine and mercapturate conjugate was significantly higher in Group D', the patients with hepatocellular carcinoma. The mean percentage recovery in this group was $18.39 \pm 5.08\%$ as compared to $5.05 \pm 1.60\%$, $6.69 \pm 2.85\%$, $6.51 \pm 3.52\%$, $7.96 \pm 3.57\%$ and $6.20 \pm 2.16\%$ in Groups A, B, C, D and R, respectively.

The mean cumulative recovery of paracetamol and its metabolites in the urine is shown in Table 2.38 and Fig. 2.22. Individual urinary excretion data are shown in Appendices 2.52–2.57.

2.4.6.3 Pharmacokinetic Results

The pharmacokinetic parameters calculated for the different study groups are shown in Table 2.39 to Table 2.43, including AUC, Cl, terminal $t_{1/2}$, MRT and V_d. Individual data are listed together with the mean value of each study group. Scattergraph of these parameters are shown in Fig. 2.23. It can be seen that both intra-group and inter-group variations were observed. The mean values of AUC varied from 64.4 ± 29.0 g ml^{-1} hr (Group

Table 2.37 Urinary Recovery of Paracetamol and Its Glucuronide, Sulphate, Cysteine and Mercapturate Metabolites in 24 h in Different Study Groups Following Ingestion of a 20 mg kg^{-1} Body Weight Dose

Group	Subject							Total
		Percentage of Total Amount Recovered in Urine Over 24 hours						Recovery as
		G	S	C	P	M	M+C	% of Dose
A	1	64.53	27.09	1.84	4.28	2.25	4.10	92.6
	2	62.04	25.55	3.52	4.14	4.75	8.27	88.5
	3	52.70	38.81	2.49	3.70	2.29	4.78	99.0
	4	54.89	37.79	2.39	3.21	1.71	4.10	94.0
	5	55.12	36.50	1.94	4.27	2.18	4.12	68.9
	6	65.04	25.94	1.75	5.08	2.19	3.94	100.4
	7	55.18	34.63	3.66	4.17	2.37	6.02	85.1
	Mean	58.50	32.33	2.51	4.12	2.54	5.05	89.8
	SD	5.18	5.90	0.78	0.57	1.00	1.60	10.7
B	1	68.70	24.57	2.12	2.48	2.12	4.24	102.7
	2	59.60	29.07	3.20	4.95	3.17	6.37	64.9
	3	55.81	30.43	3.63	5.15	4.99	8.61	70.2
	4	73.66	19.64	1.59	2.29	2.82	4.41	114.8
	5	57.01	34.60	2.27	3.72	2.40	4.67	109.5
	6	50.27	34.64	4.55	5.64	4.90	9.45	104.0
	7	37.13	56.12	2.53	2.55	1.67	4.20	84.0
	8	65.55	20.67	7.39	2.19	4.20	11.59	104.9
	Mean	58.47	31.22	3.41	3.62	3.28	6.69	94.4
	SD	11.46	11.58	1.86	1.44	1.27	2.85	18.8
C	1	43.79	39.00	4.42	7.58	5.22	9.64	80.0
	2	41.28	44.46	4.65	6.91	2.70	7.35	80.0
	3	64.01	27.77	2.57	3.98	1.67	4.24	100.0
	4	38.08	41.46	8.11	6.12	6.23	14.35	71.7
	5	59.76	30.58	2.49	4.96	2.22	4.70	69.5
	6	75.27	15.90	2.28	4.63	1.92	4.20	104.6
	7	58.80	33.17	2.49	3.29	2.25	4.74	50.4
	8	54.55	35.08	2.74	4.34	3.29	6.03	101.4
	9	72.17	21.73	1.44	2.76	1.90	3.34	115.3
	Mean	56.41	32.13	3.47	4.95	3.04	6.51	85.9
	SD	13.26	9.28	2.02	1.62	1.62	3.52	20.8
D	1	42.46	45.34	6.38	2.48	3.34	9.72	110.8
	2	59.26	32.92	1.96	4.18	1.68	3.64	94.2
	3	60.17	32.42	2.36	3.31	1.75	4.10	136.0
	4	53.34	33.80	4.51	2.24	6.11	10.62	38.9
	5	66.91	23.78	1.70	5.74	1.87	3.57	119.8
	6	31.26	52.47	7.04	5.17	4.06	11.10	88.6
	7	58.92	25.67	6.60	3.54	5.27	11.87	104.6
	8	41.71	43.50	5.45	5.74	3.59	9.04	104.7
	Mean	51.75	36.24	4.50	4.05	3.46	7.96	99.7
	SD	12.06	9.98	2.21	1.39	1.66	3.57	28.6
R	1	43.17	42.41	4.98	4.36	5.08	10.07	34.6
	2	49.47	38.98	1.80	2.49	1.52	3.32	64.7
	3	49.79	30.94	2.52	1.64	2.31	4.83	55.5
	4	47.94	24.29	1.79	2.68	1.67	3.46	55.8
	5	68.48	18.86	3.80	2.59	2.73	6.53	59.2
	6	53.84	35.16	3.11	2.76	3.07	6.19	107.5
	Mean	57.04	33.37	3.25	3.39	2.95	6.20	62.9
	SD	9.31	8.26	1.05	0.63	1.15	2.16	24.1
D'	1	23.01	48.82	19.25	0.21	8.70	27.96	74.7
	2	60.58	23.22	7.49	2.23	6.48	13.97	71.4
	3	41.79	32.03	12.22	6.48	7.48	19.71	90.3
	4	37.45	41.04	10.63	3.84	7.05	17.68	66.8
	5	40.60	37.00	12.62	2.53	7.24	19.86	86.8
	6	41.80	33.42	12.66	3.18	8.94	21.60	84.8
	7	50.49	32.67	8.73	4.11	4.01	12.74	76.1
	8	47.57	35.12	8.05	3.69	5.57	13.62	73.5
	Mean	42.91	35.41	11.46	3.28	6.94	18.39	78.1
	SD	10.86	7.42	3.77	1.79	1.61	5.08	8.3

Table 2.38 Mean Cumulative Percentage Recovery of Paracetamol and Metabolites in Different Study Groups Following Ingestion of a 20 mg kg^{-1} Body Weight Dose

	Time After Ingestion (hr)	Group A Mean	Group A SD	Group B Mean	Group B SD	Group C Mean	Group C SD	Group D Mean	Group D SD	Group R Mean	Group R SD	Group D' Mean	Group D' SD
						Mean Cumulative Percentage Recovery							
Glucuronide	Predose	0	0	0	0	0	0	0	0	0	0	0	0
	4	20.3	9.2	17.9	11.1	22.1	14.2	18.9	11.9	4.0	3.3	8.6	5.8
	8	43.6	4.2	42.8	14.4	38.4	16.1	32.8	18.9	20.8	9.9	24.1	8.4
	24	58.5	4.8	58.5	11.5	56.4	13.3	51.8	12.1	52.1	8.7	42.9	10.9
Sulphate	Predose	0	0	0	0	0	0	0	0	0	0	0	0
	4	14.3	6.9	13.8	10.9	12.5	5.7	15.9	8.4	3.8	3.6	8.0	4.6
	8	25.4	5.3	24.2	10.9	21.1	5.1	24.8	12.3	16.0	8.1	21.6	4.1
	24	32.3	5.5	31.2	11.6	32.1	9.3	36.2	10.0	31.8	8.9	35.4	7.4
Cysteine	Predose	0	0	0	0	0	0	0	0	0	0	0	0
	4	0.5	0.4	0.8	0.4	0.7	0.3	1.1	0.6	0.2	0.2	1.2	0.8
	8	1.4	0.4	2.2	1.5	1.5	0.4	2.1	1.1	1.2	0.6	5.0	1.5
	24	2.5	0.7	3.4	1.9	3.5	2.0	4.5	2.2	3.0	1.2	11.5	3.8
Paracetamol	Predose	0	0	0	0	0	0	0	0	0	0	0	0
	4	1.8	1.0	1.0	0.4	1.7	0.9	1.6	0.7	0.5	0.4	0.8	0.6
	8	3.1	0.6	2.3	0.7	3.1	1.3	2.7	1.5	1.4	0.7	2.0	1.3
	24	4.1	0.5	3.6	1.4	5.0	1.6	4.1	1.4	2.8	0.9	3.3	1.8
Mercapturate	Predose	0	0	0	0	0	0	0	0	0	0	0	0
	4	0.5	0.3	0.7	0.4	0.6	0.3	0.7	0.3	0.1	0.1	0.7	0.5
	8	1.5	0.4	2.0	0.8	1.3	0.3	1.4	0.6	1.0	0.6	3.0	0.8
	24	2.5	0.9	3.3	1.3	3.0	1.6	3.5	1.7	2.7	1.3	6.9	1.6
Cysteine + Mercapturate	Predose	0	0	0	0	0	0	0	0	0	0	0	0
	4	1.0	0.7	1.5	0.8	1.2	0.5	1.8	0.8	0.4	0.3	1.9	1.4
	8	2.8	0.7	4.1	2.1	2.8	0.6	3.5	1.6	2.2	1.2	8.0	2.1
	24	5.0	1.5	6.7	2.9	6.5	3.5	8.0	3.6	5.7	2.5	18.4	5.1

Figure 2.22   Cumulative Urinary Recovery of Paracetamol and Its Metabolites in 24 hour Urine Collection of Subjects in Different Study Groups Following Ingestion of a 20 mg kg^{-1} Body Weight Dose

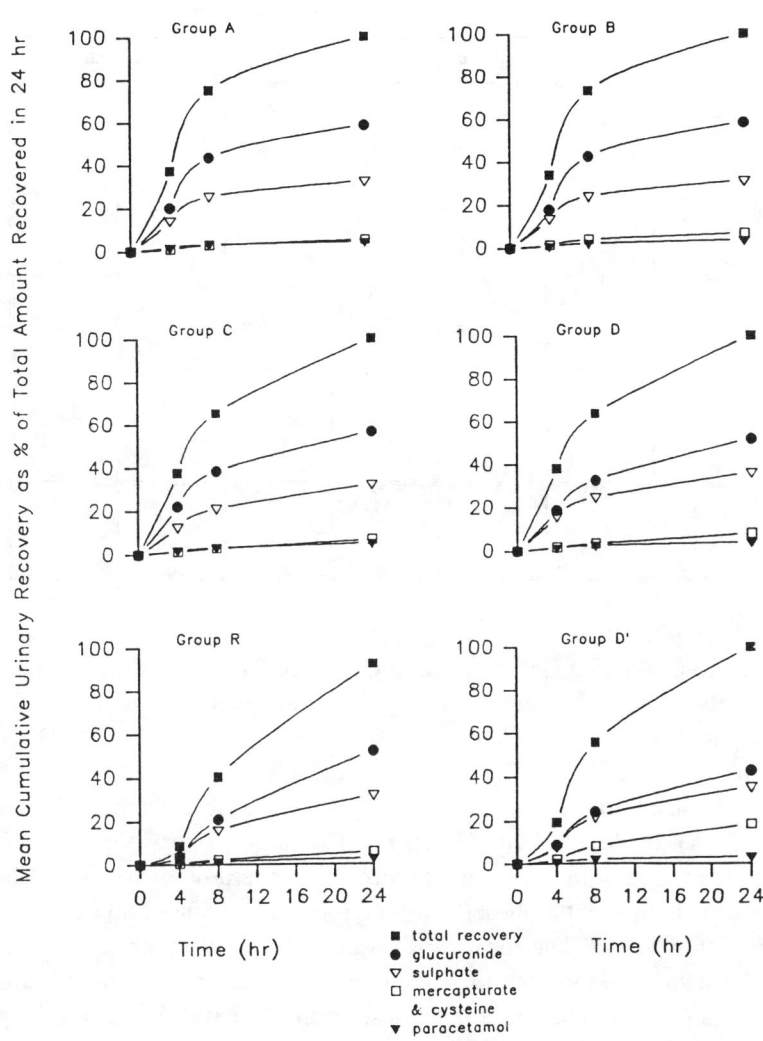

Table 2.39   Area Under Curve (AUC) of the Plasma Concentration-Time
Curves of Paracetamol in Different Study Groups Following Ingestion of
a 20 mg kg^{-1} Body Weight Dose

Subject	Area Under Curve of Study Groups (μg ml^{-1} hr)					
	Group A	Group B	Group C	Group D	Group R	Group D'
1	65.5	38.5	128.7	55.4	111.7	95.7
2	60.6	116.4	232.2	104.5	36.5	76.0
3	77.1	60.9	157.5	62.7	73.4	77.8
4	67.2	56.6	78.0	153.1	56.3	150.1
5	109.2	85.7	62.2	137.5	23.8	63.0
6	86.2	137.9	87.7	80.6	72.1	122.2
7	70.5	93.6	61.2	89.6	77.3	84.4
8		52.4	162.2	90.6		115.0
9			47.2			
Mean	76.6	80.2	113.0	96.7	64.4	98.0
SD	16.6	34.4	61.5	34.1	29.0	29.0

R) to 113.0 ± 61.5 g ml^{-1} hr (Group C). Since Cl is related to AUC by an inversely proportional relationship, the highest mean Cl value was found in Group R (6.51 ± 3.84 ml min^{-1} kg^{-1}) but the lowest was in Group D', after having taken the body weight into account, at 3.66 ± 1.02 ml min^{-1} kg^{-1}.

The mean terminal $t_{1/2}$ in the study groups ranged from 2.1 ± 0.2 hr (Group A) to 3.2 ± 1.4 hr (Group C). The largest inter-subject variation was also found within Group C, with the standard deviation at 1.4 hr as compared to the next highest 0.7 hr in Group R. Within Group C, $t_{1/2}$ ranged from 1.9 to 5.7 hr. The mean MRT values in the study groups reflects a similar pattern to those of $t_{1/2}$. Again the lowest mean value was found in Group A (3.3 ± 0.3 hr) and the highest mean MRT was 5.1 hr in Group C, with a standard deviation of 2.2 hr.

The low mean AUC value in Group R was a result of the overall lower plasma concentrations achieved in the subjects studied. The high mean V_d value in this group (1.23 ± 0.45 l kg^{-1}) was thus a related finding. The lowest mean V_d was found in Group A, at 0.97 ± 0.12 l kg^{-1}.

Table 2.40 Clearance (Cl) of Paracetamol in Different Study Groups Following Ingestion of a 20 mg kg^{-1} Body Weight Dose

Subject	Clearance of Paracetamol in Different Study Groups (ml min^{-1} kg^{-1})					
	Group A	Group B	Group C	Group D	Group R	Group D'
1	5.09	8.66	2.59	6.02	2.98	3.48
2	5.50	2.86	1.44	3.19	9.14	4.39
3	4.32	5.47	2.12	5.32	4.54	4.28
4	4.96	5.89	4.27	2.18	5.92	2.22
5	3.05	3.89	5.36	2.42	14.02	5.29
6	3.87	2.42	3.80	4.14	4.63	2.73
7	4.73	3.56	5.44	3.72	4.31	3.95
8		6.36	2.05	3.68		2.90
9			7.06			
Mean	4.50	4.89	3.79	3.83	6.51	3.66
SD	0.83	2.09	1.90	1.32	3.84	1.02

The mean metabolic clearances to the various metabolites of paracetamol in the study groups are shown in Table 2.44. The metabolic clearance of a particular metabolite is a function of the plasma clearance of paracetamol and the urinary fractional excretion as that metabolite. Its value will be affected by both these factors. The scattergraph of the individual metabolic clearance values are placed together with the scattergraph of the percentage recovery for each metabolite, in Fig. 2.24 to 2.29.

2.4.6.4 Statistical Results

Each of the pharmacokinetic parameters was first compared by a global analysis of variance (ANOVA). The post hoc multiple range test for all possible comparisons between 2 groups was the Scheffe test. Significant results ($p < 0.05$) are indicated by asterisks in the scattergraphs, Fig. 2.23. C_{max} and t_{max} are not significantly different among the study groups. For

Table 2.41   Terminal Elimination Half-life of Paracetamol in Different Study
Groups Following Ingestion of a 20 mg kg^{-1} Body Weight Dose

Subject	Terminal Elimination Half-Life of Paracetamol (hr)					
	Group A	Group B	Group C	Group D	Group R	Group D'
1	2.3	1.7	3.7	1.9	3.0	2.8
2	1.8	2.8	5.7	3.2	2.2	2.3
3	2.0	2.4	4.6	2.0	2.5	2.5
4	1.7	1.4	2.2	3.4	1.9	3.2
5	2.4	2.3	2.3	2.3	1.6	2.6
6	2.1	3.3	2.2	2.5	3.8	3.0
7	2.0	2.8	1.9	3.1	2.3	3.2
8		2.0	4.5	2.8		3.1
9			1.6			
Mean	2.1	2.3	3.2	2.6	2.5	2.8
SD	0.2	0.6	1.4	0.6	0.7	0.4

the pharmacokinetic parameters Cl, AUC, terminal $t_{1/2}$ and MRT, there was
also no statistically significant difference found. The only significant difference was in the V_d of Group R, the renal impairment group, which was
significantly higher than that of the control group at 1.25 l kg^{-1} *vs* 0.79 l
kg^{-1} ($p < 0.05$).

   The percentage recovery of the different metabolites of paracetamol in
the 24 hour urine collection and the corresponding metabolic clearance
were also compared among the study groups. The percentage recovery of
the oxidative metabolites, cysteine and mercapturate, in the 24 hour urine
collection, was much higher in Group D', patients with hepatocellular
carcinoma. The mean percentage recovery as the mercapturate and cysteine conjugates was $18.39 \pm 5.08\%$ as compared to $5.05 \pm 1.60\%$ in the
control group. In fact the mean value in Group D' was significantly higher
than every other study group. The partial metabolic clearance to the
oxidative metabolites was, as expected, also high among the hepatocellular
carcinoma patients. The mean metabolic clearance to the oxidative

Table 2.42 Mean Residence Time of Paracetamol in Different Study Groups Following Ingestion of a 20 mg kg^{-1} Body Weight Dose

Subject	Mean Residence Time of Paracetamol (hr)					
	Group A	Group B	Group C	Group D	Group R	Group D'
1	3.6	2.7	5.9	3.1	4.8	4.9
2	3.1	4.7	8.8	4.9	3.9	3.6
3	3.3	4.0	7.1	3.2	4.2	3.9
4	2.8	2.3	3.6	5.5	3.2	4.9
5	3.7	3.6	3.6	3.7	2.7	5.5
6	3.4	5.2	3.6	3.9	5.7	4.5
7	3.2	4.3	3.1	5.2	4.0	4.9
8		3.4	7.4	4.3		4.7
9			3.1			
Mean	3.3	3.8	5.1	4.2	4.1	4.6
SD	0.3	1.0	2.2	0.9	1.0	0.6

metabolites was 0.67 ± 0.26 ml min^{-1} kg^{-1} in Group D' compared to 0.23 ± 0.11 ml min^{-1} kg^{-1} in the control group. Again, the mean value in Group D' was significantly higher than every other study group.

2.4.7   Discussion

This study was designed to find out the difference in the pharmacokinetics of paracetamol in different groups of subjects who excreted different proportions of oxidative metabolites, the cysteine and mercapturate conjugates. Previous work in the Department of Clinical Pharmacology at The Chinese University of Hong Kong has shown that the percentage of urinary recovery of the oxidative metabolites of paracetamol in the 24 hour urine collection was much greater in patients with hepatocellular carcinoma (Leung & Critchley, 1991). Due to the limitations of this study, it was not able to address any fundamental changes in the pharmacokinetics of paracetamol leading to the finding of this altered metabolism in patients

Table 2.43 Volume of Distribution of Terminal Elimination Phase of Paracetamol in Different Study Groups Following Ingestion of a 20 mg kg^{-1} Body Weight Dose

Subject	Volume of Distribution of Terminal Elimination Phase of Paracetamol (l kg-1)					
	Group A	Group B	Group C	Group D	Group R	Group D'
1	1.00	1.26	0.84	0.97	0.78	0.85
2	0.87	0.68	0.70	0.87	1.72	0.87
3	0.76	1.13	0.84	0.90	0.98	0.91
4	0.74	0.70	0.83	0.64	0.99	0.62
5	0.62	0.79	1.08	0.49	1.88	1.19
6	0.71	0.69	0.72	0.89	1.51	0.70
7	0.83	0.86	0.89	1.00	0.86	1.08
8		1.13	0.80	0.88		0.78
9			1.00			
Mean	0.79	0.91	0.86	0.83	1.25	0.88
SD	0.12	0.23	0.12	0.17	0.45	0.19

with hepatocellular carcinoma. This study aimed to find out if there were any changes in other pharmacokinetic parameters including clearance, elimination half-life, volume of distribution and metabolic clearances of various metabolites, which might offer clues to the mechanisms of the altered metabolism of paracetamol in these patients.

For this comparative pharmacokinetic study of paracetamol, subjects were recruited in 5 groups. Group A served as the control group. Group B and Group C consisted of patients with some degree of liver function impairment due to alcoholism and chronic hepatitis B infection, respectively. The diagnoses were confirmed by patient history and biochemical tests. In addition, patients in Group C were all sero-positive for the surface antigen of the hepatitis B virus (HBsAg +ve). Group D patients were confirmed to have hepatocellular carcinoma by patient history, ultrasound scan, raised plasma α-foetoprotein level and/or liver biopsy. Group R was added on as a group of patients with renal function impairment, as

Figure 2.23   Scattergraphs of AUC, Cl, $t_{1/2}$, MRT and V_d of Paracetamol of Subjects in Different Study Groups Following Ingestion of a 20 mg kg^{-1} Body Weight Dose

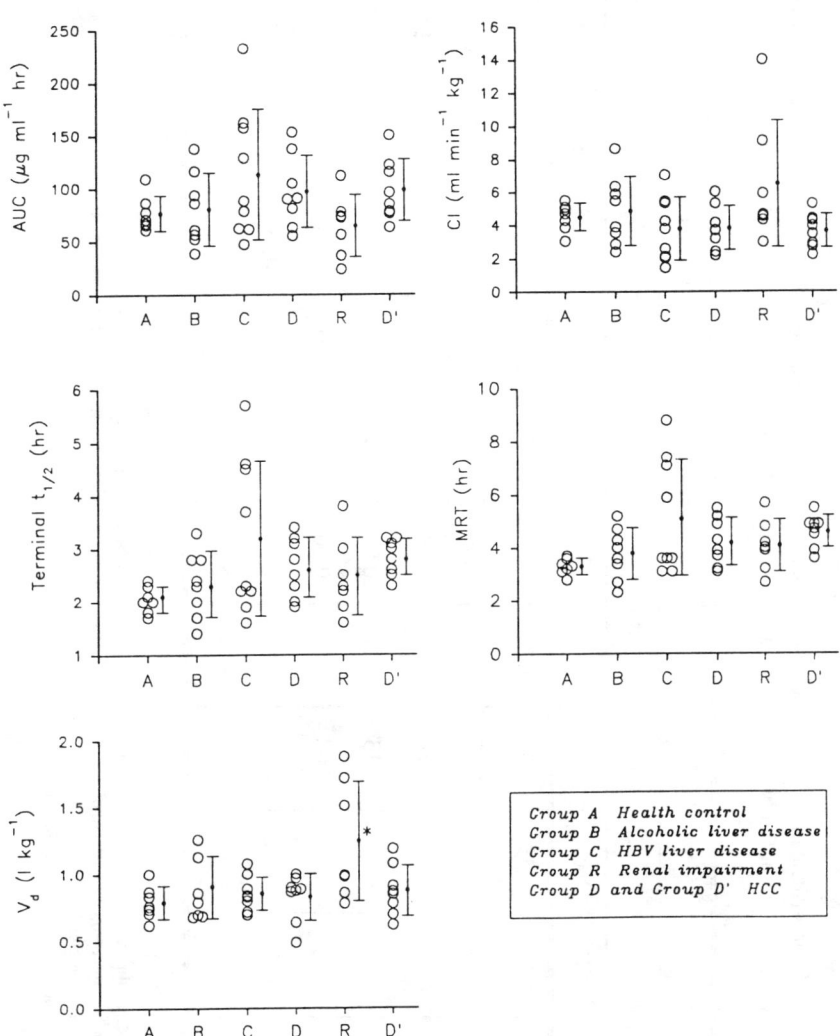

* Significantly different from Group A by multiple comparison Scheffe test, p < 0.05

Table 2.44 Mean Metabolic Clearance of Paracetamol and Its Glucuronide, Sulphate, Cysteine and Mercapturate Conjugates in Different Study Groups Following Ingestion of a 20 mg kg^{-1} Body Weight Dose

| | Mean Metabolic Clearance of Paracetamol and Metabolites (ml min-1 kg-1) | | | | | | | | | | | |
| | Group A | | Group B | | Group C | | Group D | | Group R | | Group D' | |
	Mean	SD	Mean	SD	Mean	SD	Mean	SD	Mean	SD	Mean	SD
T	4.50	0.83	4.89	2.09	3.79	1.90	3.83	1.32	6.82	4.10	3.66	1.02
G	2.64	0.59	3.00	1.70	2.31	1.49	1.93	0.69	4.13	3.09	1.59	0.67
S	1.44	0.31	1.41	0.49	1.12	0.46	1.44	0.75	2.07	0.92	1.27	0.39
C	0.12	0.05	0.17	0.13	0.11	0.02	0.18	0.12	0.21	0.16	0.42	0.18
P	0.18	0.04	0.16	0.06	0.17	0.06	0.15	0.05	0.23	0.14	0.12	0.08
M	0.12	0.07	0.16	0.08	0.10	0.03	0.13	0.06	0.18	0.10	0.25	0.09
M+C	0.23	0.11	0.32	0.20	0.20	0.05	0.31	0.18	0.40	0.26	0.67	0.26

T = Total clearance
S = Metabolic clearance to the sulphate conjugate
P = Metabolic clearance to unchanged paracetamol
M+C = Sum of the metabolic clearances
    to the cysteine and mercapturate conjugate

G = Metabolic clearance to the glucuronide conjugate
C = Metabolic clearance to the cysteine conjugate
M = Metabolic clearance to the mercapturate conjugate

Figure 2.24   Percentage Recovery of Paracetamol Glucuronide in 24 hour Urine
Collection and Its Metabolic Clearance in Subjects of Different Study Groups
Following Ingestion of a 20 mg kg^{-1} Body Weight Dose

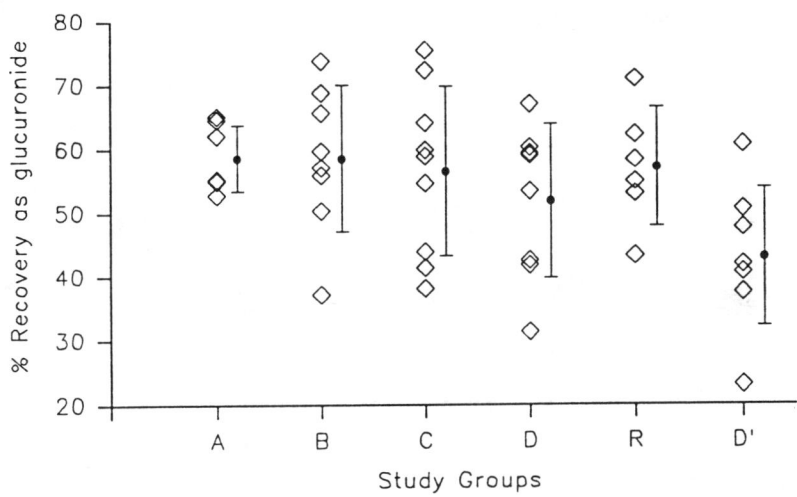

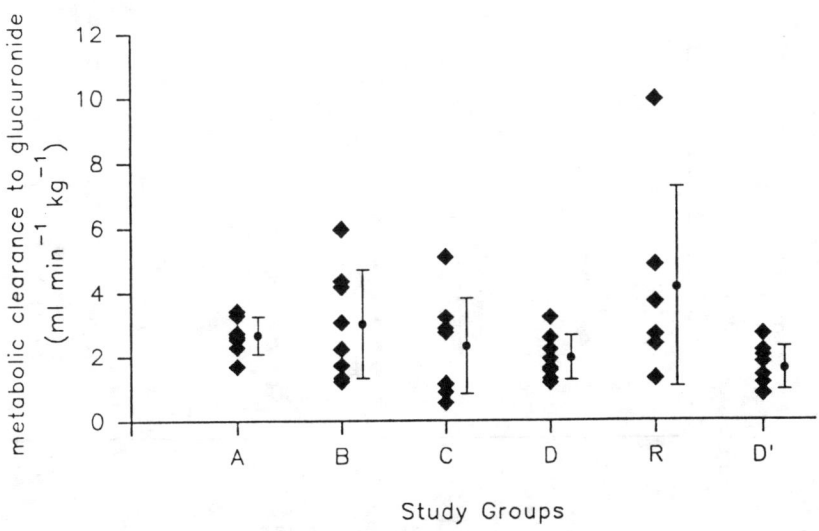

Figure 2.25   Percentage Recovery of Paracetamol Sulphate in 24 hour Urine
Collection and Its Metabolic Clearance in Subjects of Different Study Groups
Following Ingestion of a 20 mg kg^{-1} Body Weight Dose

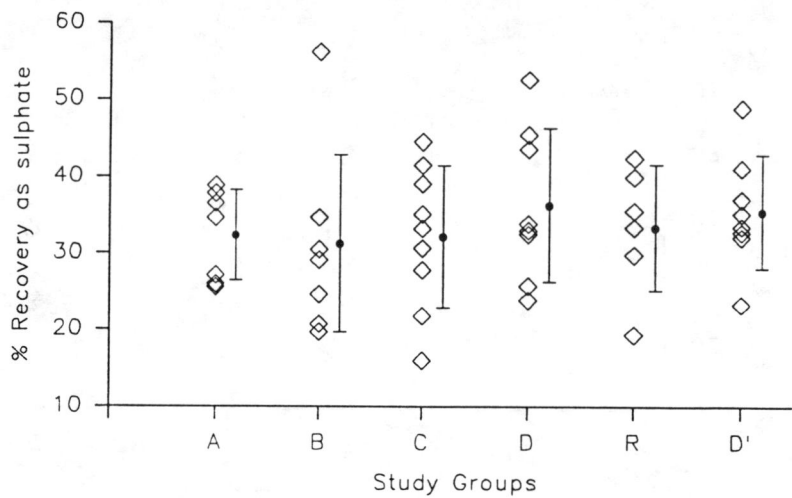

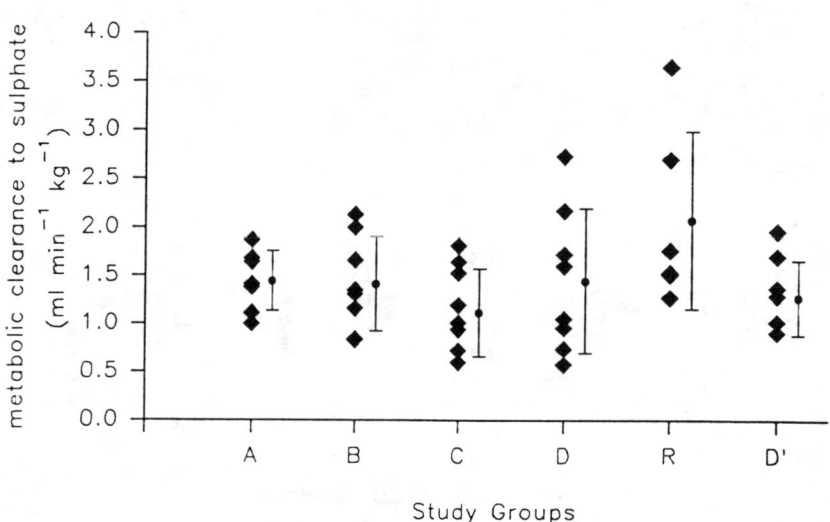

Figure 2.26   Percentage Recovery of Paracetamol Cysteine in 24 hour Urine
Collection and Its Metabolic Clearance in Subjects of Different Study Groups
Following Ingestion of a 20 mg kg^{-1} Body Weight Dose

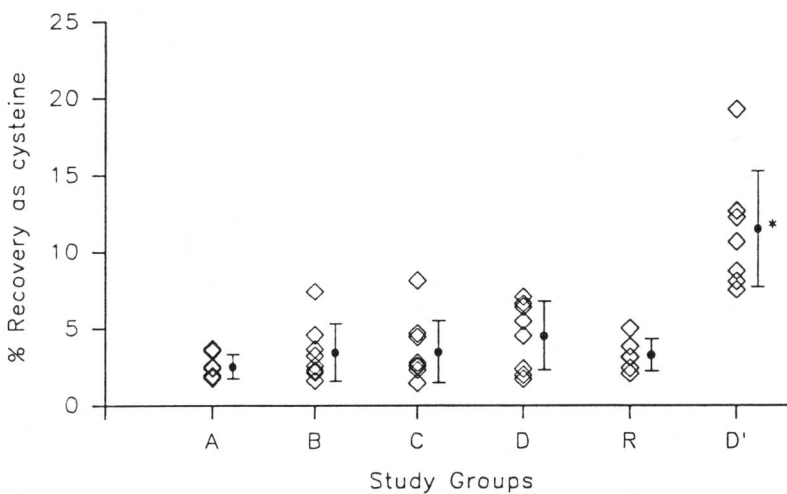

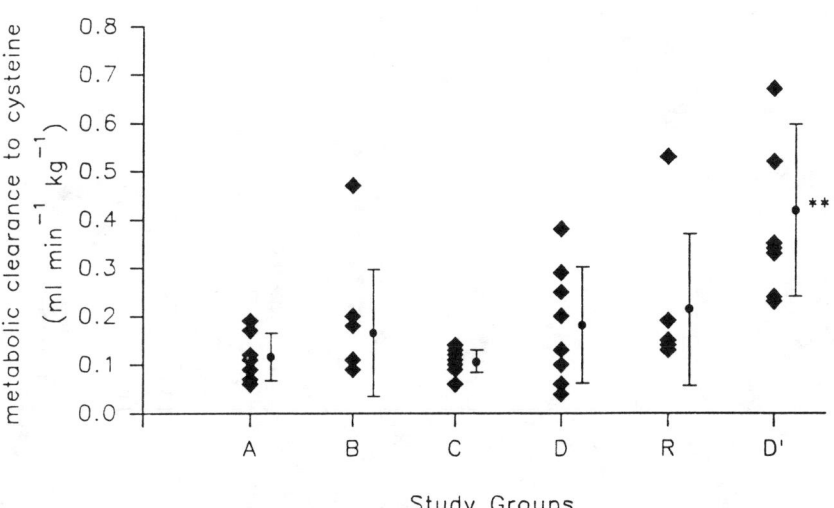

* / **   Significantly different compared to all other
study group, p<0.05 by Scheffe Multiple Range Tests

Figure 2.27   Percentage Recovery of Unchanged Paracetamol in 24 hour
Urine Collection and Its Metabolic Clearance in Subjects of Different Study
Groups Following Ingestion of a 20 mg kg^{-1} Body Weight Dose

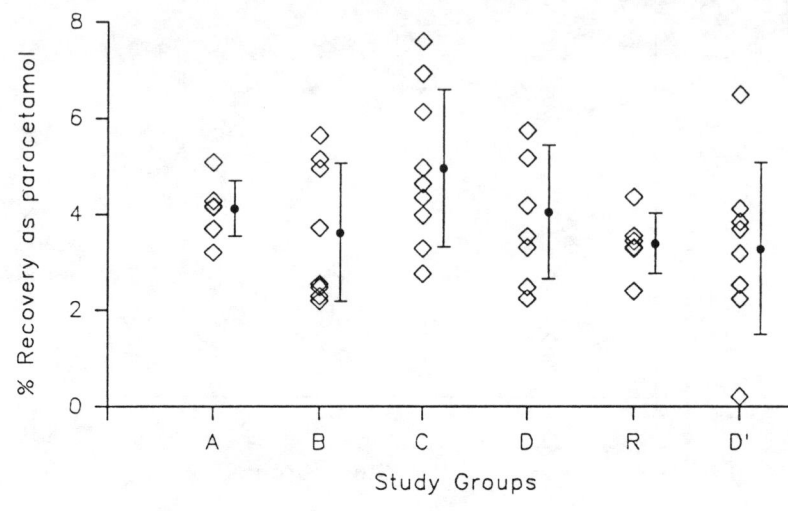

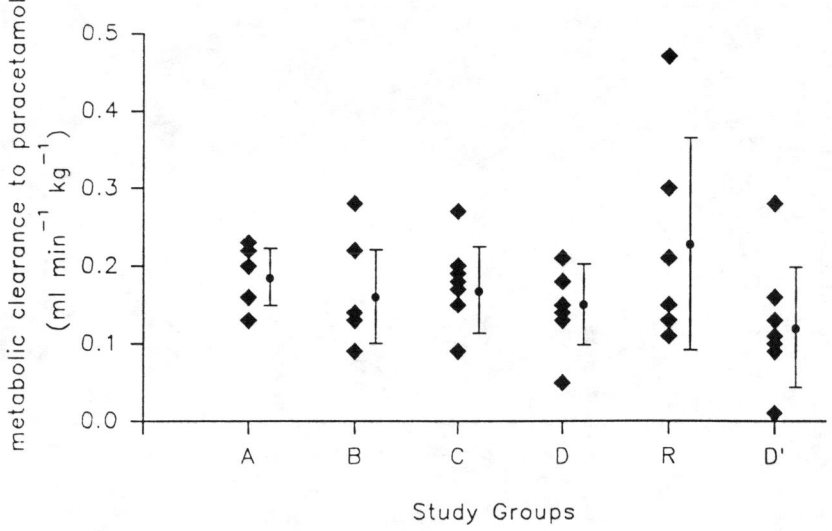

Figure 2.28 Percentage Recovery of Paracetamol Mercapturate in 24 hour
Urine Collection and Its Metabolic Clearance in Subjects of Different Study
Groups Following Ingestion of a 20 mg kg^{-1} Body Weight Dose

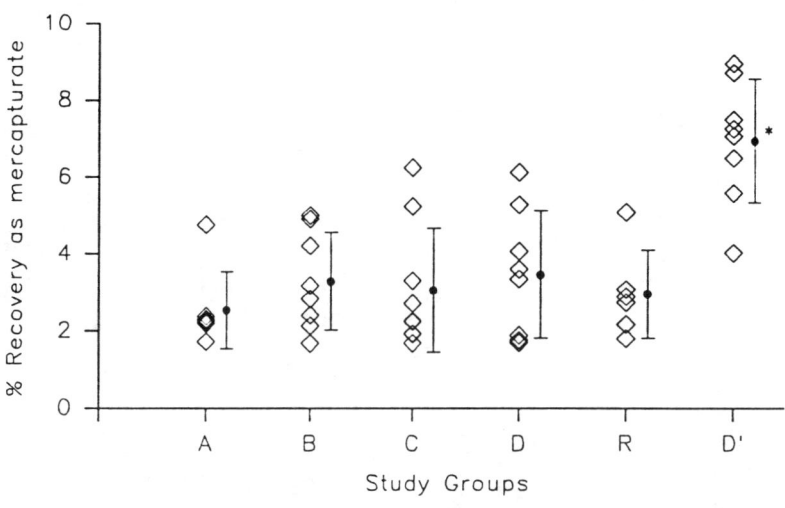

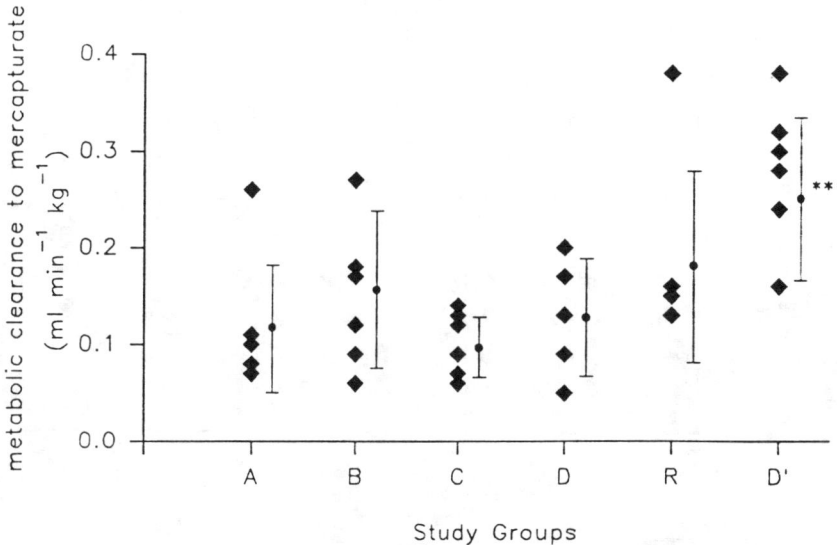

* / **   Significantly different compared to all other
            study groups, p<0,05 by Scheffe Multiple Range Tests

Figure 2.29   Percentage Recovery of Paracetamol Cysteine & Mercapturate in 24 hour Urine Collection and Its Metabolic Clearance in Subjects of Different Study Groups Following Ingestion of a 20 mg kg^{-1} Body Weight Dose

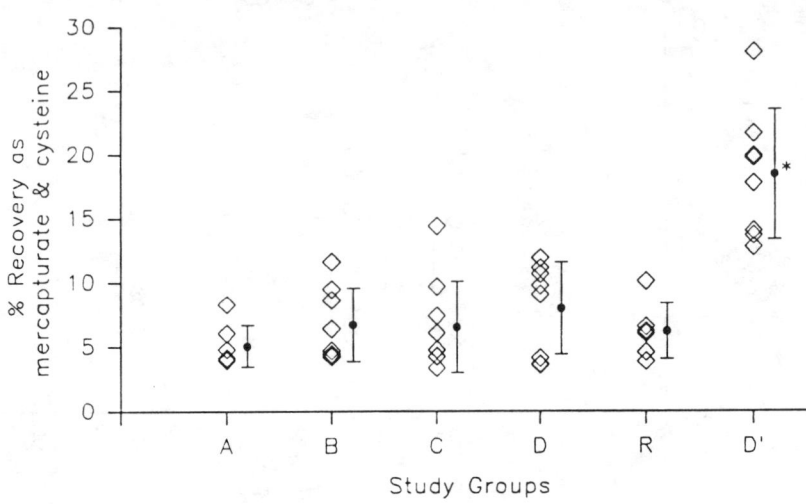

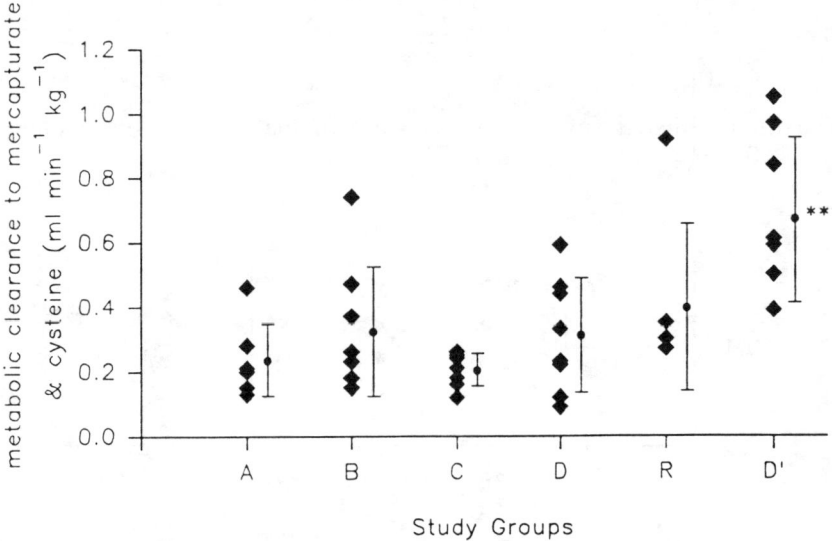

$*$ / $**$ Significantly different compared to all other
study groups, $p < 0.05$ by Scheffe Multiple Range Tests

confirmed by the plasma urea and creatinine levels, for comparison. It was intended to recruit 8 subjects in every group.

As the study proceeded and some of the results were analysed, it was found that though some of the patients in Group D did have an increased recovery of the oxidative metabolites, in some of them, it was only slightly raised. The mean percentage recovery of the oxidative metabolites in Group D, though higher than the control, was not statistically different. It was known that some patients with hepatocellular carcinoma do have near to normal recovery of the oxidative metabolites. It was not known, however, the reason for a number of the subjects in Group D to have fallen into this category. As the main objective of the study was to look at the pharmacokinetics of paracetamol in a group of hepatocellular carcinoma patients with enhanced oxidative metabolism, it was decided to recruit a further 8 patients with hepatocellular carcinoma patients as Group D'. As a result, there were all together 6 study groups instead of 5. At the close of the study, the number of subjects recruited for each group was not 8. Only 7 subjects were recruited for both Group A and Group R and 9 were recruited for Group C.

In this study, the only difference in the pharmacokinetics of paracetamol between patients with hepatocellular carcinoma and other subjects was the enhanced oxidative metabolic pathway and thus increased metabolic clearance to the cysteine and mercapturate conjugates. There was no significant difference found in other pharmacokinetic parameters. The finding that the percentage recovery of the oxidative metabolites among patients with impaired liver function, including alcoholic liver disease and chronic hepatitis B infection, was not different from healthy subjects, was a confirmation of the our previous work (Leung & Critchley, 1991). Forrest *et al.* also found no evidence of a significant alteration in the fractional urinary recovery of paracetamol metabolites (Forrest *et al.*, 1979). However, they did find a prolongation of plasma paracetamol half-lives in patients with severe but not with mild liver disease. Patients in our study, including those with liver function impairment and hepatocellular carcinoma, had plasma total protein and albumin levels within the normal range, indicating that their liver disease was not as severe as those in Forrest *et al.*'s study with prolonged paracetamol half-lives. In fact, the pharmacokinetic results showed that the mean elimination half-lives of paracetamol in all the study groups were not significantly different although there were a couple of outliers in Group C with much prolonged elimination half-lives. There was also a significant correlation between the percentage recovery of the oxidative metabolites and the elimination half-life of paracetamol with $p < 0.001$ when Group D' was excluded. The much raised percentage recovery of the oxidative metabolites in Group D' did not match proportionally with the prolongation of the elimination half-life. When the values in Group D' were also taken into account, there was still a significant correlation but p was only < 0.05 (Fig. 2.30).

The plasma clearance of paracetamol was comparable in all study groups, indicating no impairment of clearance even in those subjects with liver diseases. The 24 hour urinary recovery of unchanged paracetamol is a direct function of the plasma clearance of paracetamol and this was shown by a significant correlation (Fig. 2.31). Although the average weight in other study groups was lower than the control groups and a smaller volume of distribution might be expected, the V_d values calculated were not lower. There was, however, a significantly higher mean V_d in Group R, patients with impaired renal function. It has been demonstrated that significant sodium and water retention can take place in patients with diabetic renal disease. This leads to increased exchangeable sodium and total body water and hence volume of distribution. This may explain the finding of increased V_d of paracetamol among patients with impaired renal function. Although mean C_{max} was lower in Group R compared to other groups, it did not reach a statistical significance (17.64 ± 8.15 in Group R vs 22.91 ± 4.57 in Group A). The reduced C_{max} in patients with renal impairment may be a result of a combination of delayed gastric emptying due to diabetic autonomic neuropathy and increased V_d. It was thus consequential that there was a tendency for the AUC to be lower in Group R. Paracetamol clearance and elimination half-life were not affected by renal function since paracetamol is primarily metabolised in the liver, as shown by comparable elimination half-lives. On the other hand, the plasma concentration-time curves (Fig. 2.17–Fig. 2.20) showed significant retention of the polar conjugates of paracetamol which were inefficiently excreted by the kidneys in patients with renal impairment. These findings were in agreement with previous similar studies (Lowenthal *et al.*, 1976; Martin *et al.*, 1991).

The fractional recovery of the metabolites of paracetamol was not different in Group R as compared to the healthy controls, though the total amount recovered in 24 hours was lower. The comparable fractional recovery of the different metabolites suggested that despite the presence of renal impairment, paracetamol was handled similarly and that the

Figure 2.30   Correlation between Percentage Recovery of Paracetamol Cysteine and Mercapturate in 24 hour Urine Collection and Paracetamol Half-life in Subjects of Different Study Groups Following a 20 mg kg^{-1} Body Weight Dose

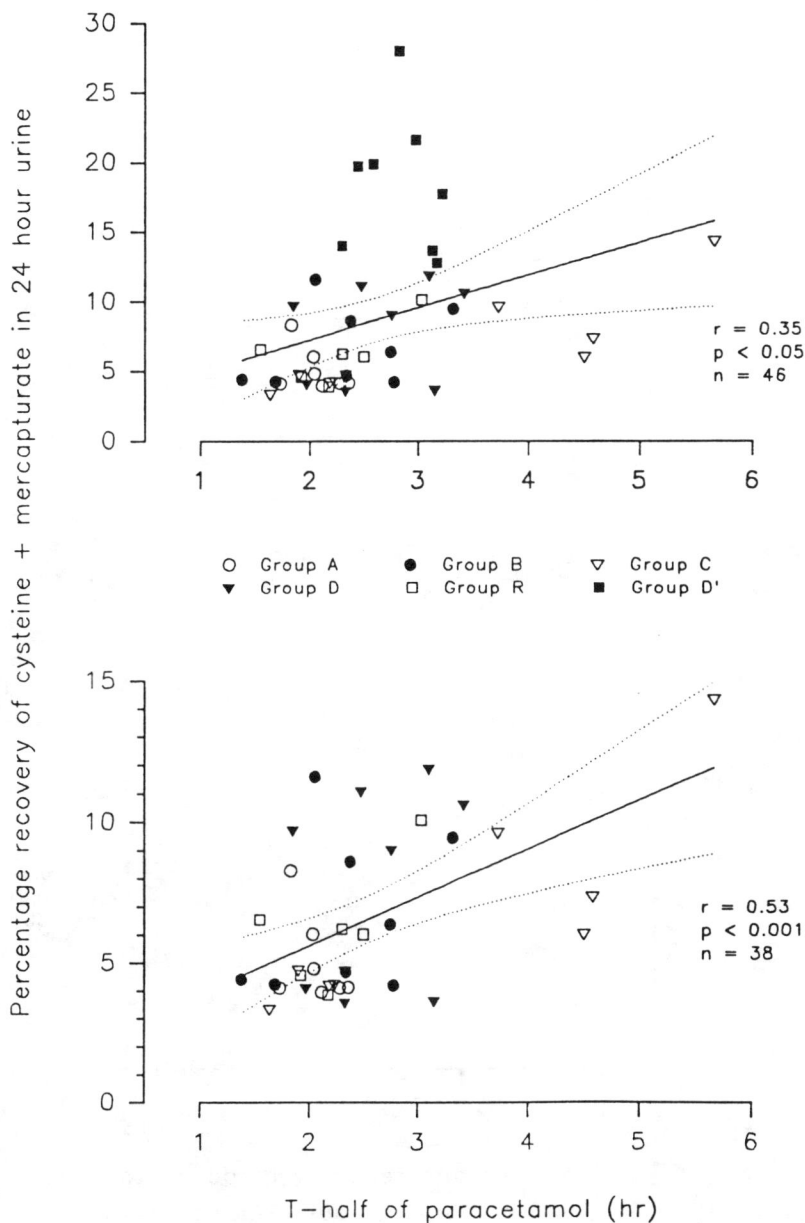

Figure 2.31   Correlation between Clearance of Paracetamol and Percentage Recovery of Unchanged Paracetamol in 24 Hour Urine Collection in Subjects of Different Study Groups Following a 20 mg kg^{-1} Body Weight Dose

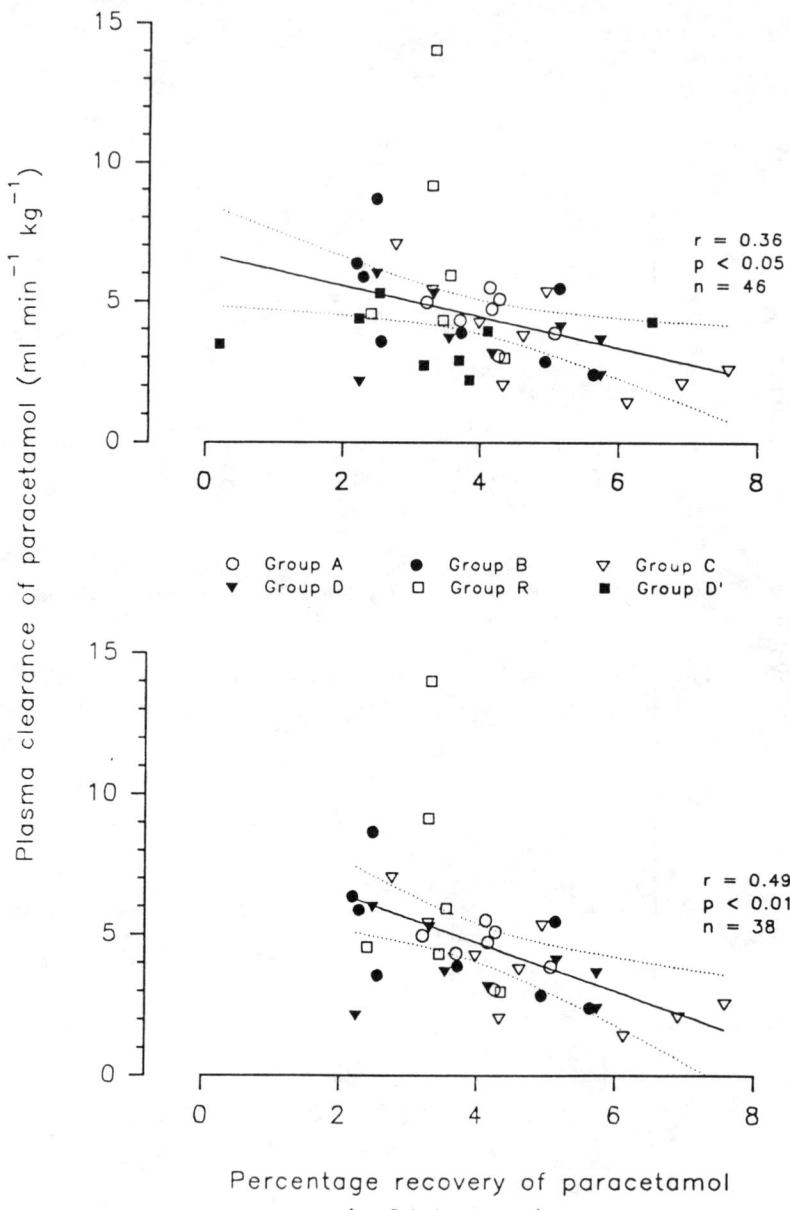

metabolic activation of paracetamol was of little clinical significance. These findings were in accordance with previous reports in non-diabetic patients with renal impairment (Prescott *et al.*, 1989), that glucuronide and sulphate conjugation remain as the predominant route of metabolism in these patients. These metabolites are inert and no adverse effect is expected. However, these data probably carry more significance for other drugs or chemicals dependent on metabolic activation. For agents that are biotransformed to active metabolites, accumulation of these toxic substances in patients with renal impairment could lead to serious adverse reactions.

In this study, although the patients in different study groups were older than the control subjects, this is unlikely to have affected the results. Triggs *et al.* found only a modest increase in the plasma half-life in geriatric subjects with a mean age of 81 years compared with subjects of mean age 24 years (Triggs *et al.*, 1975). In addition, another *in vitro* study using liver fractions from subjects of a wide range of age also did not show fall in the glucuronidation and sulphation activities of paracetamol with increasing age (Herd *et al.*, 1991). Therefore, age alone can not account for the differences in metabolism of paracetamol among healthy subjects and patients with hepatocellular carcinoma. The overall pattern of the urinary excretion of metabolites in patients with impaired liver function but not hepatocellular carcinoma (Group B and Group C) did not differ from that observed in the healthy subjects. It was of particular significance that there was normal excretion of the cysteine and mercapturate conjugates. These two metabolites reflect conversion of paracetamol to the reactive hepatotoxic intermediate which undergoes conjugation with reduced glutathione (Jollow *et al.*, 1973; Mitchell *et al.*, 1973a; Mitchell *et al.*, 1973b; Potter *et al.*, 1973). These findings are in support of the suggestion that a therapeutic dose of paracetamol is unlikely to cause liver damage in patients with mildly impaired liver function when the plasma albumin level is within the normal range. However, other factors may also contribute to the threshold dose of paracetamol required to produce liver damage e.g. the rate of paracetamol absorption, the rate of production of the toxic intermediate, hepatic glutathione stores and the rate of glutathione synthesis and all these factor may be affected in liver diseases. Repeated doses of paracetamol may be potentially even more damaging. Nevertheless, based on these findings, it seems unnecessary to implement dosage reduction in patients with mildly impaired liver function with normal serum albumin.

Patients in Group D', the hepatocellular carcinoma patients, had greatly enhanced oxidative metabolism. The increase in the fractional recovery of the oxidative metabolites seemed to be at the expense of the fractional recovery of the glucuronide conjugate. The mean recovery of the glucuronide conjugate in Group D' was $42.91 \pm 10.86\%$ while that in Group A was $58.50 \pm 5.18\%$. This difference, though substantial, did not reach a statistical significance as the low mean value in Group D' was attributed, to a large extent, to one single low value of 23.01%. The mean fractional recovery of the sulphate conjugate was not very different in all the study groups with a narrow range of 31.22 ± 11.58 to $36.24 \pm 9.98\%$. As the recovery of the sulphate conjugate was not increased significantly in Group D', it suggested that the increased production of the oxidative metabolites was not a consequence of a primary impairment in glucuronidation as a corresponding increase in sulphate conjugation would be expected. Epileptic patients on anticonvulsant therapy have enhanced glucuronidation and correspondingly reduced sulphate conjugation with decreased plasma paracetamol half-lives (Prescott *et al.*, 1981). In this study, the elimination half-lives of paracetamol in all the study groups were comparable and no statistical significance was found, indicating that there was no fundamental impairment in paracetamol metabolism. Furthermore, plasma clearance of paracetamol was shown to be normal in patients with hepatocellular carcinoma by the plasma data and also by unaltered fractional recovery of unchanged paracetamol in the 24 hour urine collection. This again suggests that there was no significant primary impairment of glucuronidation. All these data seem to indicate that there is a genuine increase in the oxidative metabolic pathway of paracetamol via the action of microsomal cytochrome P_{450} mixed function oxidase and thus the metabolic activation of paracetamol to the toxic intermediate, is enhanced in patients with hepatocellular carcinoma.

Among patients in Group B and Group C, there are a few outliers with the fractional recovery of the oxidative metabolites extending up into the range of the hepatocellular carcinoma patients. These elevated levels of mercapturate and cysteine conjugates in the 24 hour urine collection again reflect enhanced metabolic activation by microsomal cytochrome P_{450}. This is of particular interest since the metabolic activation of xenobiotics by microsomal enzymes has been implicated in the formation of carcinogenic substances (Gonzalez, 1989) and possibly involved in the pathogenesis of hepatocellular carcinoma.

2.4.8   Summary

The pharmacokinetics of paracetamol was studied in different categories of subjects including healthy controls, alcoholic patients, patients with chronic hepatitis B infection, hepatocellular carcinoma and renal function impairment after a single oral 20 mg kg^{-1} dose, given as a syrup. Pharmacokinetic parameters estimated included the area under the plasma concentration-time curve from zero hour to infinity, plasma clearance, terminal elimination half-life, volume of distribution, mean residence time and the metabolic clearance to the various metabolites. Other parameters also compared were maximum concentration, the time to reach maximum concentration and the fractional recovery of the various metabolites in the 24 hour urine collection.

Apart from much enhanced oxidative metabolism of paracetamol among patients with hepatocellular carcinoma, there were virtually no significant difference in all the parameters studied among the different groups. The mean percentage recovery of the cysteine and mercapturate metabolites in the 24 hour urine collection was $18.39 \pm 5.08\%$ among patients with hepatocellular carcinoma and only $5.05 \pm 1.60\%$ among healthy subjects. There was a tendency for the fractional recovery of the glucuronide conjugate to be reduced among the hepatocellular carcinoma patients but the difference did not reach a statistical significance. There was no significant difference in the fractional recovery of the sulphate conjugate and unchanged paracetamol, nor was there any significant difference in any of the pharmacokinetic parameters estimated among the different study groups.

Metabolic activation of paracetamol to the toxic intermediate seemed to be genuinely enhanced among patients with hepatocellular carcinoma and a small proportion of patients with chronic liver diseases e.g. chronic hepatitis B infection. It was postulated that metabolic activation by microsomal enzymes might be involved in the formation of carcinogenic substances from xenobiotics with some implications in the pathogenesis of hepatocellular carcinoma.

CHAPTER 3

Metabolic Activation of Aflatoxin B$_1$ in Healthy Subjects and in Patients with Liver Disease & Hepatocellular Carcinoma

3.1 General introduction

Aflatoxins are a group of bisfuranocoumarin metabolites isolated from strains of the fungi *Aspergillus* flavus and *A. parasiticus*. This group of mycotoxins was first discovered in 1960 during the investigation of a dramatic form of mouldy feed toxicosis in England, which became known as "Turkey-X" disease. The early signs of disease were anorexia, lethargy and muscular weakness. Within a few days the birds died in opisthotonus. At autopsy, haemorrhages were seen in the liver, which was also necrotic. The kidneys were often engorged. Histopathological examination revealed parenchymal cell degeneration and extensive proliferation of bile duct epithelial cells.

Apart from turkeys, there were also reports of other poultry, cattle, pigs and sheep being affected. Every outbreak was traced to flocks that had been fed rations containing groundnut meal newly imported from Brazil. The toxic substance isolated was found to be associated with *A. flavus* and this toxin was later named aflatoxin. They were found to be natural contaminants in many types of food, e.g. peanut, cottonseed meal, corn and rice (Shank & Wogan, 1972a; Shank & Wogan, 1972b), particularly in tropical countries. For more history and progress on the research of aflatoxin, see Goldblatt and *Wyllie et al.* (Goldblatt, 1969; Wyllie & Morehouse, 1977). Gradually over the years the motivation for research has shifted away from the purely animal production problem caused by aflatoxin poisoning to the greater concern for the potential hazard to human health, including its carcinogenicity. The hazard posed to human may either be direct, where there is direct consumption of human foodstuff spoilt by the fungi; or indirect, where aflatoxin in animal feedstuff and its metabolites accumulate in the milk and meat for human consumption.

3.1.1   Chemical structures and properties

The aflatoxins are a group of bisfuranocomarin metabolites isolated from strains of the *Aspergillus flavus* group of fungi. There are 4 main naturally occurring aflatoxins (Fig. 3.1), designated AFB_1, AFB_2, AFG_1 and AFG_2. The aflatoxins fluoresce strongly in ultraviolet light; B_1 and B_2 produce a blue fluorescence whereas G_1 and G_2 produce a greenish yellow fluorescence (Nesbitt, O'Kelly, Sargeant & Sheridan, 1962; Asao, Buchi, Abdel-Kader, Chang, Wick & Wogan, 1965). Four other minor metabolites were also isolated in small amounts from cultures of *A. flavus* and *A. paraciticus*: AFM_1, M_2, B_{2a} and G_{2a}. In some animal species, e.g. dairy cattle, AFB_1 and AFB_2 are partially metabolised to give the hydroxylated derivatives AFM_1 and AFM_2, respectively.

The aflatoxins are soluble in methanol, chloroform, dimethyl sulphoxide and other organic solvents but only sparingly soluble in water (10–30 µg/ml). They are very stable in dry heat up to the melting point. However, in the presence of moisture, there is a destruction of aflatoxin over a period of time, most likely involving the opening up of the lactone ring. They are also deactivated by extremes of pH (<3 or >10), oxidizing agents and ultraviolet radiation. A review of the chemical properties of the aflatoxins is given by Wyllie and Morehouse (Wyllie & Morehouse, 1977).

AFB_1 and to a lesser extent, AFG_1 were responsible for the extreme biological potency of aflatoxin-contaminated foodstuff and feeds. These two aflatoxins possess an unsaturated bond at the 8,9-position on the terminal furan ring. For AFB_2 and AFG_2, the bonds at this position are saturated and they are essentially biologically inactive unless these agents are first metabolically oxidized to AFB_1 and AFG_1 (Asao *et al.*, 1965; Groopman, Cain & Kensler, 1988).

3.1.2   Contamination of food by aflatoxins

Many foodstuff have been shown to be contaminated by aflatoxins. The most commonly implicated commodities include peanuts, cassava, dried fish, rice and some alcoholic beverages fermented from maize (Shank &

Figure 3.1 Chemical and physical properties of aflatoxins

Aflatoxin	Molecular formular	Molecular weight	Melting point (°C)	Ultraviolet absorbance (362-363 nm)	Fluorescence emission
B_1	$C_{17}H_{12}O_6$	312	268 - 269	21,800	425
B_2	$C_{17}H_{14}O_6$	314	286 - 289	23,400	425
G_1	$C_{17}H_{12}O_7$	328	244 - 246	16,100	450
G_2	$C_{17}H_{14}O_7$	330	237 - 240	21,000	450
M_1	$C_{17}H_{12}O_7$	328	299	19,000	425
M_2	$C_{17}H_{14}O_7$	330	293	20,400	-

AFB1

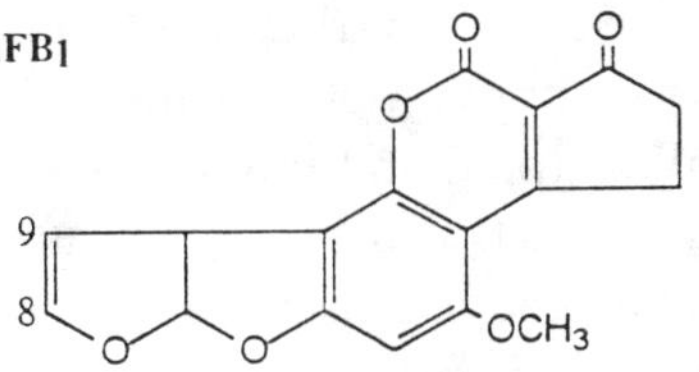

AFB2

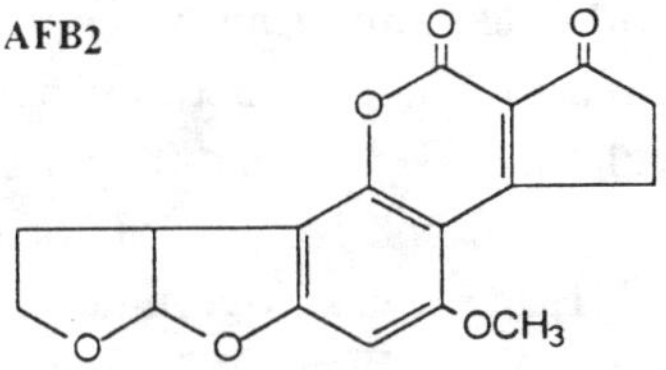

AFM1

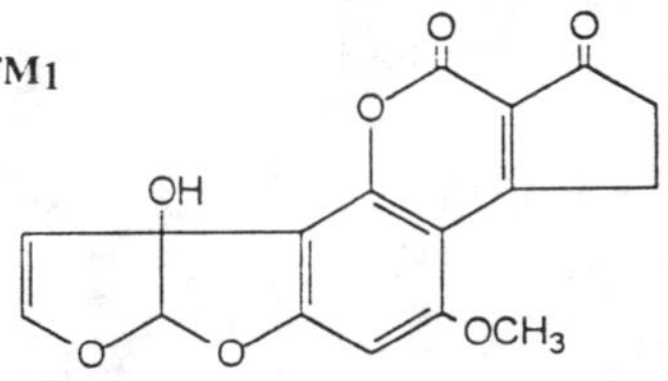

AFM2

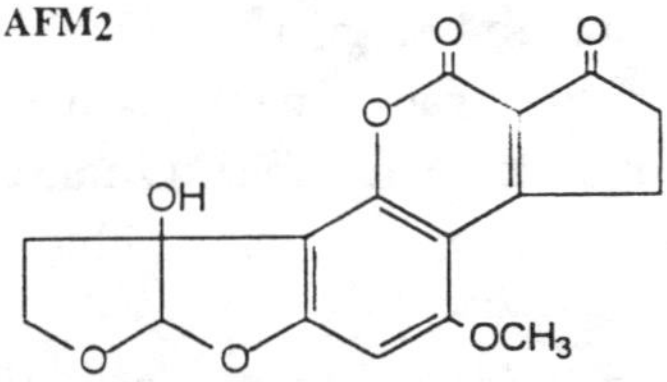

AFG1

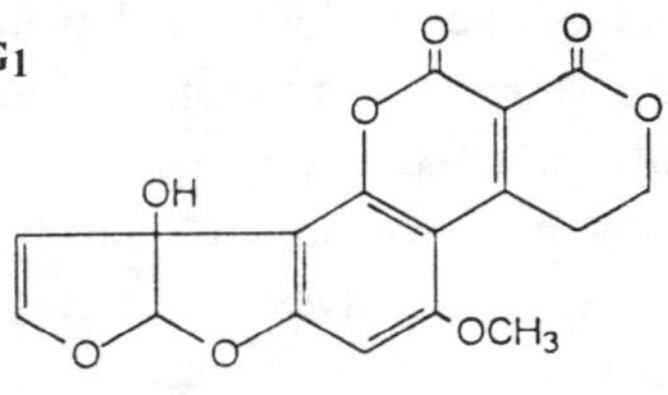

AFG2

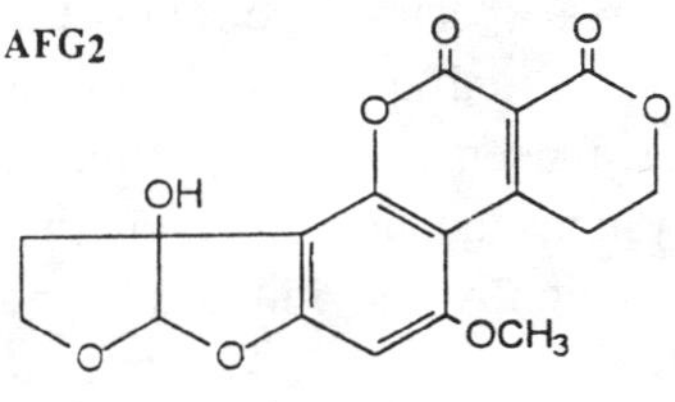

Wogan, 1972b; Shank & Wogan, 1972a; Chu, 1991). These are usually a result of inadequate food storage facilities and preservation techniques, combined with hot, and humid weather and unhygienic environmental conditions, all of which are conducive to the growth of the fungus and the elaboration of aflatoxins on foodstuff. Apart from direct consumption of food spoiled by toxigenic strains of *A. flavus* or *A. paraciticus*, exposure to the mycotoxin can also result from consumption of products derived from animals fed aflatoxin-contaminated feeds. These include meat and milk. Milk from village dairies in Iran has been found to contain high levels of AFM_1 (Suzanger, Emami & Barnett, 1976) and it has been found that some women from villages in Sudan and Zimbabwe excreted aflatoxins in breast-milk at levels similar to or higher than those considered safe in animal milk, for human consumption (Coulter, Lamplugh, Suliman, Omer & Hendrickse, 1984; Wild, Pionneau, Montesano, Mutiro & Chetsanga, 1987).

The potential hazard of aflatoxins to human health has led to worldwide monitoring programmes of the toxin in various commodities as well as regulatory actions by most countries. Most countries have a regulatory level around 20 parts per billion (ppb). In Hong Kong, the limit is set at 20 ppb for peanuts or peanut products and 15 ppb for any other food (Hong Kong Government, 1990). Preventive measures for controlling mycotoxin problems include use of resistant crops, crop rotation, avoiding mechanical damage and damage by birds or insects and drying the crop quickly to less than 10–30 % moisture content after harvesting. A number of detoxification methods have been used but may be difficult and not economically feasible in some cases. These methods include ammoniation, treatment with ozone and chlorine, etc (Chu, 1991).

3.1.3   *Metabolism of aflatoxins*

AFB_1 is actively metabolised by a variety of mechanisms in different animal species. The relative importance of each pathway is dependent on the animal species as well as the experimental conditions. Metabolites have been recovered from urine, milk and various *in vitro* incubation systems containing liver slices, homogenates or sub-cellular fractions. Essentially the initial metabolism of AFB_1 involves hydroxylation by the cytochrome P450 microsomal mixed-function oxidase system and a cytosolic nicotinamide adenine dinucleotide phosphate (NADPH)-dependent reductase. These enzymes are localized mainly on the endoplasmic reticulum of liver cells, but are also present in kidney, lungs, skin and other organs. Various hydroxylated derivatives result from the oxidative metabolism catalyzed by these enzymes and these metabolites may undergo phase II metabolism to glucuronide or sulphate conjugates which are excreted in urine or bile (Wyllie & Morehouse, 1977; Metcalfe & Neal, 1983; Groopman *et al.*, 1988). The major metabolic pathway of AFB_1 is shown in Fig. 3.2.

Early studies on the metabolism of AFB_1 were based on animal species whose metabolic pathways were subsequently found to be quite different from those of man and are therefore of limited help in understanding the relationship between its metabolism and toxicity in man. It was then found that the metabolic pathways in monkeys were similar to those of man and thus these have been used in later studies of aflatoxin metabolism. More recent research has used *in vitro* systems employing cultured tissue preparations especially those of the presumed target tissue, the liver, in the form of isolated hepatocyte cultures or subcellular fractions (Neal, 1987).

The individual metabolism of AFB_1 is largely dependent on the cytochrome P450 content, which is controlled by both endogenous and exogenous factors. Apart from inter-species and inter-strains differences, there is increasing evidence for polymorphism in the cytochrome P450 contents of human liver, in which the types of cytochrome present or their expression are genetically segregated in the general population (Clark, 1985; Jacqz, Hall & Branch, 1986; Horai & Ishizaki, 1988).

Apart from genetically pre-determined factors which affect the susceptibility of humans to aflatoxins, environmental and other exogenous factors can also exert their effects. Diet is known to affect the general cytochrome P450 levels in animals and presumably humans. The influence of specific dietary constituents, tobacco smoking, alcohol intake and other xenobiotics, including drugs, can potentially modify the intrinsic capacity to metabolize environmental pollutants, including the aflatoxins.

Hydroxylation of the AFB1 molecule can take place at various positions. Although described many years after the isolation of other metabolites of AFB1, the hydroxylation product at the cyclopentone ring (3-carbon), named AFQ1, has frequently been reported as the major metabolite in humans (Masri, Haddon, Lundin & Hsieh, 1974; Roebuck & Wogan, 1977; Moss & Neal, 1985), though this is contradicted in one study (Merrill & Campbell, 1974). AFQ1 was first identified in monkeys. The high metabolic production of this metabolite seems to be specific to

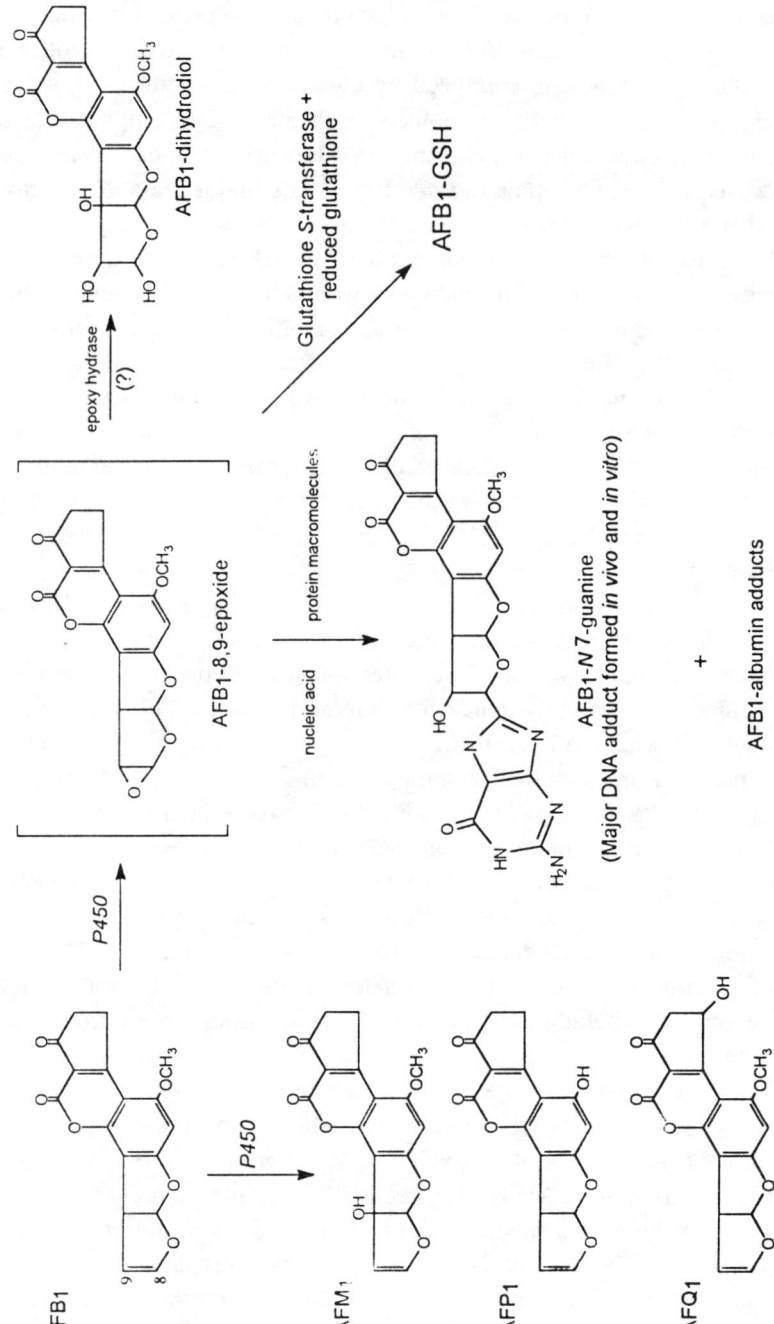

Figure 3.2 Primary metabolic pathways of AFB_1

primates as similar high metabolic production were also demonstrated in in vitro studies using hepatic microsomal fractions from rhesus and marmoset monkeys (Masri *et al.*, 1974; Makarananda, 1989). The percentage conversion to AFQ1 from AFB1 metabolism in human microsomal fractions was 60–90% (Moss & Neal, 1985). Ramsdell and Eaton suggested that the high conversion to AFQ_1 by primate microsomes divert a significant portion of the AFB1 dose away from more toxic intermediates (see below for epoxide formation), providing a protective effect (Ramsdell & Eaton, 1990b).

Early in the study of aflatoxin metabolism, it was found that a toxic metabolite was excreted into the milk when cows were fed rations known to contain aflatoxin. This was not a detoxification product because when the milk was fed to ducklings, the pathological changes induced in the liver were indistinguishable from those caused by aflatoxin itself (Allcroft & Carnaghan, 1966). This was referred to as the milk toxin and was later found to be the 10-hydroxylated metabolite of AFB_1, named AFM_1. AFM_1 has generally been regarded as a minor metabolite in human liver systems with some individual variation (Moss & Neal, 1985). It probably comprises 1–4% of consumed AFB_1 (Campbell, Caedo, Bulatao-Jayme, Salamat & Engel, 1970; Sun & Chu, 1984) but despite the low level of production, AFM_1 appears to be the only primary metabolite of AFB_1 to be excreted in an unconjugated form and may therefore be useful in assessing aflatoxin consumption (Denning, 1987).

AFP_1 is formed by oxidative demethylation of AFB_1, catalysed by mixed-function oxidase. Oxidative demethylation of AFB_1 has been shown in in vitro studies using liver tissue from goats, sheep, rats, mice, rabbits and golden hamsters but not from guinea pigs or dogs (Bassir & Emafo, 1970). Studies using liver slices and liver microsomes from these animal species demonstrated that oxidative demethylation was the major metabolic pathway, whereas 10-hydroxylation was the minor. In the rat, 88.8% of the metabolism of AFB_1 was via oxidative demethylation and only 1.7% via 10-hydroxylation (Bassir & Emafo, 1970). In human *in vitro* studies, results were more variable. AFP_1 was found to be a principal metabolite in some studies, but only a minor one, if present at all, in others (Merrill & Campbell, 1974; Roebuck & Wogan, 1977; Moss & Neal, 1985). Inter-individual sample variation within a single study was also high. Nevertheless, the conjugated forms of AFP_1, the glucuronide and sulphate, were frequently detected in the urine of animals treated with AFB1, especially in rhesus monkeys (Bassir & Emafo, 1970; Dalezios & Wogan, 1972).

AFB_{2a} (or 8-hydroxyaflatoxin B_1), a minor metabolite dependent on hepatic NADPH, was found to be a relatively non-toxic metabolite of AFB$_1$ in both animal and human studies, but a later study suggested that it might be a misidentification of another metabolite, .8,9-dihydro-8,9-dihydroxy-aflatoxin B$_1$, also known as the dihydrodiol (Patterson & Roberts, 1972; Neal, Judah, Stripe & Patterson, 1981). AFB$_1$ was also found to be metabolised by cytosol fractions to aflatoxicol, the formation of which was also NADPH-dependent. This reduction process was first reported by Patterson and Roberts and was also demonstrated in human *in vitro* studies (Patterson & Roberts, 1971; Salhab & Edwards, 1977). The process was found to be reversible with AFB$_1$ and AFM$_1$ as the metabolism products (Patterson & Roberts, 1972).

Probably the most important AFB$_1$ metabolism pathway involves the epoxidation at the 8,9 position. There is much evidence to indicate that AFB$_1$ requires metabolic activation to exert its biological and biochemical effects as a potent hepatocarcinogen and toxin (Campbell & Hayes, 1976). This epoxidation is considered an activation rather than detoxification process in the metabolism of AFB$_1$. During the course of AFB$_1$ metabolism, the reactive electrophilic epoxide can covalently react with various nucleophilic centres in cellular macromolecules including DNA, RNA and proteins. This poses a potential biological hazard to the cell or organism, and constitutes a putative mechanism by which AFB$_1$ and other xenobiotics exert toxic, carcinogenic and genotoxic effects.

Following the formation of the AFB$_1$-8,9-epoxide, the only detoxification pathway, other than possible macromolecular binding not involving a toxic response, is by conjugation with glutathione to form AFB$_1$-glutathione (AFB$_1$-GSH). A very minor pathway may involve the spontaneous or epoxide hydrolase-catalysed reaction of the epoxide with water, producing 8,9-dihydro-8,9-dihydroxy-AFB$_1$ (AFB$_1$ dihydrodiol). This reaction is probably not catalysed by epoxide hydrolase as induction of this enzyme in rats by pre-treatment with antioxidants did not result in corresponding decreased DNA-binding (Kensler, Egner, Trush, Bueding & Groopman, 1985). The dihydrodiol is not a predominant metabolite in laboratory animals and has not been detected in human urine (Gorelick, 1990). It has been suggested that the capacity of humans for to detoxify AFB1 by conjugation with glutathione is low, as very little AFB$_1$-GSH is produced (Moss & Neal, 1985). In AFB$_1$-treated marmoset monkeys in which a similar low level of AFB$_1$-GSH was found, the mercapturate conjugate of AFB$_1$ has been detected in the urine but this has not been the case in humans (Moss, Neal & Judah, 1985).

Using human microsomal systems *in vitro* and assaying for AFB_1-dihydrodiol, it was found that 10–20% of the soluble metabolites of AFB_1 were formed via epoxidation (Moss & Neal, 1985). The first AFB_1-DNA adduct was identified by Essigmann *et al.* as the 8,9-dihydro-8-(N^7-guanyl)-9-hydroxy AFB_1 (AFB_1-N^7-Gua), the major product liberated from DNA modified *in vitro* with AFB_1 and a rat liver microsomal activation system (Essigmann, Croy, Nadzan, Busby Jr, Reinhold, Buchi & Wogan, 1977). This has been subsequently confirmed *in vivo* (Croy, Essigmann, Reinhold & Wogan, 1978). The structure and properties of the AFB_1-DNA adduct were studied by *in vitro* formation by incubation of calf thymus DNA with activated AFB_1. Using UV spectra, proton NMR spectroscopy and mass spectroscopy, it was confirmed that the major AFB_1-DNA adduct was the N^7-guanine adduct (Wood, Smith & Garner, 1988; Shaulsky, Johnson, Shockcor, Taylor & Stark, 1990).

The most studied animal model for the formation of AFB_1-DNA adducts has been the rat, using DNA extracted from liver tissues of treated animals and subsequent detection by following radioactivity, immunological detection (ELISA and immunocytochemistry) and synchronous fluorescence spectrophotometry (Harris, Laveck, Groopman, Wilson & Mann, 1986; Nakatsuru, Qin, Masahito & Ishikawa, 1989; Wild, Montesano, Van Benthem, Scherer & Den Engelse, 1990c; Zhang, Chen, Haghighi, Yang, Hsieh, Wang & Santella, 1991). Other animals susceptible to AFB_1 have also been studied, including rainbow trout and coho salmon (Nakatsuru et al., 1989). Specific monoclonal antibodies have been produced (Hertzog, Smith & Garner, 1982). The formation of AFB_1-DNA adducts was shown to be a dose-dependent response (Appleton, Goetchius & Campbell, 1982; Wild, Garner, Montesano & Tursi, 1986; Buss, Caviezel & Lutz, 1990) over a dose range of $10–1000$ ng kg^{-1}. The responses were not found to be different between rats depleted of glutathione by diethyl maleate pre-treatment and control rats, indicating hepatic glutathione offered little protection against DNA-binding of AFB1 (Appleton et al., 1982); but in another study, DNA-binding was increased in rats pretreated 6 hours ahead (the time of maximal glutathione depletion) with a toxic dose of ethanol but not 18 hours (time with approximately normal glutathione levels) before AFB_1 administration (Wang, Wang, Shiah & Lin, 1990). DNA-binding of AFB_1 seemed also to be highly specific to liver tissues, where detection of the DNA adduct by immunocytochemical methods showed much more homogeneous binding than kidney tissues. In the same study, no adducts were detected in other organ tissues studied, including the oesophagus, forestomach, colon, spleen and testes (Wild *et al.*, 1990c).

DNA binding has been demonstrated in cultured human bronchus and colon tissues incubated with AFB_1 (Autrup, Essigmann, Croy, Trump, Wogan & Harris, 1979) and binding was shown to be dose-dependent. The AFB_1-N^7-guanine adduct could be detected in the urine of people who had dietary exposure to the carcinogen, including people from Kenya and China (Groopman, Donahue, Zhu, Chen & Wogan, 1985; Autrup, Seremet, Wakhisi & Wasunna, 1987), using affinity chromatography and high performance liquid chromatography. More recently, direct demonstration of AFB_1-DNA adducts formed *in vivo* in liver tissues were reported by many groups, either in patients known to have hepatocellular carcinoma or people accidentally poisoned by AFB1 (Hsieh, Hsu, Chen & Santella, 1988; Lee, Sarosi & Vyas, 1989; Harrison & Garner, 1991).

The binding of ^{3}H-AFB_1 to ribosomal RNA added to *in vitro* human liver microsomal incubations have also been reported and the *in vivo* binding to nucleic acid via AFB_1-epoxide was found to have a higher activity than binding to protein (Swenson, Miller & Miller, 1974; Swenson, Lin, Miller & Miller, 1977). Similar to DNA-binding, binding of AFB_1 to serum albumin has also been widely studied in both animals and human. It was shown that AFB_1 binds primarily to serum albumin and very little to other plasma proteins (Dirr & Schabort, 1986), in a dose-dependent manner (Wild *et al.*, 1986). The adducts were sufficiently stable to allow accumulation to steady-state levels upon chronic exposure. For many animal species, between 1–3% of a dose of AFB_1 was found to bind to plasma albumin. Based on the half-life of plasma albumin being around 20 days in human, AFB_1-albumin adducts was expected to be a useful tool in following AFB_1 exposure (Wild *et al.*, 1986; Groopman *et al.*, 1988).

The major serum albumin adduct of AFB_1 was isolated and characterised to be AFB_1-lysine by Sabbioni (Sabbioni, Skipper, Büchi & Tannenbaum, 1987), who later elucidated the structure, chemical and physical properties (Sabbioni, 1990). AFB_1-lysine was subsequently demonstrated in human serum from various African countries, Thailand (Wild, Jiang, Allen, Jansen, Hall & Montesano, 1990a) and the Guangxi Province of China (Sabbioni, Ambs, Wogan & Groopman, 1990). It was suggested to be an excellent dosimeter for exposure assessment as there were highly significant correlations between the adduct level following AFB_1 intake and urinary excretion of AFM_1 (Gan, Skipper, Peng, Groopman, Chen, Wogan & Tannenbaum, 1988).

A lysine adduct of AFG_1, an aflatoxin of lower biological potency than AFB_1, was also identified and was found to be formed at a level 3–6 fold lower than with equivalent doses of AFB_1 (Sabbioni & Wild, 1991). It was suggested that this AFG_1 adduct could be added as an internal standard for methods using the measurement of aflatoxin-albumin adducts to quantitate human exposure to aflatoxin.

The metabolic activation of AFB_1 to the active, DNA-binding 8,9-epoxide is now known to be mediated by cytochrome P450s. They are a large family of isoenzymes catalysing a diverse spectrum of reactions including endogenous substances and xenobiotics. Many different P450 isoenzymes have been purified from human liver, their corresponding cDNAs cloned and classified into families and subfamilies. For a detailed review, see that by Gonzalez (Gonzalez, 1989). Those P450 enzymes that catalyze the metabolic activation of AFB_1 to the reactive 8,9-epoxide have been identified primarily in livers from humans, rodents and fish. Even in a single tissue, multiple P450s have been shown capable of activating AFB_1. Before studies on specific cytochrome P450s, the activation of AFB_1 was investigated using microsomes or their partially purified fractions. A lot of these studies employed microsomes from animals pretreated with P450 inducers e.g. 3-methylcholanthrene (Neal, Judah & Green, 1986) or phenobarbitone (Metcalfe, Colley & Neal, 1981), in which only certain P450 activities were specifically, but not always selectively, amplified. The usefulness of these studies was limited by the fact that concurrent expression or induction of multiple metabolic activities might result and hence limit their usefulness for assigning aflatoxin activation to specific P450 isoenzymes. Although the available data seemed to indicate that phenobarbitone-induced microsomes mediated the highest rate of binding of DNA by AFB_1, the relative lack of selectivity for mediating DNA binding and the presence of multiple isoenzymes in these preparations prevented the identification of the most effective isoenzyme.

Studies with specific cytochrome P450s help provide more information on the relative importance of various cytochrome P450s in the bioactivation of AFB_1 but quantitative comparisons are still restricted to comparing the metabolism *between* different species and only qualitative comparisons can be made for individual pathways of AFB_1 metabolism. As a result, a quantitative assessment of the relative risk to people from the carcinogenic effect of AFB_1 based on estimates of its metabolism could not be made. An epidemiological study reported a possible association between the poor metaboliser phenotype for debrisoquine oxidation and resistance to the formation of hepatic tumours presumed to be caused by the ingestion of AFB_1 in the diet (Idle, Mahgoub, Sloan, Smith, Mbanefo & Bababunmi, 1981). One possible explanation for this observation was that the specific cytochrome P450 which was impaired in poor metabolisers of debrisoquine was also responsible for the metabolic activation of AFB_1 to a carcinogenic intermediate. This was refuted by Plummer *et al.* who concluded different isoenzymes of cytochrome P450 were responsible for the metabolic activation of AFB_1 and the 4-hydroxylation of debrisoquine in both the rat and in man. This was based on evidence that the addition of debrisoquine to incubation systems did not alter the rate of covalent binding of activated AFB_1 to microsomal proteins (Plummer, Boobis & Davies, 1986).

On the other hand, evidence was provided for nifedipine oxidase, now known as CYP3A4 in the nomenclature recommended by Nebert *et al* (Nebert, Nelson, Coon, Estabrook, Feyereisen, Fujii-Keriyama, Gonzalez, Guengerich, Gunsalus, Johnson, Loper, Sato, Waterman & Waxman, 1991), being the principal enzyme involved in the metabolic activation of aflatoxins in human liver (Shimada & Guengerich, 1989). Various P450 isoenzymes were purified from human liver samples. There were good correlations between levels of immunochemically determined CYP3A4 and rates of metabolic activation of AFB_1 which was also inhibited by polyclonal antibodies raised against this isoenzyme. The use of an assay for CYP3A4 activity as an indication of the relative extent of potential metabolic activation of AFB_1 in different species or individuals, is only valid if other isoenzymes of P450 do not significantly or variably contribute to the metabolic activation of AFB_1. As research in this area continued, it was found not to be the case. Not only was there evidence emerging for the involvement of multiple forms of cytochrome P450 in the metabolic activation of AFB_1 (Aoyama, Yamano, Guzelian, Gelboin & Gonzalez, 1990; Forrester, Neal, Judah, Glancey & Wolf, 1990), but also that CYP3A isoenzymes on the whole as a family, could only effectively catalyze the formation of AFB_1-8,9-epoxide from AFB_1 at relatively high substrate concentration (Ramsdell, Parkinson, Eddy & Eaton, 1991). Ramsell and Eaton concluded from their study that at tissue levels expected from dietary AFB_1 exposure, CYP3A enzymes, including CYP3A4, would not be expected to substantially contribute to the metabolic activation of AFB_1 to AFB_1-8,9-epoxide. Another isoenzyme(s) of cytochrome P450 appeared to be principally responsible at low AFB_1 levels (Ramsdell *et al.*, 1991). Although the study of Forrester *et al.*, using antibodies against specific cytochrome P450s to inhibit metabolic activation of AFB_1, provided data on the strong correlation with CYP3A expression, it was thought to be only because they represent the major cytochrome P450 forms in the human liver. The correlation between CYP3A3 and CYP3A4 expression and AFB_1 metabolism was due to the fact that they are present in high concentration and not because they are the only P450 with the capacity to metabolize this substrate. In addition, antibodies against CYP3A1, CYP2A1 and CYP1A2 also inhibited AFB_1-8,9-epoxide formation but there was significant variability in the effectiveness of these antibodies (Forrester *et al.*, 1990). These data seemed to support the involvement of multiple forms of P450 in the metabolic activation of AFB_1 in human liver. Although the CYP3A gene family plays an important role in the metabolic activation of AFB1, other species of cytochrome can also play a major role. Different levels of expression may account for the variability in the relative roles of different isoenzymes. Since the expression of these cytochromes are highly inducible by environmental and/or hormonal factors, these factors would play a part in determining the metabolism of AFB_1 in an individual. Involvement of genetic factors has yet to be established.

On a similar line but using a different study method, Aoyama reported contribution to the metabolic activation of AFB_1 by five isoenzymes of cytochrome P450: CYP1A2, CYP2A3, CYP2B7, CYP3A3 AND CYP3A4 (Aoyama *et al.*, 1990). Using human cell lines that stably expressed human cytochrome P450s, Crespi et al. were able to confirm the role of metabolic activation of AFB_1 by CYP3A4, CYP1A2 and CYP2A3 (Crespi, Penman, Steimel, Gelboin & Gonzalez, 1991).

Conjugation with glutathione has been regarded as a detoxification pathway of AFB_1 as AFB_1-GSH is non-reactive. The conjugation of AFB_1-8,9-epoxide with glutathione is catalyzed by glutathione S-transferases (GST). The GST comprise a large family of enzymes divided into 5 classes: alpha, mu, pi, theta and microsomal. Little is known about the identity of the GST which are responsible for the detoxification of activated AFB_1. At present, the study of the catalytic conjugation of AFB_1-8,9-epoxide with glutathione has mainly been done with GST isolated from rat and mouse, and studies of GST from other animal species in this area have been few. By modifying the diet, levels or activities of GST could be altered in experimental animals and it has been shown that feeding with ethoxyquin, an antioxidant, increased GST activity in rats and resulted in reduced in vivo binding of AFB_1 to DNA of liver and kidney (Mandel,

Manson, Judah, Simpson, Green, Forrester, Wolf & Neal, 1987). This was also accompanied by reduced hepatocarcinogenesis which was attributed to a reduction in DNA-adduct formation resulting from increased detoxifying metabolism. Other dietary antioxidants also shown to induce GST and mitigate the tumourigenic effect of AFB_1 include 2(3)-tert-butyl-hydroxyanisole (BHA), butylated hydroxytoluene (BHT) and oltipraz see (Gorelick, 1990). These all had similar effects on the metabolism of AFB_1 to ethoxyquin and induced the biliary excretion of the AFB_1-GSH conjugate.

Studies with cytosolic fractions from different species suggest that activities of cytosolic GST for AFB_1 conjugation are higher in species which are more resistant to the carcinogenic effects of AFB_1, such as the mouse and the hamster, compared to rats. GST *in vitro* activity towards AFB_1-8,9-epoxide has been associated with multiple isoenzymes from the alpha class including YaYa, YaYc and YcYc (Coles, Meyer, Ketterer, Stanton & Garner, 1985). Quinn *et al.* showed that purified GST from normal rat liver, rainbow trout liver and human liver had much less AFB_1-specific DNA protective activity than GST from mouse liver preparations (Quinn, Crane, Kocal, Best, Cameron, Rushmore, Farber & Hayes, 1990). It was also demonstrated that the resistance of mouse liver to AFB_1 could be explained by a single GST isoenzyme of the alpha class (YaYa) with a relatively high activity towards DNA-binding metabolites of AFB_1, but GST with such high DNA protective activity against AFB_1 was not evident in humans. The finding of GST of the alpha class having the highest AFB_1-8,9-epoxide conjugating activity was also confirmed by Ramsell and Eaton (Ramsdell & Eaton, 1990a). In another study, cytosolic glutathione transferase activity toward microsomally activated AFB_1 was studied. They found that human microsomes were only one-fourth as efficient in activating AFB_1 to the 8,9-epoxide as rat microsomes, which was still less than mouse microsomes. But mice are resistant to the carcinogenic effects of AFB_1 due to efficient conjugation of the epoxide with GSH. In contrast, humans appear to lack substantial capacity for GSH conjugation with AFB_1-8,9-epoxide and so human liver tissue may be relatively efficient at generating AFB_1-DNA adducts when exposed to dietary levels of AFB_1 (Moss & Neal, 1985; Ramsdell & Eaton, 1990b).

In contrast to the relatively large amount of information from *in vitro* studies of GSH activities in AFB_1-epoxide conjugation, *in vivo* studies are few. By studying breakdown products of AFB_1-GSH in body fluids e.g. urine, a useful method may be provided for the study of the relative formation of the GSH conjugate in different species or different subjects. However, few studies has been done in this area, especially, as we would expect, in humans. The mercapturate conjugate of AFB_1 has been detected in the urine of AFB_1-treated marmoset monkeys but this has not been the case in human systems (Moss *et al.*, 1985).

One study addressed the possible genetic pre-disposition of humans towards AFB_1 susceptibility. It was found that GST of the mu class was also active in AFB_1-GSH conjugation and the mu form is polymorphic in human liver, characterised by high or low rates of conjugation of trans-stilbene oxide or benzo[a]pyrene-4,5-oxide. The results of this study showed that human liver cytosols prepared from individuals with a high rate of glutathione conjugation inhibited AFB_1-DNA adduct formation in vitro, while those prepared from individuals with low GST mu activity did not inhibit adduct formation (Liu, Miller, Taylor, Nagorney, Lucier & Thompson, 1990).

Since GST activities are apparently inducible by exogenous factors, extrapolation of animal studies to man may not be substantiated as humans may be exposed to various environmental inducing or inhibitory factors that would affect the conjugation of AFB_1-epoxide by GST, analogous to the metabolic activation of AFB_1.

3.1.4   Human diseases possibly related to exposure to aflatoxins

3.1.4.1 Acute aflatoxicosis

Outbreaks of acute poisoning in specific communities have been rare. There are several well documented reports which provide evidence of acute aflatoxicosis in man. One of these came from an occurence in two Taiwanese farming villages (Ling, Wang, Wu, Tung, Lin, Lin & Lin, 1967). A total of 27 people became ill with 3 deaths and it was traced back to mouldy rice found to contain approximately 200 µg AFB_1/kg. As postmortem examinations could not be done, the histopathological changes were not known and thus AFB_1 could only be suspected of being causally related to the illness. A similar report came from Uganda in which mouldy cassava found to contain 1.7 mg aflatoxins/kg was involved in the acute death of a 15-year old boy (Serck-Hanssen, 1970). In 1981, 12 people from nearby area in Kenya died after eating maize which contained up to 12,000 ppb of AFB_1 (Ngindu, Johnson, Kenya, Ngira, Ocheng, Nandwa, Omondi, Jansen, Ngare, Kaviti, Gatei & Siongok, 1982). Liver tissue at necropsy was found to contain up to 89 ppb of AFB_1. In these reports, the affected individuals suffered from vomiting, abdominal pain, pulmonary oedema and fatty infiltration and necrosis of the liver.

A more extensive report came from western India in which a total of 397 patients were involved with 106 deaths, mainly due to massive gastrointestinal bleeding (Krishnamachari, Bhat, Nagarajan & Tilak, 1975). Males were affected twice as much as were females. Maize was found to be heavily contaminated with *Aspergillus flavus*. Analysis showed that the average consumption of aflatoxin could be up to 2–6 mg over a period of a month. Liver biopsies showed bile duct proliferation and giant cells.

3.1.4.2 Reye's syndrome

Reye's syndrome is an acute, often fatal disease affecting infants and young children. It is largely of unknown etiology which involves encephalopathy and fatty degeneration of the viscera. The disease often progresses from a mild prodromal viral illness to severe cerebral involvement with coma (Reye, Morgan & Baral, 1963). The aetiology is unknown but current postulates incriminate the interaction of a reaction to viral infection, environmental factors and a genetic predisposition. Salicylates, aflatoxin, insecticides, outdated tetracyclines, valproate, warfarin, etc, have all been implicated by epidemiological observations which have many imperfections (Mowat, 1987). Nevertheless, the association with Reyes's syndrome has led to the withdrawal of aspirin products for children in both the U.K. and the U.S.A.

The evidence for aflatoxins to be associated as one of the factors in the causation of Reye's syndrome is mainly circumstantial. There has been clusters of Reye's syndrome observed in northeast Thailand, predominantly in rural areas, and which were geographically and seasonally related to heavy contamination of food with aflatoxins (Olson, Bourgeois, Cotton, Harikal, Grossman & Smith, 1971; Shank, Bourgeois, Reschamras & Chandavimol, 1971). Incidentally Thailand is one the countries in the world where exposure to aflatoxins is very high. In some studies, presence of aflatoxins was demonstrated in autopsy specimens (Shank *et al.*, 1971).

3.1.4.3 Kwashiorkor

Kwashiorkor is a disease of young children in some developing countries where malnutrition is a problem. It affects mainly recently weaned children, typified by oedema, hypoalbuminaemia, skin and hair changes and an accompanying immune deficiency leading to susceptibility to infections. Patients often also have hepatomegaly and fatty changes in the liver. It was believed to be a result of protein deficiency in the presence of energy sufficiency in the diet but that is no longer widely supported (Jackson & Golden, 1987). Epidemiological evidence indicated that the geographical and seasonal variation in the incidence of kwashiorkor parallels aflatoxin contamination of foodstuffs (Hendrickse, 1984). The possible involvement of aflatoxins in the condition has also been indicated by the presence of aflatoxins in biospy or autopsy liver specimens from affected individuals (Coulter *et al.*, 1984; Hendrickse, 1984). Nevertheless, the relationship between aflatoxins and kwashiorkor is still unclear (Editorial, 1984).

3.1.4.4 Impaired immune function

In experimental animals, ingestion of aflatoxin has been found to exert modifications on the immune system, including depressed antibody formation, complement and phagocytosis, as well as cell-mediated immunity (Wyllie & Morehouse, 1977). These findings were probably related to the inhibitory effects of aflatoxins on protein synthesis. These findings bear rather significant implications on human health especially when considering the factors associated with the development of hepatocellular carcinoma. Infection with the hepatitis B virus (HBV) is highly associated with the development of hepatocellular carcinoma. An efficient cell-mediated immune system is required for the elimination of this virus. If the immune system is impaired due to aflatoxin ingestion, there would be an additive effect of aflatoxin in the aetiology of hepatocellular carcinoma in areas of high HBV prevalence since AFB₁ itself is also considered a factor in hepatocarcinogenesis. Prolonged persistence of the HBV may be enhanced due to the immunosuppression with the consequent development of cirrhosis, which could facilitate further carcinogenic changes.

Immunosuppression due to the presence of aflatoxins could influence the pattern of infection with other infectious diseases, including the human immunodeficiency virus (Hendrickse & Maxwell, 1988).

3.1.4.5 Hepatocellular carcinoma

The association of exposure to aflatoxins and the development of hepatocellular carcinoma (HCC) has been studied in many populations.

Evidence of aflatoxin cancer risk for humans has been issued by various institutions including the International Agency for Research on Cancer (IARC) and the World Health Organisation (WHO).

In 1976, the IARC suggested "a causal relationship" between liver cancer and aflatoxin intake (IARC, 1976) and WHO concluded in 1979 that "aflatoxin ingestion may increase the risk of liver cancer" (World Health Organization Task Group on Environmental Health Criteria for Mycotoxins, 1979). In 1987, another working group of the IARC, based on more recent information, produced the statement that there was "sufficient evidence that aflatoxin is a probable human carcinogen" (IARC, 1987). This conclusion would mean that "a positive relationship has been observed between exposure to the agent and cancer in studies in which chance, bias and confounding, could be ruled out with reasonable confidence". Most of the evidence implying the causative role of aflatoxins in HCC came from epidemiological studies, which established a positive association between the geographic distribution of areas/countries of high incidence of HCC and the level/prevalence of aflatoxin-contaminated foodstuffs. Evidence from such studies and studies on the monitoring of aflatoxin metabolites excretion are now available from Uganda (Alpert, Hutt, Wogan & Davidson, 1971), Swaziland (Peers, Gilman & Linsell, 1976; Peers, Bosch, Kaldor, Linsell & Pluijmen, 1987), Kenya (Peers & Linsell, 1973; Autrup et al., 1987), Mozambique (van Rensburg, Cook-Mozaffari, van Schalkwyk, van der Watt, Vincent & Purchase, 1985), Thailand (Shank & Wogan, 1972b; Shank & Wogan, 1972a; Wild et al., 1990a), the Philippines (Bulatao-Jayme, Almero, Castro, Jardeleza & Salamat, 1982) and China (Gan et al., 1988). Although information on the latent period is lacking such that definite proof of a principal aetiologic role for aflatoxins in HCC is not possible, there is strong circumstantial evidence.

There is, however, some lingering scepticism regarding the agreement to this certainty (Campbell, Chen, Liu, Li & Parpia, 1990). The reservations about the change of the strength of the evidence from "circumstantial" to "sufficient" by the IARC seemed to centre around the failure to take into account the contribution by persistent infection with hepatitis B virus. There seemed to be equally compelling epidemiological evidence for the involvement of chronic HBV infection in the aetiology of HCC and it is likely that the different factors act synergistically. The demonstration of the N^7-guanyl adduct of AFB_1 in urine and liver tissues of populations exposed to AFB_1 and patients with HCC add to the evidence that not only has exposure to AFB₁ taken place, but also that it has been metabolically activated and covalently bound to genetic material (Groopman *et al.*, 1985; Autrup *et al.*, 1987; Hsieh *et al.*, 1988; Lee *et al.*, 1989).

A detailed discussion on the aetiological factors for hepatocellular carcinoma including chronic HBV infection, dietary aflatoxins, cirrhosis, cigarette smoking and alcohol intake is given in Chapter 1 of this thesis.

3.1.5 *Biochemical and molecular epidemiology of aflatoxins*

Hepatocellular carcinoma is one of the leading causes of cancer mortality in Asia and Africa. In China, it is the third leading cause of cancer deaths in males and accounts for more than 120,000 deaths per year. The incidence is highest around the southeast coast, particularly the Shanghai, Guangxi, Fujian, Jiangsu and Guangdong provinces where the mortality rate of HCC can be up to 300 per 100,000/year for males (Yeh, Yu, Mo, Luo, Tong & Henderson, 1989). Similar high rates have been reported for some parts of western Africa. In contrast, the incidence of HCC in the U.S.A. is very low, around 2.6 cases per 100,000/year for males. Thus, the incidence of HCC around the world varies by at least 100–10,000 fold. The incidence of HCC is also high in Hong Kong. The rate for males in 1987 was about 30/100,000 per year.

Since many studies have provided data on the positive association between high intakes of aflatoxin and high incidence rates of HCC and that dosimetry data are also available, there is a strong motivation to investigate further the circumstantial relationship between aflatoxin ingestion and HCC incidence by monitoring aflatoxins and its metabolites in human body fluids (Garner, Ryder & Montesano, 1985). The application of these monitoring methods to field studies would generate further biochemical and molecular epidemiological data. The main goal of such field studies would be to identify individuals at high risk of HCC by obtaining evidence of high exposure to AFB₁. The latter may lead to pathobiological lesions in target cells and/or increased oncogenic susceptibility due to host factors.

Methods have been developed for the study of AFB₁, its metabolites (e.g. AFM₁) and adducts (protein and nucleic acid) in human body fluids and tissues, including chemical and immunological assays (Campbell *et al.*, 1970; Siraj, Hayes, Unger, Hogan, Ryan & Wray, 1981; Tsuboi, Nakagawa, Tomita, Seo, Ono, Kawamura & Iwamura, 1984; Groopman *et al.*, 1985; Autrup *et al.*, 1987; Wild *et al.*, 1987; Hsieh *et al.*, 1988; Wilkinson, Denning & Morgan, 1988; Lee *et al.*, 1989; Wild, Jiang, Sabbioni, Chapot & Montesano, 1990b; Harrison & Garner, 1991; Olubuyide, Makarananda, Judah & Neal, 1991). These methods could be applied to populations with possible exposure to AFB_1 and patients with HCC with regard to possible previous AFB1 exposure.

In China, there is geographical variation in the incidence of HCC. The provinces along the southeast coast have the highest clustering of cases. In Fusui County in southern Guangxi, the HCC rate among men is 120/ 100,000 per year and role of the dietary AFB_1 has been studied in this endemic area. Urinary excretion of AFM_1 from local inhabitants was found to be significantly elevated compared to other areas in the country with lower HCC rates. There was an almost perfect linear relationship between the estimated AFB_1 in the diet of each subpopulation and the respective HCC rates. Furthermore, the level of serum albumin adducts correlated highly with urinary excretion of AFM_1, as well as the estimated AFB_1 intake (Gan *et al.*, 1988; Yeh *et al.*, 1989). Yeh *et al.* did not find any significant association between the prevalence of hepatitis B surface antigen (HBsAg) positivity in the subpopulations and the corresponding HCC mortality rates. It was estimated that about 10% of adults living in the endemic areas had an intake of more than 1mg of AFB_1 per year. The primary source of contamination was corn and rice; the second was the local undistilled alcoholic beverage produced from these grains. Since men generally consumed more food and alcohol than women, it seemed that the higher prevalence of HCC among males and in the age group between 40–50 could partly be attributed to exposure to AFB_1 and could not be explained by viral aetiology alone. In addition, AFB_1-N^7-Gua, the major AFB_1-nucleic acid adduct was identified in the urine samples of people from the Guangxi province (Groopman *et al.*, 1985).

An epidemiological study conducted in Swaziland, a country where HCC is one of the commonest malignancies, was published by Peers *et al.* in 1987 (Peers *et al.*, 1987). Data were collected to assess the relationship between aflatoxin exposure, HBV infection and the incidence of HCC. Across 4 broad geographic regions, there was a more than 5-fold variation in the estimated daily intake of aflatoxins but the proportion of HBsAg carriers varied very little. It was found that the HCC incidence varied by 5-fold and was strongly associated with the estimated level of aflatoxin intake. In an analysis involving 10 smaller subregions, aflatoxin exposure emerged as a more important determinant of the variation in HCC incidence than the prevalence of HBV infection.

The problem of food stuff contamination by aflatoxins in relation to HCC was also addressed in Kenya. A population based study was carried out by Peers and Linsell (Peers & Linsell, 1973). Food samples collected in Murang'a District were demonstrated to be contaminated with aflatoxins and there was a statistically significant association between aflatoxin ingestion levels and the number of liver cancer cases, but the authors did recognise certain limitations in the study e.g. data obtained from cancer registries might not be complete. Nevertheless, AFB_1-N ^{7}-Gua has also been detected in human urine collected in this region of high cancer risk (Autrup *et al.*, 1987). The seasonal variation in aflatoxin exposure was most probably due to extended storage of foodstuffs under improper conditions favouring the growth of *A. flavus*. Continuing biochemical epidemiological investigation showed a corresponding seasonal variation in the urinary excretion of AFB_1-N ^{7}-Gua adducts. More recently, antibody activity against an aflatoxin epitope has been detected in serum from inhabitants in Kenya who had experienced high exposure to AFB_1, though the biological consequences of these antibodies remain known (Autrup, Seremet & Wakhisi, 1990).

The importance of the presence of AFB_1-DNA adducts in human tissues and body fluids is that they are an indication that not only was exposure to AFB_1 demonstrated, but also its metabolic activation and interaction between the ultimate carcinogenic form of AFB_1 and genetic material *in vivo*.

Since AFB_1 is a procarcinogen which requires metabolic activation before exerting its biological potency in attacking cellular macromolecules, including protein and genetic material, the inter-individual variation in this specific enzymic activity would have an influence on the susceptibility to AFB_1. Similarly, conjugation of AFB_1-8,9-epoxide with glutathione is a detoxification pathway and inter-individual variation in the activity of this metabolism may also be a determinant in AFB_1 susceptibility. It would be of considerable interest to compare the rates of metabolic activation of AFB_1 in individuals with normal livers with those in patients with chronic HBV infection, which has a close association with the development of HCC, and also with patients with HCC. These studies may help provide information on possible synergism between HBV and AFB_1 in HCC (Ayoola, 1984).

3.2 Development of an ELISA method to monitor AFB$_1$ exposure in human serum

3.2.1 Introduction

Various methods of aflatoxin exposure assessment have been used. In a number of AFB$_1$ exposure-HCC incidence correlation studies, the methods used for the estimation of exposure were based on those for the monitoring of food sample contamination (Peers & Linsell, 1973; Peers *et al.*, 1987; Yeh *et al.*, 1989). Common methods used to analyse samples for the presence of aflatoxins include TLC or HPLC of extracted samples. Although the methodology for measuring aflatoxin levels in food by TLC and HPLC is well established, it can be time consuming, costly and requires technical skill. Thus, these methods have not been widely applied to the measurement of aflatoxin metabolites in the human body. In addition, these data provide no information on the biologically effective dose of aflatoxin at the individual level i.e. the amount of the activated agent that has actually reacted with critical cellular targets, such as DNA, protein or RNA, which may be influenced by intake, distribution, metabolic (in)activation and excretion of aflatoxin.

One of the desirable features of a laboratory assay for aflatoxin exposure would be that of providing a long-term exposure assessment in a sample obtained non-invasively. With the development of more sensitive assays using immunological methods, it has been possible to measure aflatoxin metabolites and nucleic acid adducts in human urine, serum and milk (Sizaret, Malaveille, Montesano & Frayssinet, 1982; Groopman *et al.*, 1985; Wild *et al.*, 1987; Gan *et al.*, 1988). However, rapid excretion means that their measurements reflect only exposure over a very short period of time prior to the measurement. Therefore, it is necessary to look for a more stable marker of exposure.

It has been demonstrated that AFB$_1$ binds to peripheral plasma albumin in a dose related manner and the accumulated binding level after repeated exposure parallels the binding to liver DNA (Dirr & Schabort, 1986; Sabbioni, *et al.*, 1987; Wild *et al.*, 1986). A good correlation was also seen between AFB1 intake, calculated from food analysis, and AFB$_1$-albumin addduct levels (Gan *et al.*, 1988). The major aflatoxin-albumin adduct was characterised to be an AFB$_1$-lysine residue (Sabbioni, 1990). As the half-life of albumin in human is about 20 days, aflatoxin-albumin seems to be a promising long term marker of aflatoxin exposure which took place during the prior weeks (Groopman *et al.*, 1985; Wild *et al.*, 1990b).

Since 1980, the development of immunoassays for the detection of AFB$_1$ and its metabolites have been promising with various antibodies being successfully raised against the different immunogens. Polyclonal antibodies appear to be particularly suitable for the measurement of exposure since various aflatoxin-derived materials can be assayed, giving a more representative picture of the exposure. On the other hand, a range of monoclonal antibodies might be advantageous in determining at an individual level the pattern of aflatoxin metabolites present.

Both radioimmunoassay (RIA) and enzyme-linked immunosorbent assays (ELISA) have been used to assay aflatoxins in biological samples. Despite the high specificity of antibodies and the sensitivity afforded by radiolabelled tracers permitting the use of RIA to measure very low levels of aflatoxins, this technique has several drawbacks. It requires radiolabelled substrates, access to scintillation counters and skilled personnel. The short half life of the isotopes used limits the shelf life of the reagents. The need for γ-emitting isotopes also subjects the operators of RIA to radiation hazards. In comparison, ELISA requires no radioactivity, expensive analytical equipment or highly trained technical personnel. It is just as sensitive, if not more sensitive, than RIA. It is generally agreed that the development of ELISA methods should be concentrated on for routine monitoring work.

The principles of ELISA depends on the reaction between an antigenic compound and an antibody with specificity against a particular part of the antigenic molecule. In the double sandwich technique, a secondary antibody is then added which has specificity against the primary antibody. This secondary antibody is conjugated with an enzyme. Upon the addition of a chromogenic substrate for the enzyme, the colour produced will be used for the quantification of the original antigen. When this technique is used, the intensity of the colour produced will be proportional to the original amount of antigen present and this is termed 'non-competitive'. In 'competitive ELISA', the intensity of the colour produced is inversely proportional to the original amount of antigen present. This involves a pre-incubation step of the sample under study with a fixed amount of the primary antibody and the ligand is immobilised on ELISA plates.

The sensitivity of ELISA is partly attributed to the ability of a molecule of the conjugated enzyme catalysing the reaction of many substrate molecules, thus amplifying the reaction signal. This technique of double sandwich competitive ELISA is used in this study.

Aflatoxin B_1 after transformation by the mixed function oxidase cytochrome P450s, forms the reactive 8,9-oxide. This was found to be the reactive species that binds to serum albumin. The chemistry of the adduct and its formation was elucidated by Sabbioni *et al* (Sabbioni, 1990). The adduct is formed by the binding of AFB_1-8,9-epoxide, forming initially the dihydrodiol with sequential oxidation to the dialdehyde and condensation with the ε-amino group of lysine. The structure of this adduct is shown in Fig. 3.3. Though the aflatoxin structure of this adduct is highly modified, what remain are the coumarin and cyclopentenone rings which are still recognised by the antibody raised. An analysis of human serum samples obtained from an exposed population revealed a highly significant correlation coefficient between aflatoxin-lysine adduct levels and AFB_1 consumption (Gan *et al.*, 1988). Therefore, estimation of aflatoxin-albumin adducts is a good dosimeter for exposure over the previous few weeks. It was estimated that 1–3% of ingested AFB_1 becomes covalently bound to serum albumin. This value was very similar to that observed when rats were administered AFB1 (Wild *et al.*, 1986).

It has been found that the detection of the intact AFB_1-albumin by

Figure 3.3   Structure of AFB_1-lysine

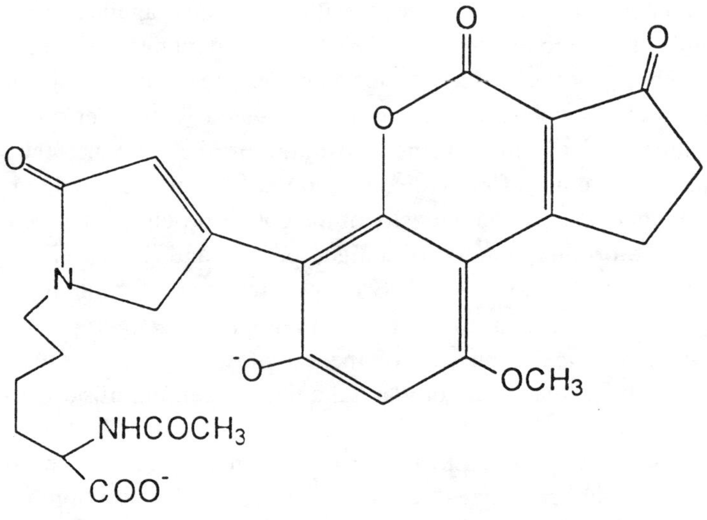

ELISA was not very sensitive. The recognition of isolated AFB_1-lysine residues is about 30 fold greater (Wild *et al.*, 1990b). A more sensitive assay for the detection of AFB_1 albumin adducts would be to subject the modified albumin to hydrolysis to release AFB_1-lysine residues employing a suitable hydrolytic enzyme. Although AFB_1-lysine is probably not the only aflatoxin molecule present after hydrolysis (e.g. AFB_1-peptides may occur), it has been observed that a dilution curve of a digested rat albumin sample in ELISA had a very similar slope to AFB_1-lysine itself, suggesting similar antigenicity of all residues after hydrolysis (Wild *et al.*, 1990b).

This approach is in contrast to the measurement of AFB_1-lysine adducts following enzyme digestion of serum albumin by HPLC and fluorescence detection. By HPLC and fluorescence detection, only one precise species of AFB_1-lysine can be measured at a particular retention time and not other hydrolysis products. Thus it is expected that ELISA apparently detects higher levels of adducts when compared to fluorescence and that some positive samples by ELISA may be determined as negative by fluorescence. It is possible to combine the two methods. Initially, samples will be screened by ELISA after hydrolysis of albumin. HPLC fluorescence detection can then be used to confirm the presense of AFB_1-lysine.

To avoid non-specific inhibition in ELISA, digested albumin samples must be subjected to clean-up procedures. These may include Sep-pak C_{18} cartridge and specific immunoaffinity column purifications.

The objective of this study is to develop a protocol to study the presence of AFB_1-lysine adduct in human serum sample using ELISA on digested serum albumin with clean-up steps, as an index to both AFB_1 exposure and its *in vivo* metabolic activation. The antibody eventually used was a monoclonal one but preliminary studies with a polyclonal antibody raised in rabbits was also used (see discussion section 3.2.5.13). Both of them were able to recognise a range of aflatoxins, metabolites and adducts, giving a representative estimation of exposure. It was also hoped that the level of aflatoxin exposure could be correlated to other parameters of the human subjects e.g. the hepatitis B virus status, alcohol and cigarette consumptions, etc.

3.2.2 *Preparation of all the components necessary for analysing AFB₁-albumin adducts by ELISA*

3.2.2.1 Materials

AFB_1 was purchased from Sigma Chemical Company (St. Louis, USA).

^{3}H-AFB$_1$ was purchased from Morevak Biochemicals (Brea, California, USA). AFB$_1$-lysine was kindly supplied by Dr. G.E. Neal, Toxicology Unit, Medical Research Council, Carshalton, Surrey, England.

Bovine serum albumin (BSA), Tween 20, 3,3',5,5'-tetramethylbenzidine (TMB), trichloroacetic acid, proteinase K (Protease Type XXVIII) and gelatin were obtained from Sigma Chemical Company (St. Louis, USA). PBS (phosphate buffered saline) tablets were purchased from Oxoid Ltd (Basingstoke, Hants, U.K.) and dimethyl sulphoxide (DMSO) of 'Spectrosol' grade was from BDH Chemicals Ltd. (Poole, Dorset, U.K.). All other chemicals and organic solvents used in all experiments were of analytical or HPLC grade.

3.2.2.2 Preparation of rabbit AFB1 antiserum

Sandy half-lop female rabbits were immunised with AFB$_1$ conjugate by injecting 500 g protein of immunogen (prepared from AFB$_1$ bound to quail liver microsomal protein by metabolic activation (Makarananda, 1989)) mixed 50/50 (v/v) with Freund's complete adjuvant intramuscularly into the front and hind limbs of each animal. Subsequent injections were given four weeks apart on 3 occasions, each of 500 μg protein of immunogen mixed with an equal volume of Freund's incomplete adjuvant. Each animal was bled via an ear vein to obtain 30 ml blood samples ten days after the last injection.

After collection, the blood was allowed to clot for 2 hours at room temperature. The clot was loosened from the sides of the collection vessel using a Pasteur pipette and placed at 4°C overnight to allow it to contract. The serum was then removed from the clot and the insoluble material was removed further by centrifugation at 10,000 xg for 10 minutes at 4°C.

The antibody titre of the antiserum obtained was evaluated using the competitive ELISA binding assay (section 3.2.3.1). Every six months, each animal was given a booster dose of 500 μg protein of immunogen mixed with an equal volume of Freund's incomplete adjuvant. Each batch of antiserum collected was tested for its antibody titre.

3.2.2.3 Preparation of the rat monoclonal antibody

Three rats were immunised with AFB$_1$ conjugate by injecting 100 g protein of immunogen (prepared from AFB$_1$ bound to quail liver microsomal protein by metabolic activation (Makarananda, 1989)) mixed 50/50 (v/v) with Freund's complete adjuvant subcutaneously. Subsequent injections were given 2 weeks apart on 2 occasions, each of 100 μg protein of immunogen mixed with an equal volume of Freund's incomplete adjuvant. After each immunisation, blood was drawn to assay for antibody titre by ELISA. After 8 weeks, the animal which consistently showed the highest titre was given an intravenous booster dose and the spleen was removed 3 days later for fusion with a myeloma cell line, Y_3-Ag 1.2.3, a myeloma tumour cell line from the Lou strain of rat. This myeloma cell line secretes κ light chain immunoglobulin and has been used successfully in the derivation of rat x rat hybrid myelomas (Galfrè, Milstein & Wright, 1979). Before fusion, the myeloma cells were grown continuously in a spinner flask and about 5×10^7 cells were used in fusion.

The spleen from the selected immunised rat was removed rapidly and asecptically, and rinsed in serum free medium. It was gently teased to free cells which were transferred to a tube and spun at about 2,000 xg for 5 minutes. The supernatant was removed and the pellet of cells resuspended in serum free medium and spun again. After this wash, the cells were resuspended in 10 ml of serum free medium and mixed with the myeloma cells which were also suspended in 10 ml of the same medium. The ratio of myeloma cells to spleen cells should be about 1:5. The mixture of cells was spun to remove the medium and with a pasteur pipette, 50% polyethylene glycol (1 ml/10^8 cells) was added drop by drop over 1 minute with contant stirring with the pipette. It was then incubated for 30 seconds at 37°C. The cell suspension was diluted 1:1 with prewarmed serum free medium every minute to a final volume of 20 ml.

These cells were then spun to remove the supernatant and resuspended in HAT (Hypoxanthine Aminopterin Thymidine) medium to give a concentration of 5×10^5 to 10^6 cells/ml. Two 24-well culture plates were half-filled with this cell suspension, topped up with HAT medium and incubated. The HAT medium was used to select out successful hybridomas. Aminopterin inhibits the *de novo* synthesis of purines by impairing tetrahydrofolate metabolism. In normal cells a second scavenging pathway of purine synthesis, using the enzyme hypoxanthine guanine phosphoribosyl transferase (HGPRT) is present. Hybridoma cells derived from splenocytes can thus still grow in the presence of aminopterin when the scavenging pathway is boosted by exogenous additions of hypoxanthine and thymidine. However, the myeloma cells used are deficient in the enzyme HGPRT, and they eventually die in the presence of HAT medium. Fused cells, or successful hybridomas were picked out and cultured in separate dishes. The procedures in the production of monoclonal antibody is outlined in Fig. 3.4. Cell culture supernatant of successful hybridoma was concentrated by ammonium sulphate precipitation and the antibody titre tested by ELISA.

3.2.2.4 Concentration of cell culture supernatant by ammonium sulphate precipitation

The hybridoma cell culture supernatant from section 3.2.2.3 was

Figure 3.4   Schematic Presentation of the Procedures in the Production of a Monoclonal Antibody

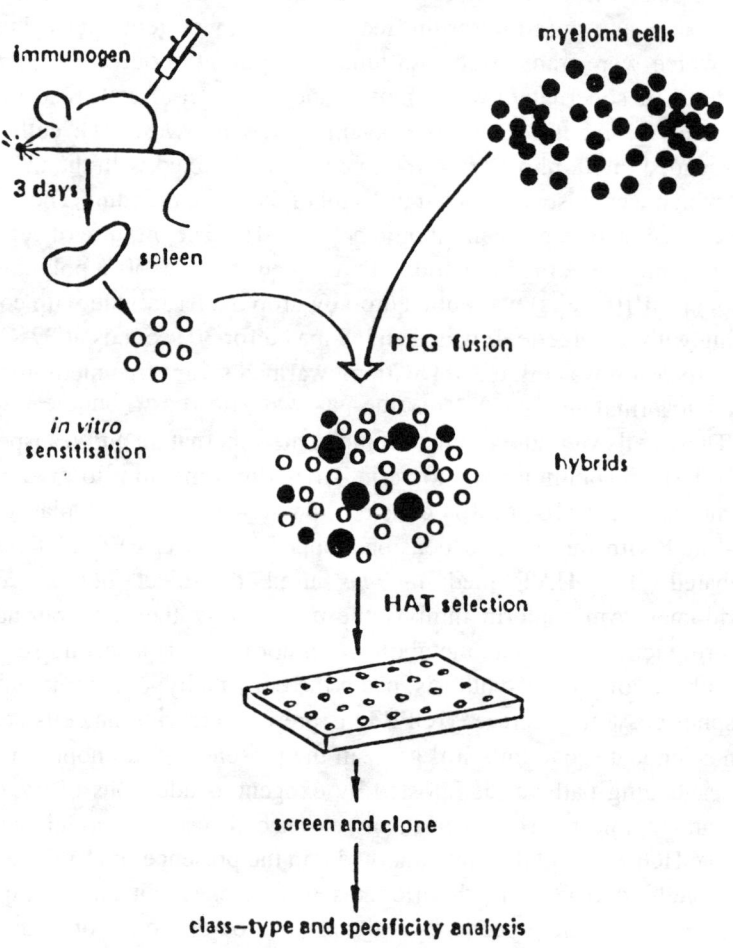

centrifuged for 30 minutes at 3,000 xg to remove debris. It was then transferred to a large beaker with a stirring bar over a magnetic stirrer. A same volume of saturated ammonium sulphate solution (761 g/L, pH 4.1M, corrected to neutral with HCl) was added slowly to avoid high local concentration. The solution was then 50% saturated with ammonium sulphate. It was kept at 4°–6°C overnight before being centrifuged at 3,000 xg for 30 minutes and the supernatant was discarded. The pellet was resuspended in the miniumum volume of PBS, usually about 0.1 volume of the starting volume, taking care to avoid frothing and bubbles. The concentrated antibody solution was transferred to a dialysis tubing and dialysed versus 3 changes of PBS over 1 day. Enough space in the dialysis tubing must be allowed for volume expansion during dialysis. The protein concentration of the final monoclonal antibody solution was determined according to the method of Lowry (Lowry, Rosenbrough, Farr & Randall, 1951) and stored in aliquots at –70°C.

3.2.2.5 Preparation of the BSA-AFB₁ conjugate

Bovine serum albumin modified by AFB₁ (BSA-AFB₁) for use as coating antigen in the ELISA binding assay was prepared according to the method of Sizaret *et al.* with further modifications (Sizaret *et al.*, 1982).

6.5 mg of AFB₁ was dissolved in 3 ml dichloromethane which had been dried overnight by molecular sieve beads type 3A (BDH Chemical Ltd., Poole, Dorset, U.K.). Chlorine gas was allowed to bubble into the AFB₁ solution in a stoppered glass tube with a side arm until a yellow colour appeared, signifying saturation of the gas. Without delay, 9.3 mg BSA in 4.5 ml 0.01M sodium phosphate buffer (pH 7.4) was added followed by 0.5 ml DMSO dropwise with magnetic stirring. The mixture was kept at 37°C with shaking for 30 minutes. The insoluble material was then removed by centrifugation at 3,500 xg for 15 minutes.

The conjugate was precipitated by the sequential addition, with magnetic stirring, of 43 mg NaCl, 6 ml ethyl acetate and 12 ml acetone. This mixture was kept on ice for 15 minutes before centrifuging again for 15 minutes at 3,500 xg. The precipitate was washed once with 22 ml ethanol, same volume of 1:1 ether and ethanol and finally same volume of ether. After each wash, the precipitate was re-dispersed and re-centrifuged. After the ether wash, the precipitate was swirled round the tube before drying overnight in a desiccator. This was to prevent it drying into a tightly-packed pellet.

After drying, the conjugate was dissolved in 10 ml PBS with the aid of sonication. The volume may have needed to be adjusted if dissolution was difficult. The BSA-AFB1 solution was stored in aliquots at −70°C.

The protein content of the conjugate was determined according to the method of Lowry *et al.* (Lowry *et al.*, 1951) using bovine serum albumin as the standard and the absorbance read by an LKB Ultrospec II with an LKB Autofill II (Pharmacia). The UV absorbance of the conjugate was scanned from 200nm–405nm (UVIKON 860, Kontron Instruments, Watford, Herts., U.K.). The ratio of the number of molecules of AFB_1 to BSA was then calculated.

3.2.2.6 Preparation of the immunoaffinity gel

The immunoaffinity gel was prepared as recommended by the literature accompanying the purchase of CNBr-activated Sepharose 4B gel from Pharmacia. Basically, the biospecific ligand, the antibody, is covalently attached to a chromatographic bed material, the matrix. The immobilised ligand should retain the specific binding affinity for the substance of interest, which can then be selectively desorbed by altering the eluting solvent.

The required amount of freeze-dried powder of CNBr-activated Sepharose 4B gel, 6 g, (Pharmacia, Milton Keynes, Herts., U.K.) was swollen in 1mM HCl for 15 minutes. One gram of freeze-dried material gave about 3.5 ml of final gel volume. The swollen gel was then washed and reswollen using the same solution on a sintered glass filter of porosity G3. About 200 ml was used per gram of dry powder in several aliquots and the supernatant was sucked off between successive additions. The use of an acidic solution preserves the activity of the reactive groups which hydrolyse at high pH.

The gel was then washed with the coupling buffer (0.1M NaHCO3 buffer, pH 8.3, containing 0.5M NaCl) using 5 ml per gram dry gel. It was then immediately transferred to a solution of 6 ml rabbit anti-AFB1 serum diluted to 18 ml with the coupling buffer or an appropriate amount of the monoclonal antibody. The coupling reaction was allowed to proceed at room temperature for 2 hours in an end-over-end rotor. The coupling reaction was then effectively completed. After coupling, residual active groups remaining on the gel were hydrolysed by standing the gel in a blocking buffer (Tris-HCl buffer, pH 8 with 0.2M glycine) for 2 hours.

After the blocking step, the gel was washed alternately with buffers of high and low pH to remove excess uncoupled ligand. 0.1M acetate buffer, pH 4 and the coupling buffer, each containing 0.5M NaCl were used, four or five cycles each. The gel was finally suspended in PBS containing 0.02% sodium azide as preservative and stored at 4°C until use.

The same procedure was followed for affinity gel coupled with the rat monoclonal antibody with 10 mg of protein for each ml of swollen gel.

3.2.2.7 Preparation of the ELISA plates

Immulon I flat bottom plates (Dynatech Laboratories Inc., Virginia, USA) were coated with 10 ng of BSA-AFB$_1$ (prepared in section 3.2.2.5) in 50 μl of PBS in each well. The outer rows of the 96 well plates were not used as they gave rise to variable results.

The plates, lightly covered with foil, were allowed to dry at 37°C overnight or longer. When they are completely dried, the plates were stored at –20°C for extended period of time without apparent loss of binding capacity. When the plates were required, they were removed from cold storage and washed with 0.05% Tween 20 in PBS (PBS-Tween 20) (8 successive wash/suck cycles using an Immunowash [NUNC, Denmark]).

Non-specific binding sites were blocked by adding 100 μl of 0.25% gelatin in PBS (PBS-gelatin) and left at room temperature for 60 minutes. The plates were then washed again with PBS-Tween 20 before use (4 successive washes).

3.2.3 General procedures used in the analysis of AFB$_1$-albumin adducts

All glass tubes used in competitive ELISA binding assays were washed with 6M HCl after normal glassware cleaning, followed by 4 rinses each of tap water and distilled water. The overall protocol of analysis was as follows:

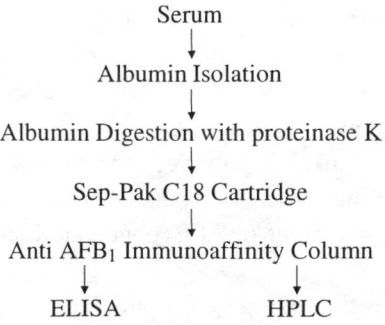

Serum
↓
Albumin Isolation
↓
Albumin Digestion with proteinase K
↓
Sep-Pak C18 Cartridge
↓
Anti AFB₁ Immunoaffinity Column
↓   ↓
ELISA   HPLC

3.2.3.1 Competitive ELISA binding assay

An aliquot of the test solution (200 µl) was incubated with the same volume of diluted rabbit anti-AFB$_1$ serum (1:2,500 with PBS-gelatin) or monoclonal antibody (1:5,000) on a shaking plate at 37°C for 60 minutes. The glass tubes should be covered to avoid evaporation. At the end of the incubation period, the contents of the glass tubes were mixed. 50 µl of each incubation mixture was dispensed into replicate of 6 wells on prepared ELISA plates which were then sealed with plate sealing tapes (Titertek, Flow Laboratories, Herts, U.K.) to prevent evaporation. They were placed on a Vari-Shaker (Dynatech Laboratories Ltd., Sussex, U.K.) with continuous shaking for 90 minutes at room temperature. After 90 minutes, the contents of the wells were discarded into a waste bucket containing bleach solution to destroy any toxin. The plates were washed using an Immunowash (NUNC, Denmark) for 10 successive wash/suck cycles.

The secondary antibody, anti-rabbit IgG-peroxidase conjugate, for the rabbit polyclonal antibody, or anti-rat IgG-perioxidase conjugate, for the monoclonal antibody (Sigma Chemical Company, St. Louis, USA) was diluted 1:5,000 with PBS-gelatin. 50 µl was added to each well and the plates were sealed again. They were incubated at room temperature for 90 minutes with continuous shaking. The plates were washed again with 10 successive wash/suck cycles, followed by 2 washes with distilled water. The substrate was prepared by warming 24.75 ml of 0.1M sodium acetate buffer, pH 6.0, to approximately 40°C for 30 minutes, then adding 250 µl of 3,3',5,5'-tetramethylbenzidine solution (10 mg in 1 ml DMSO) and warming for another 30 minutes. Just before use, 10 µl of 100 volume hydrogen peroxide was added. 50 µl of the substrate solution was dispensed into each well and the plates were left for 30 minutes at room temperature. At the end of the reaction time, 50 µl of 2M H_2SO_4 was added into each well to stop the reaction. After 15 minutes, the absorbance at 450 nm was read using a microtitre plate reader (Titertek Multiscan MCC, Flow Laboratories, Rickmansworth, Herts., U.K.).

The percentage inhibition of the sample was calculated as compared to the absorbance of a blank solution (zero inhibition). The value of AFB$_1$ equivalent present in the sample was calculated from a standard inhibition curve constructed from a range of AFB$_1$ concentrations ranging from 0.001 ng/ml to 100 ng/ml,

Each sample was diluted many fold to obtain a reading which would fall within the range of proportionality. Included in each plate were standards at 3 points of the range of proportionality and a blank. These standards helped to negate variations between the plates.

3.2.3.2 Sep-pak C₁₈ cartridge

Sep-pak C_{18} cartridges (Millipore UK, Middlesex, U.K.) were activated with 10 ml of methanol, followed by 10 ml of distilled water to dilute the concentration of methanol. The sample (usually 1 ml) was loaded onto the cartridge which was then washed with 5 ml of distilled water. The retained material was then eluted with 5 ml of methanol.

The cartridge could be reused by reactivating with 10 ml methanol and 10 ml distilled water. It could be reused up to 4 times.

3.2.3.3 Immunoaffinity column

Disposable polystyrene columns (Pierce & Warriner (U.K.) Ltd., Chester, U.K.) of 2 ml size were filled with 1 ml bed volume of immunoaffinity gel as prepared in section 3.2.2.6. The gel was washed with 20 ml of PBS to remove sodium azide which was present as a preservative.

The sample (usually 1 ml) was loaded onto the column and washed with 5 ml PBS. The retained material was then eluted with 5 ml 85% methanol in PBS. The column was washed again with 20 ml PBS before reusing once more.

3.2.3.4 Evaporation process

In most of the procedures mentioned in the above sections, the study sample was contained in a volume of about 5 ml. This needed to be concentrated in order to be presented for the next step. In other cases, the organic solvents required to be removed to prevent interference in the other analytic steps. The evaporation process was carried out in a vacuum concentrator (HS-1-110, Heto Lab Equipment, Denmark) at 40°C.

When evaporating samples in 100% methanol, 0.5 ml PBS was added to each tube to prevent rapid evaporation to dryness and thus avoid variable recoveries.

3.2.3.5 HPLC

Samples for HPLC were introduced into the system via a Rheodyne 7120 injection valve (Berkeley, California, USA). The system consisted of two chromatographic pumps Model 6000 and a solvent programmer Model

660 (Waters Associate, Millipore UK, Middlesex, U.K.). The column used was a Chromsphere C_{18} 8μm (Chrompack UK, Ltd.). The column was eluted with a linear 15–40% methanol in water gradient containing 0.02% phosphoric acid and 8% acetonitrile at a flow rate of 1 ml min^{-1}. The gradient elution took 6 minutes followed by maintenance of 40% methanol for 3 minutes. The gradient was then reversed to 15% methanol in 1 minute. The system was kept at 15% methanol to equilibrate for 3 minutes before the next injection.

Fluorescence was monitored by a fluorescence detector Model 420 (Waters Associates, Millipore UK, Middlesex, U.K.) with excitation at 365nm and emission at 425nm.

1 ml (1 minute) fractions were collected from the HPLC using an LKB 2112 Redirac Fraction Collector (Bromma, Sweden) in 5 ml plastic scintillation minivials. 13 fractions were collected for each sample.

3.2.3.6 Radioactive counting

Samples were counted in 5 ml plastic scintillation minivials. 4 ml of scintillant (Monofluor, National Diagnostic, Aylesbury, Bucks., U.K.) was added to each vial and counted in a Wallac 1410 liquid scintillation counter (Pharmacia Diagnostic). Counting time was 10 minutes for each sample. All samples were counted in duplicate.

3.2.3.7 Albumin isolation

Albumin was isolated essentially by the method of Quinn *et al.*, with further modifications (Quinn, Gamble & Judah, 1975). 0.5 ml of serum was routinely used as the starting material. 1% trichloroacetic acid in ethanol was added to make up to 10 ml. The precipitated immunoglobulins were removed by centrifuging at 10,000 x*g* for 20 minutes. To the supernatant was added 2 volumes (20 ml) of ether. The albumin was precipitated and was collected by centrifuging at 10,000 x*g* for 10 minutes. The precipitate was washed once with 2 volumes of 1:1 ether and ethanol and the suspension was again centrifuged to collect the albumin. It was drained and kept briefly in a desiccator to remove most of the volatile solvents. The albumin was dissolved in 10 ml PBS. The protein content was determined by the method of Lowry (Lowry *et al.*, 1951), using BSA as standard and the absorbance read by an LKB Ultrospec II with an LKB Autofill II (Pharmacia).

3.2.3.8 Digestion of albumin

1.5 mg albumin in 1.0 ml PBS was digested with proteinase K. 200 μl of a 5 mg/ml solution was added at 0 hr and 4 hr. The samples were incubated at 37°C for a total of 24 hours. 200 μl of isopropanol was also added to each digestion. Following hydrolysis, 2 mg of BSA was added to improve precipitation and removal of excess enzyme, followed by 2 volumes of cold ethanol. The samples were kept at –20°C for 2 hours and then centrifuged at 1,500 xg for 15 minutes. The precipitate was removed and ethanol in the supernatant was removed by a vacuum concentrator (Heto Lab. Equipment, Denmark). The sample was reconstituted to 1 ml with PBS, ready for the next step.

3.2.3.9 Animal procedures

Male Porten-Wistar rats (approx. 250g each) were injected with ^{3}H-AFB₁ to obtain radiolabelled serum albumin for use in the development of a method to monitor AFB₁-albumin adducts. Three dosage regimens were used to obtain adequately modified rat serum albumin:

AFB₁ Dose ($\mu g\ kg^{-1}$)	Radioactivity ($\mu Ci\ kg^{-1}$)	Treatment Time (hrs)
100	20	24
100	100	4
400	600	4

The animals were housed in grid-bottomed cages and received food and water *ad libitum*. The animals (2 in each dosage regimen) were given the dose by intra-peritoneal injection. At the end of the treatment time, the animals were anaesthetised by exposure to diethyl ether until respiration stopped. The thorax was opened up quickly and blood was collected by cardiac puncture. The serum was prepared as in section 3.2.2.2. Blood from animals in each dosage regimen was pooled and albumin prepared from each sample.

The ^{3}H-AFB₁ solutions used to inject the animals, the serum samples and the prepared albumin solutions were all counted for radioactivity. The protein concentration of serum albumin solution was estimated by the method of Lowry's (Lowry *et al.*, 1951). The level of modification of rat serum albumin by ^{3}H-AFB₁ was calculated for each dosage regimen.

3.2.4 Validations

3.2.4.1 Analysis of standard AFB1 and AFB1-lysine in ELISA

Standard solutions of AFB₁ ranging in concentration from 0.01 ng/ml to

100 ng/ml were prepared in PBS, using a stock solution of 10 μg/ml. The concentration of standard AFB_1-lysine solutions ranged from 0.001 ng/ml to 100 ng/ml and were prepared from a stock of 17.5 μg/ml stock solution. Competitive ELISA (section 3.2.3.1) were performed on these samples and the percentage inhibition was calculated with reference to PBS control.

3.2.4.2 Optimisation of antiserum dilution and concentration of coating antigen in ELISA

Each ELISA plate was coated with $BSA-AFB_1$ (prepared as in section 3.2.2.5), the concentration of which varied in each row of the plate as shown in Fig. 3.5. The plates were allowed to dry completely and prepared as in section 3.2.2.7. Rabbit anti-AFB_1 serum was diluted in concentrations from 1:5,000 to 1:20,000. The diluted antiserum solutions were added to the plates directly (50 μl/well) and the ELISA procedures were carried out

Figure 3.5   Optimisation of antiserum dilution and concentration of coating antigen in ELISA

'Checker Board'

Amount of coating antigen/well

	X	X	X	X	X	X	X	X	X	X	X	X
20 ng	X											X
15 ng	X											X
12.5 ng	X											X
10 ng	X											X
7.5 ng	X											X
5 ng	X											X
	X	X	X	X	X	X	X	X	X	X	X	X

Rabbit antiserum dilution   *1:20,000   1:15,000   1:10,000   1:7,500   1:5,000*

as described in section 3.2.3.1. ELISA was done in 4 replicate plates. From this 'checker board', the optimal concentrations of the coating antigen and anti-AFB₁ serum were selected.

3.2.4.3 Elution characteristics and capacity of the immunoaffinity column

Disposable plastic columns of 2 ml capacity were packed with immunoaffinity gel (prepared as in section 3.2.2.6) to 1 ml bed volume. Each column was washed with 20 ml PBS to remove sodium azide. Standard ^{3}H-AFB₁ solutions were prepared in two concentrations –20 ng/ml and 40 ng/ml, each containing about 5×10^5 DPM/ml. The columns were loaded with 1 ml of the ^{3}H-AFB₁ sample and then washed with 20 ml of PBS and 15 ml of 85% methanol. The void volume and washings were collected in 2 ml fractions. They were dried in a vacuum concentrator to less than 1 ml and then the volume was adjusted to 1 ml with PBS. 250 μl of each fraction was taken for radioactivity counting. Each column was washed with 20 ml of PBS and the experiment repeated with the other concentration of ^{3}H-AFB₁ sample.

Immunoaffinity gels prepared with both rabbit antiserum and rat monoclonal antibody were tested.

3.2.4.4 Comparison of immunoaffinity gels prepared with different affinity gels

Immunoaffinity gel was prepared using two different types of affinity gels — CNBr-Sepharose 4B gel and EAH-Sepharose 4B gel. Coupling of rabbit anti-AFB1 serum with CNBr-Sepharose 4B gel was as described in section 3.2.2.6. The coupling procedures of antiserum with EAH-Sepharose 4B gel was carried out following instructions accompanying purchase. It required a carbodiimide coupling reaction. The gel was supplied pre-swollen in 0.9% NaCl. The required amount of gel, 6 g dry powder or 24 ml swollen gel volume, was washed on a sintered glass filter, porosity G3, with 0.5M NaCl, using 50 ml per gram of gel, followed by the same volume of distilled water adjusted to pH 4.5. The required amount of EDC (1-ethyl-3-(dimethylaminopropyl)-carbodiimide), 10 mg/ml of swollen gel, was dissolved in water and the pH adjusted to 4.5. 6 ml of rabbit anti-AFB₁ serum, the EDC solution and gel suspension were mixed to give a total volume of about 50 ml. It was mixed in an end-over-end mixer at room temperature for 24 hours. After the coupling period, the gel was washed alternately with 0.1M sodium acetate buffer (pH 4.0) and 0.1M bicarbonate buffer (pH 8.3), each containing 0.5M NaCl to remove excess ligand, urea derivatives and unreacted carbodiimide. The gel was suspended in PBS containing 0.02% sodium azide and stored at 4°C.

Four immunoaffinity columns were prepared, two with immunoaffinity gel prepared from CNBr-Sepharose 4B gel and two with immunoaffinity gel prepared from EAH-Sepharose 4B gel, each of 1 ml bed volume, prepared according to section 3.2.3.3. One of each type of the immunoaffinity column was loaded with 1 ml of a 20 ng/ml ^{3}H-AFB$_1$ solution and the other with 1 ml of a 40 ng/ml solution, each solution containing about 5 $\times$ 10^5 DPM/ml. Each column was eluted with 20 ml of PBS, followed by 15 ml of 85% methanol. The void volume and all washings were collected in 2 ml fractions. They were dried in a vacuum concentrator to less than 1 ml volume and adjusted to 1 ml with PBS. 250 µl of each fraction was taken for counting for radioactivity.

3.2.4.5   Immunoaffinity column experiment of AFB$_1$-lysine

An immunoaffinity column was prepared using antibody coupled CNBr-Sepharose 4B gel. A sample of 40 ng/ml of lysine-AFB1 was prepared from a stock of 17.5 µg/ml soluton. 1 ml of the sample was loaded onto the column. It was washed with 20 ml of PBS followed by 15 ml of 85% methanol. The void volume and all washings were collected in 2 ml fractions. They were dried in a vacuum concentrator to less than 1 ml volume and adjusted to 4 ml with PBS. The fractions were read by a fluorescence spectrometer (Perkin-Elmer LS-5 Luminescence Spectrometer). The excitation and emission maxima of the stock AFB1-lysine sample were determined and the fluorescence of each fraction at these settings were read.

3.2.4.6   HPLC analysis of fractions from immunoaffinity column

To investigate whether the radioactivity in the post-immunoaffinity column fractions was actually associated with AFB$_1$, these fractions were analysed by HPLC. The ^{3}H-AFB$_1$ solutions loaded onto the immunoaffinity column and other fractions under study were injected into the HPLC system as described in section 3.2.3.5. The sample size was 20 µl. 1 ml/min fractions were collected into plastic scintillation minivials. 4 ml of scintillant (Monofluor, National Diagnostic, U.K.) was added to each vial and the radioactivity counted. The percentage of radioactivity in each HPLC fraction was calculated and compared to the retention time of AFB_1.

3.2.4.7 Elution characteristic and capacity of Sep-Pak C₁₈ cartridge

Sep-pak C_{18} cartridges were prepared as in section 3.2.3.2. ^{3}H-AFB$_1$ solutions of 20 ng/ml and 40 ng/ml were prepared, each containing about 5×10^5 DPM/ml. 1 ml of the solution was loaded onto an activated cartridge using a syringe. It was then washed with 10 ml distilled water followed by 10 ml of methanol. The void volume and all washings were collected in 1 ml fractions. 250 µl of each fraction was taken for radioactivity counting with the addition of 4 ml scintillant. The percentage of radioactivity in each fracion was calculated.

3.2.4.8 HPLC analysis of fractions from Sep-Pak C18 cartridge

To investigate whether the radioactivity in the fractions eluted from Sep-Pak C_{18} cartridges was actually associated with AFB_1, these fractions were analysed by HPLC. The ^{3}H-AFB$_1$ solutions loaded onto the Sep-Pak C_{18} cartridge and other fractions under study were injected into the HPLC system as described in section 3.2.3.5. The sample size was 20 µl. 1 ml/ min. fractions were collected into plastic scintillation minivials and the radioactivity counted. The percentage of radioactivity in each HPLC fraction was calculated and compared to the retention time of AFB_1.

3.2.4.9 Digestion of serum albumin by proteinase K

A proteolytic enzyme, once activated, will begin to catalyse the hydrolysis of itself, thus terminating its action. Therefore, different digestion regimens, whereby more enzymes were added at intervals, were set up to select the most efficient digestion regimen on serum albumin.

Rat serum albumin modified by ^{3}H-AFB$_1$ (section 3.2.3.9 and section 3.2.3.7) was used. Starting material was 1.5 mg in 1 ml PBS. Four regimens were set up:

A   No proteinase K
B   proteinase K at 0hr, 4hr
C   proteinase K at 0hr, 2hr, 4hr
D   proteinase K at 0hr, 2hr, 4hr, 24hr

At the appropriate time, 200 µl of a 5 mg/ml solution of proteinase K in PBS was added to each digestion. Each digestion also contained 200 µl isopropanol and the incubation was carried out at 37°C. All samples were processed after 28 hours. At the end of the incubation, the rest of the albumin digestion was carried out as described in section 3.2.3.8. The radioactivity of the starting material and the final hydrolysates were counted by taking 50 µl samples. The recoveries were calculated.

3.2.4.10   Effect of ethanol in samples to be loaded onto Sep-Pak C_{18} cartridge

After digestion of serum albumin, BSA and cold ethanol were added to the digestion mixture to improve precipitation of excess enzyme. It was necessary to investigate the effect of ethanol in the subsequent clean-up step, whether it was necessary to remove ethanol before applying the sample onto an immunoaffinity column. An alternative might have been dilute the concentration of ethanol in the sample.

Digestion of rat serum albumin modified by ^{3}H-AFB$_1$ was as described in Regimen B in section 3.2.4.9. i.e. enzyme was added at 0 hr and 4 hr and incubated for 24 hours. BSA and cold ethanol were added to each digestion mixture as described. In regimen A, the ethanol was removed by a vacuum concentrator and the final volume adjusted to 1 ml with PBS (A). In regimen B, PBS was added to a final volume of 25 ml (B). In regimen C, PBS was added to a final volume of 50 ml (C). Samples A, B and C were loaded onto activated Sep-Pak C_{18} cartridges. In B and C, where the 'void volume' was large, it was collected in 5 ml fractions. Each cartridge was then washed with 5 ml PBS, followed by 5 ml methanol. All fractions were dried in a vacuum concentrator and the final volume adjusted to 1 ml. Aliquots were taken for radioactivity counting and the percentage recovery of radioactivity in each fraction was calculated.

3.2.4.11   Effect of drying in a vacuum concentrator on recovery of radioactivity of 3H-AFB1

During the validation process, the recovery at each step was followed by radioactive counts of ^{3}H-AFB$_1$. A concentration step was necessary in between each step to prepare the sample in a small volume, usually 1 ml, for the next step. In order to test whether drying in a vacuum concentrator would affect the recovery of readioactive counts, the following experiment was set up. Three sets of samples were set up:

A   counted directly

B   5 ml methanol and 0.5 ml PBS added to each tube and evaporated in a vacuum concentrator

C   5 ml PBS added to each tube and evaporated in a vacuum concentrator

After evaporation (not to complete dryness), the volume of each tube was adjusted to 1 ml. 200 µl was taken for counting and the recovery was calculated compared to the control (A). There were 4 tubes in each set:

1   100 µl of a sample of ^{3}H-AFB$_1$

2   50 µl

3   20 µl

4   0 µl

3.2.4.12   Evaluation of the overall procedure for the analysis of serum albumin adducts of AFB1

Digestion of rat serum albumin (modified by ^{3}H-AFB$_1$) was set up as in section 3.2.4.9 according to the 4 regimens. At the end of the incubation period, the hydrolysates were processed as described. 2×20 µl of each sample were taken for radioactivity counting. The rest of each sample was loaded onto an activated Sep-Pak C$_{18}$ cartridge. It was washed with 5 ml distilled water, followed by 5 ml methanol. 0.5 ml PBS was added to each methanol fraction and they were concentrated to less than 1 ml. The volume was adjusted to 1 ml with PBS. 2×20 µl of these methanol fractions from Sep-Pak C$_{18}$ cartridges were taken for radioactivity counting and the rest loaded onto anti-AFB$_1$ immunoaffinity columns. They were washed with 5ml PBS followed by 5ml 85% methanol. The methanol fractions were collected and evaporated to less than 1 ml. The volume was adjusted to 1 ml with PBS. 2×20 µl samples of each methanol fraction from the immunoaffinity columns were taken for radioactivity counting.

The overall recovery of the clean-up steps in these four digestion regimens were calculated.

3.2.4.13   HPLC analysis of samples obtained after digestion and all clean-up procedures

Rat serum albumin, modified by ^{3}H-AFB$_1$, was taken through the whole process of albumin isolation, digestion and clean-up by Sep-Pak C$_{18}$ cartridge and anti-AFB$_1$ immunoaffinity column as in section 3.2.4.12. The final sample obtained was injected into the HPLC system as described in section 3.2.3.5. 1 ml/min fractions were obtained and the radioactivity was counted.

3.2.5   Results and discussion

3.2.5.1 BSA-AFB$_1$ conjugate

The presumed structure of BSA-AFB$_1$ is shown in Fig. 3.6. The reaction between BSA and AFB$_1$ was found to be via one or more residues of lysine. Therefore, for each batch of BSA-AFB$_1$ prepared, the ratio of AFB$_1$ to BSA may be different. The extinction coefficient of AFB$_1$ at 363nm = 20,150 $mol^{-1}cm^{-1}$. i.e. the absorbance of 1 nmole of AFB$_1$ in 1 ml of solution is approximately 0.02. The UV scan of the BSA-AFB$_1$ prepared showed a maximum at 404 nm. This shift was due to the conjugated state and the higher pH. According to Beer-Lambert's law,

Absorbance = $\varepsilon\,c\,l$ where ε = extinction coefficient
c = concentration of sample
l = length of path

The absorbance at 404nm was 1.421. The estimated concentration of AFB$_1$ in the solution = 1.421/0.02 nmol ml
= 71.05 nmol ml^{-1}

Figure 3.6   Structure of BSA-AFB$_1$

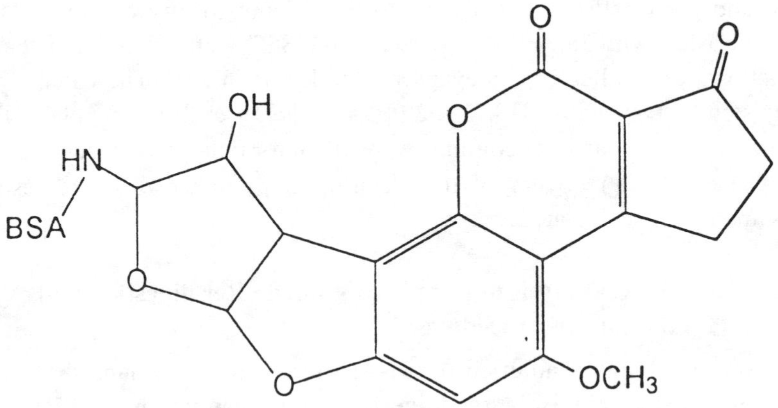

(From Sizaret *et al.*, 1982).

The protein concentration of the conjugate was estimated by the method of Lowry to be 350 µg/ml. The molecular weight of BSA is 66,200. Therefore, the concentration of BSA in the conjugate solution
$= 350 \times 1000/66{,}200$ nmol ml^{-1}
$= 5.3$ nmol ml^{-1}

Ratio of AFB$_1$: BSA $= 71.05 : 5.3$
$= 13.4 : 1$

3.2.5.2 Treatment of experimental animals with ^{3}H-AFB$_1$

The amount of AFB$_1$ associated with rat serum albumin was calculated from the radioactivity associated with the ^{3}H-AFB$_1$ solution for injection and the radioactivity of the modified rat serum albumin. The level of modification in the three dosage regimens was shown in Table 3.1.

The level of modification of rat serum albumin by ^{3}H-AFB$_1$ depends on many factors. Depending on the strain of experimental animal used, the extent of metabolic activation of AFB$_1$ to the reactive metabolite, the ability to conjugate the reactive metabolite, the turnover of serum albumin, etc, will all affect the level of modification. In the same strain of ex-perimental animal, a linear relationship was observed between the level of AFB$_1$ bound to serum albumin and the dose of AFB$_1$ administered. It was estimated in that about 2–3% of the initial dose was bound to albumin at 48 hours.

In the 3 dosing regimens in this experiment, the exposure period of the first regimen was 24 hours. It was expected that a significant proportion of the modified serum albumin would be excreted. The level of modification was thus fairly low. The objective of this dosing experiment was to obtain rat serum albumin of an adequately modified level so that it could be used as the starting material in the validation of a method to monitor plasma albumin adducts of AFB$_1$. Regimen C gave a level of modification of about 25 ng AFB$_1$/mg albumin. This was used as the starting material for other experiments.

3.2.5.3 Optimisation of antiserum dilution and concentration of coating antigen in ELISA

In the checker board described in section 3.2.4.2, a gradation of colour was observed in each ELISA plate. The general trend was that the larger amount of coating antigen used and the higher the concentration of an-tiserum, the colour produced would be more intense (higher absorbance).

Table 3.1 Level of modification of rat serum albumin in different dosage regimens

Regimen	Dosage of ^{3}H-AFB$_1$ (per kg body weight)	Specific activity of ^{3}H-AFB$_1$ injection solution (DPM/ng AFB$_1$)	Specific activity of rat serum albumin (DPM/mg)	Level of modification of rat serum albumin (ng AFB$_1$/mg)
A	100 μg AFB$_1$ 20 μCi	473	983	2.1
B	100 μg AFB$_1$ 100 μCi	1,900	7,590	4.0
C	400 μg AFB$_1$ 600 μCi	2,748	68,248	24.8

The objective of this experiment was to find the lowest amount of coating antigen and rabbit anti-AFB$_1$ antiserum that would produce the highest absorbance, thus optimising the performance of ELISA. The absorbance produced at different concentrations of coating antigen and antiserum diluton was shown in Fig. 3.7. It was expected that as the amount of coating antigen used was increased, at a given dilution of antiserum, the absorbance would also increase as more antigen would react with the antibodies. Similarly, at fixed amount of coating antigen, when the concentration of antiserum was increased, the absorbance produced was also expected to rise. But these increases were not expected to be infinite. The rise in absorbance would be proportional to the increase in antigen/antiserum concentration over a certain range and then it would reach a plateau. This was because there were other constraints such as the capacity of the ELISA wells to adsorb coating antigen, the concentration of the secondary antibody and the concentration of the substrate. Therefore, within the constraints of these other conditions, it was able to select the optimal concentrations of coating antigen and antiserum dilution. i.e. the lowest amounts of these that could be used to produce the highest absorbance. A high absorbance is desirable as during competitive ELISA, the inhibition would be much more pronounced.

From Fig. 3.7, it could be observed that there was a general trend for the absorbance to rise as the concentration of the antiserum was increased and it began to level off at dilution 1:7,500 and above. But at antiserum dilution 1:5000 and coating antigen concentration at 10 ng/well, the absorbance seemed to be at the maximal. Therefore, these conditions were selected as the experimental conditions for future ELISA.

In this 'checker board' exercise, antiserum was added directly onto the coated ELISA plates. i.e. the competition step was omitted. In the analysis employed for the study of AFB$_1$ albumin adducts, competitive ELISA was used. The sample under study was first incubated with an anti-AFB$_1$ antiserum or monoclonal antibody in equal volumes before the mixture was loaded in ELISA wells. This step effectively doubled the dilution of the antiserum used. Therefore, when we have selected an antiserum dilution of 1:5,000 from this 'checker board' exercise, in practice, a dilution of 1:2,500 would be required in future ELISA. The condition selected for competitive ELISA for the study of AFB1 albumin adducts were thus:

Coating antigen BSA-AFB$_1$ 10 ng/well
Rabbit anti-AFB$_1$ antiserum   1:2,500

Figure 3.7 Optimisation of ELISA Conditions — Absorbance in ELISA Wells at Different Amounts of Coating Antigen and Dilutions of Rabbit Anti-AFB$_1$ Antiserum

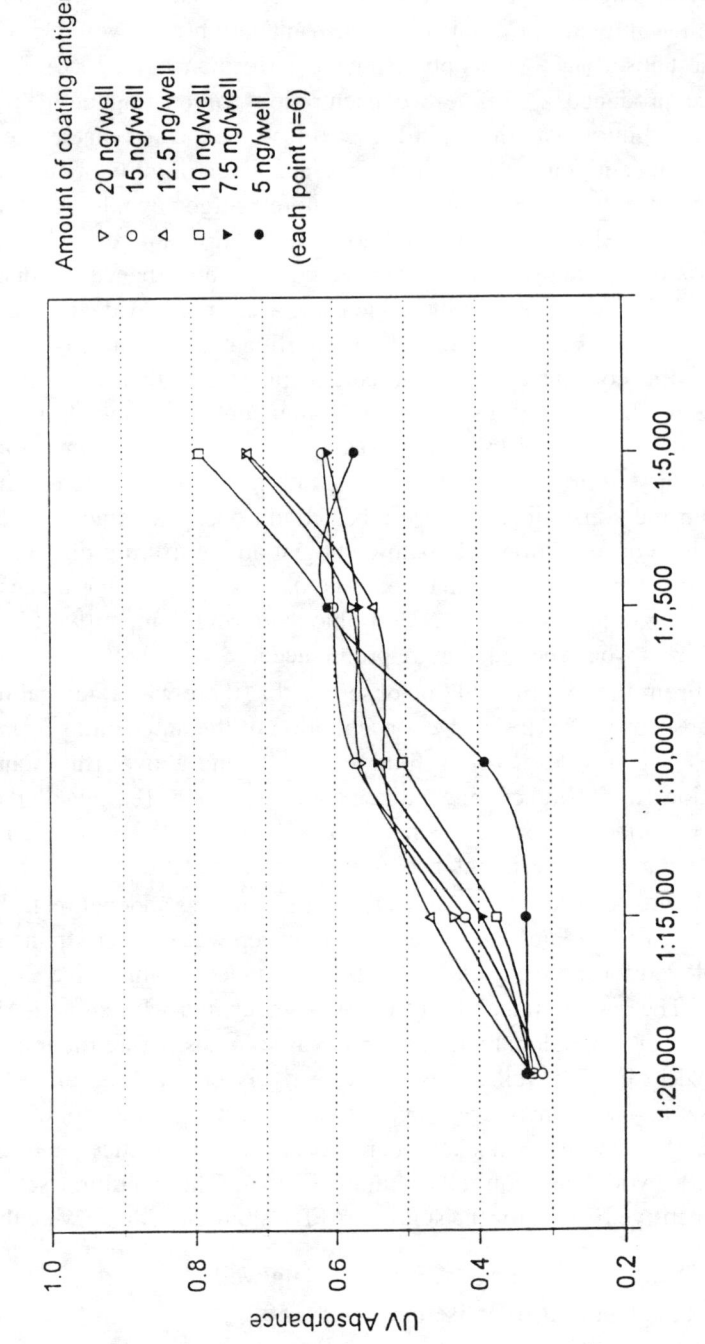

Amount of coating antigen

▽	20 ng/well
○	15 ng/well
△	12.5 ng/well
□	10 ng/well
▶	7.5 ng/well
●	5 ng/well

(each point n=6)

This exercise was not repeated completely for the rat monoclonal antibody as the optimum amount of coating antigen was already determined to be 10 ng/well. This amount was also used in ELISA with the rat monoclonal antibody and the optimal monoclonal antibody dilution for ELISA was determined to be 1:5,000 using a range of dilution of the monoclonal antibody from 1:10 to 1:1,000,000 (Fig. 3.8).

3.2.5.4   Analysis of standard AFB₁ and AFB1-lysine in ELISA

The digestion end product of AFB₁ serum albumin adducts was putatively AFB₁-lysine if digestion was, in the ideal case, complete. In practice, it was expected that a range of AFB₁-peptides as well as AFB₁-lysine were released from the modified serum albumin. The immunogen used for the immunisation of rabbits to produce anti-AFB₁ serum was AFB₁ bound to microsomal proteins. Thus the antibody produced was a polyclonal antibody, capable of recognising a range of AFB₁-related structures. In actual fact, it was shown that the major epitope for antibody recognition of aflatoxin lies in the coumarin and cyclopentonone rings of the aflatoxin molecules. A previous study indicated that the rabbit anti-AFB₁ serum could detect other metabolites of AFB₁, including AFB₁-NAcCys, AFB₁-GSH, AFB₁-FAPy, AFB₁-Cys, AFM₁, AFB₁-CysGly and AFB₂, all with approximately the same sensitivity as it detected AFB₁ (Makarananda, 1989).

In another study, rabbit anti-AFB₁ serum was obtained by injecting animals with a similar immunogen (Sizaret *et al.*, 1982). It was found that AFB₁-lysine adduct was approximately 6-fold more reactive with the antiserum than was AFB₁ itself. As in our study, AFB₁-lysine and other modified peptides were the anticipated end products of digestion, it was essential that they were recognised by the antiserum. The ELISA competition curves for AFB₁ and lysine-AFB₁ are shown in Fig. 3.9a. The recognition of AFB₁-lysine by the rabbit antiserum was slightly more sensitive compared to AFB1 itself. A good steep slope of proportionality was obtained.

Although AFB₁-lysine could be successful recognised by the rabbit anti-AFB₁ serum, the recognition of other AFB₁-modified peptides may not be of the same order of sensitivity. This was because, though the epitope for antibody recognition was identical (the coumarin and cyclopentenone rings), in these larger molecules of peptides, the epitope may be partially obstructed due to the stereochemistry of the attached groups.

Figure 3.8 Absorbance in ELISA Wells at Different Dilutions of Rat Monoclonal Antibody

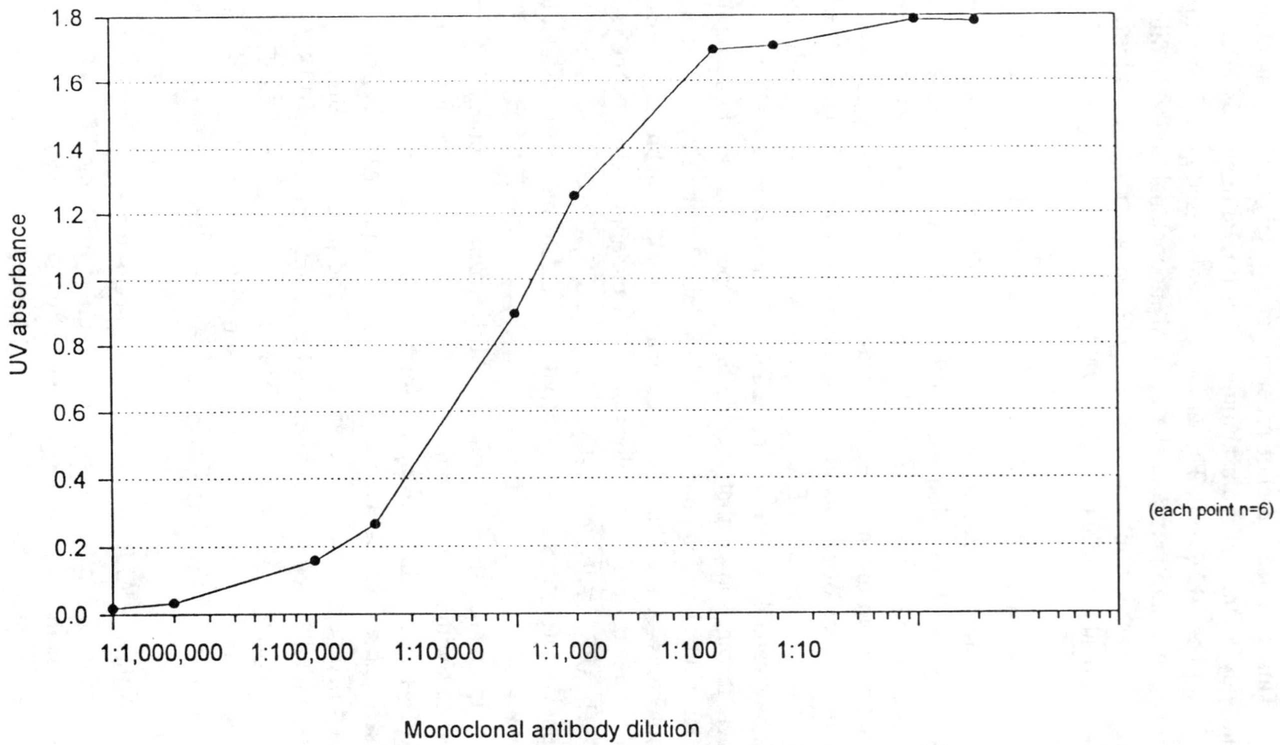

(each point n=6)

Figure 3.9 Standard ELISA Inhibition Curves Using AFB_1 and AFB_1-lysine as Substrates with a) Rabbit Antiserum and b) Rat Monoclonal Antibody

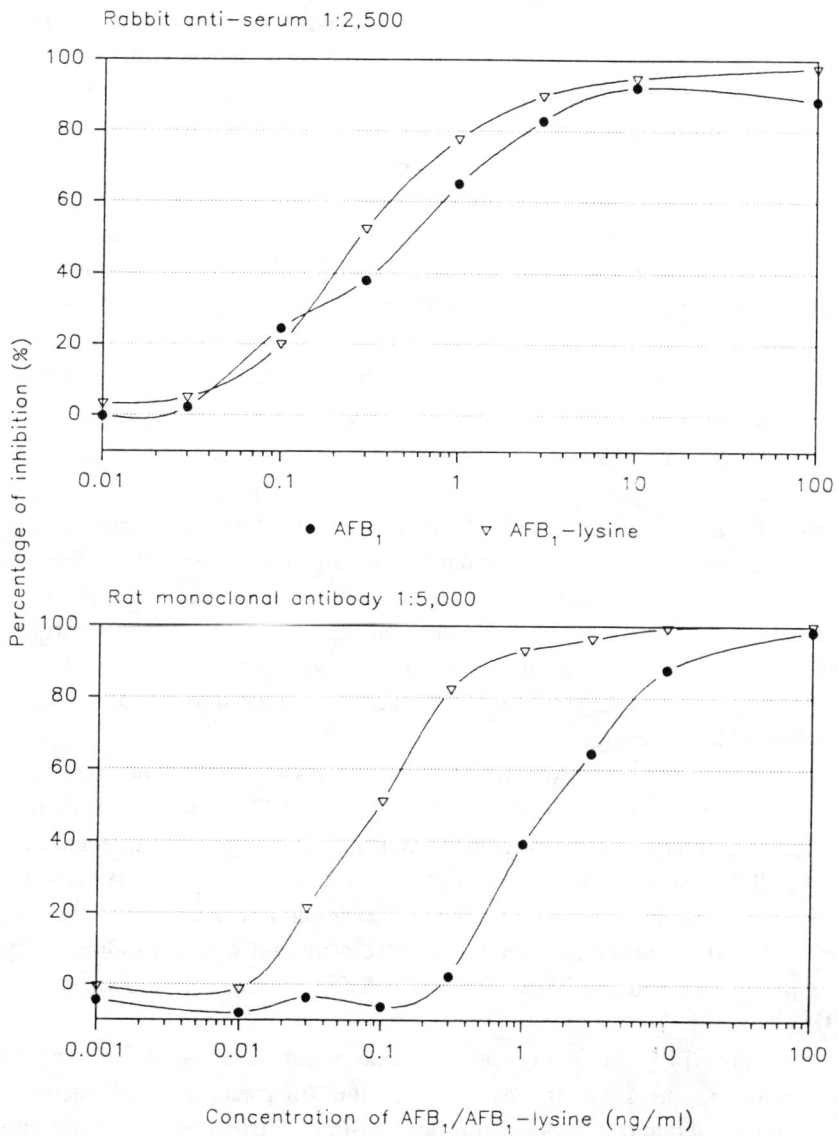

Therefore, in future ELISA studies, the AFB_1 content of the samples would be expressed in lysine-AFB_1 equivalents.

The recognition of AFB_1 and AFB1-lysine by the rat monoclonal antibody was also very sensitive, even more so than the rabbit anti-serum (Fig. 3.9b). The sensitivity to AFB_1-lysine was approximately 10 times that of AFB_1 itself. This was as expected as the original immunogen was an AFB_1-protein. The proportional part of the ELISA competition curve of the rat monoclonal antibody has a steeper slope than that of the rabbit anti-serum. This indicated that the monoclonal antibody was more specific against the two substrates tested — AFB_1 and AFB_1-lysine. The dilution of the monoclonal antibody used in ELISA (1:5,000) was also higher than that of the rabbit anti-serum (1:2,500).

3.2.5.5 Sep-Pak C_{18} cartridge — elution characteristics and capacity

The elution profile of AFB_1 from Sep-Pak C_{18} cartridges was shown in Fig. 3.10. It can be seen that when a sample of ^3H-AFB_1 was loaded onto a Sep-Pak C_{18} cartridge, it was retained on the cartridge even after being washed with 10 ml of PBS. About 95% of the total radioactivity was recovered in the first 2 ml of methanol washing. There was little difference between the elution profile obtained for a 20 ng/ml sample and a 40 ng/ml sample, indicating that the AFB_1 retention capacity of the cartridge was not exceeded even at 40 ng/ml. In practice, it was expected that quantities exceeding 40 ng of AFB_1 would seldom be encountered in the samples that we would be handling.

The radioactivity of the methanol fraction was shown to be associated with AFB_1 by HPLC analysis. Fraction 2 (first PBS fraction) and fraction 12 (first methanol fraction) from the Sep-Pak cartridge were injected into the HPLC system as described in section 3.2.3.5 for analysis. A standard ^3H-AFB_1 sample was also injected for comparison. Each 1 ml fraction from the HPLC was collected into mini scintillation vials for radioactivity counting. The radioactivity of these HPLC fractions are shown in Fig. 3.11.

In this HPLC set up, the retention time of a standard AFB_1 sample was about 6.6 minutes. i.e. it was eluted in the 7th fraction (1 ml/fraction). When the methanol fraction from the Sep-Pak cartridge was injected into the HPLC, it has a profile corresponding to that of a standard sample of ^3H-AFB_1. The fraction with the highest percentage of radioactivity of both of these samples being the 7th HPLC fraction, corresponding to the

Figure 3.10 Elution Characteristics of ^{3}H-AFB$_1$ from Sep-Pak C$_{18}$ Cartridges

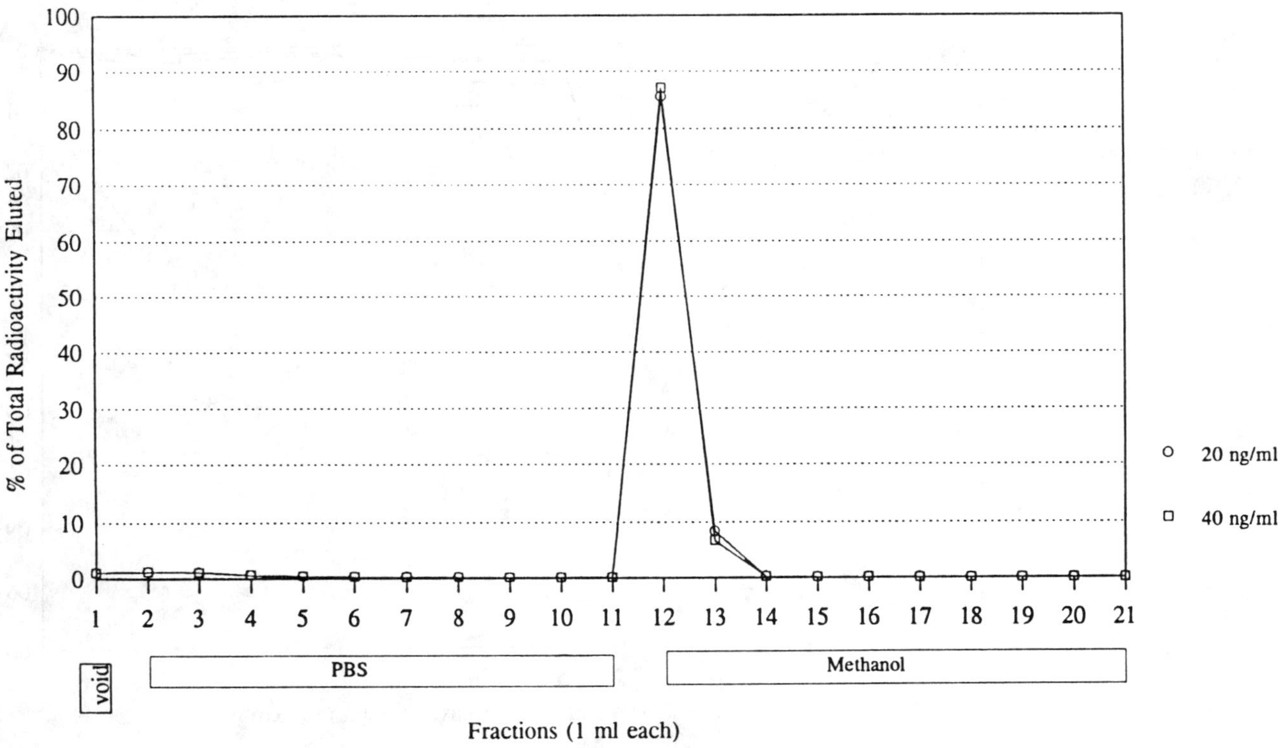

% of Total Radioactivity Eluted

Fractions (1 ml each)

Void

PBS

Methanol

○ 20 ng/ml

□ 40 ng/ml

Figure 3.11 HPLC Analysis of Fractions Obtained from Sep-Pak C$_{18}$ Cartridges

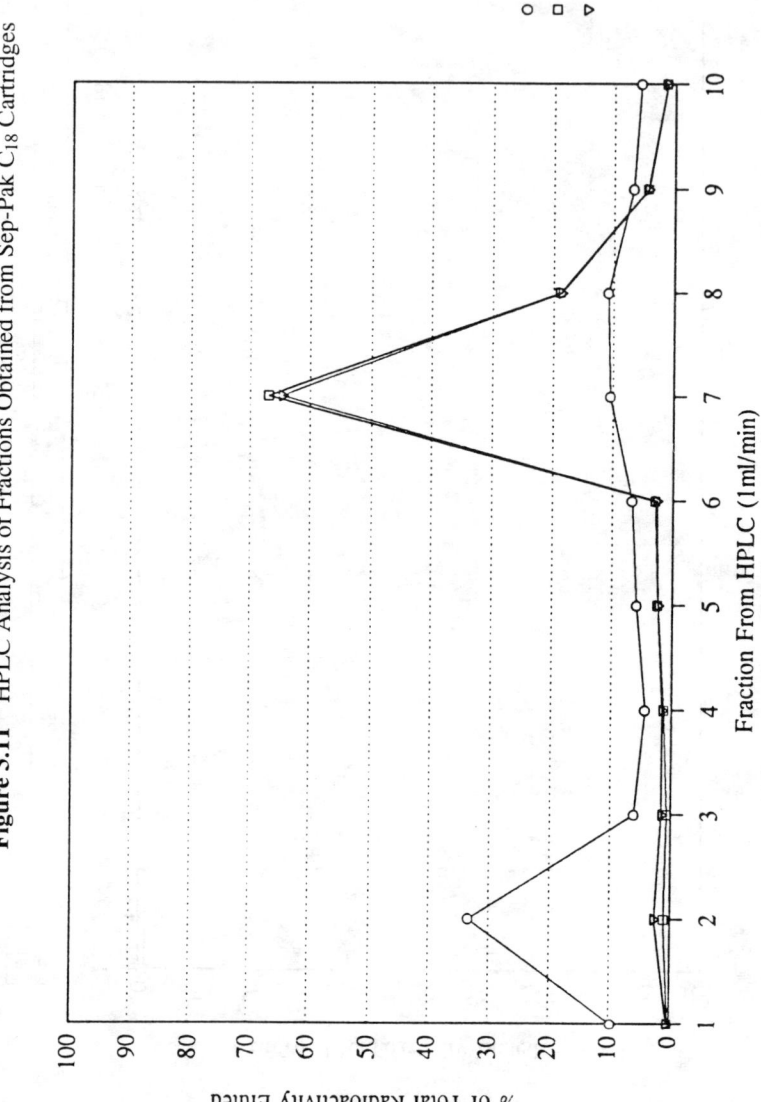

o   unretained fraction
□   methanol fraction
▵   standard 3H-AFB1

retention time of AFB_1. When the unretained fraction from the Sep-Pak cartridge was injected into the HPLC, most of the radioactivity was eluted in the first two fractions. This radioactivity represented tritium exchanged from the AFB_1. Therefore, although the radioactivity in the first few ml of methanol washing was about 95% of the total radioactivity, it represented almost 100% retention of AFB_1.

In this elution experiment, 10 ml of PBS and 10 ml of methanol were used to characterise the whole elution profile of ^3H-AFB_1 from a Sep-Pak C_{18} cartridge. In practice, to prepare the sample for the next step, it was necessary to reduce the volume of the methanol fraction to below 1 ml. It was much more convenient to handle a volume of 5 ml instead of 10 ml in a vacuum concentrator. From Table 3.2, it was shown that if only 5 ml PBS and methanol were used, the percentage of radioactivity recovered in these two fractions were 3.8% and 94.1% respectively. Thus, it was decided that in future studies, 5 ml of PBS and 5 ml of methanol would be used.

Table 3.2   Radioactivity in fractions from Sep-Pak C_{18} cartridges obtained after loading with 1 ml sample containing 40 ng of ^3H-AFB_1

Fraction from Sep-Pak	Radioactivity	
	Total eluted (DPM)	% of total eluted
Void (unretained)	6,099	1.07
PBS washing (first 3 ml)	21,713	3.82
Methanol washing (first 5 ml)	53,484	94.13

3.2.5.6   Elution characteristics of immunoaffinity columns

Different affinity gels are available for immobilising ligands. The correct choice of coupling method depends on the substance to be immobilised. Two gels were chosen for the coupling of rabbit anti-AFB_1 serum. CNBr-activated Seharose 4B gel enables ligands containing primary amino groups to be rapidly immobilised by a spontaneous reaction, whereas EAH-Sepharose 4B gel requires cyanogen bromide activation. This latter gel has a six-carbon long spacer arm and permits coupling via a carboxyl groups. Cyanogen bromide is an extremely toxic and unpleasant chemical. The use of CNBr-activated gel will negate the need for handling this chemical in the laboratory.

Cyanogen bromide reacts with hydroxyl groups on sepharose and converts these groups into imidocarbonate which can then react with nucleophiles. The activated groups react with primary amino groups of the ligand to form isourea linages. The activation procedure also cross-links sepharose and thus enhances its chemical stability.

EAH-Sepharose 4B gel has free primary amino groups at the end of 6-carbon spacer arms for coupling ligands containing free carboxyl groups. It is formed by covalent linkage of 1,6-diaminohexane to sepharose 4B gel using cyanogen bromide. The coupling of ligands with EAH-Sepharose gel requires a carbodiimide which promotes condensation between a free amino and a free carboxyl group to form a peptide link. The carbodiimide yields an isourea upon hydration. Therefore, EAH-Sepharose 4B gel, which contains a free amino group, can be coupled with carboxyl-containing ligands.

Since the rabbit anti-AFB_1 serum and rat monoclonal antibody were shown to have high affinity for AFB_1, it was expected that AFB_1 would be retained on a column packed with this immunoaffinity gel if the coupling reaction was successful. With the right solution, the immobilised AFB_1 would be desorbed and eluted.

The elution profiles of AFB_1 from the two kinds of immunoaffinity columns are shown in Fig. 3.12. In CNBr-Sepharose 4B gel (Fig. 3.12a), over 90% of the total radioactivity was eluted in the first two methanol fraction. A very small amount of radioactivity (about 4%) appeared in the first PBS fraction. There was virtually no difference observed between the elution profiles of a 20 ng/ml sample and a 40 ng/ml sample, indicating that even at the higher amount of sample, the capacity of the immunoaffinity column was not exceeded.

Fraction 2 (first PBS fraction) and Fraction 12 (first methanol fraction) were analysed by HPLC to confirm the association of radioactivity with AFB_1. These two fractions and a standard AFB_1 sample were injected into the HPLC system and fractions were collected at 1 ml/min into mini scintillation vials for radioactivity counting. The percentage of radioactivity of these HPLC fractions are shown in Fig. 3.13. It can be seen that the profile of the methanol fraction corresponded to that of the standard AFB_1 sample, whereas the PBS fraction produced a very different profile. This represented exchanged radioactivity material from AFB_1. Therefore, an immunoaffinity column prepared from CNBr-Sepharose gel was able to retain AFB_1 successfully even when the loading sample size was 40 ng. Although it retained about 95% of the total radioactivity, this represented almost 100% retention of AFB1 as verified by HPLC.

Figure 3.12 Elution Characteristics of ³H-AFB₁ from Immunoaffinity Columns Prepared from Two Different Kinds of Affinity Gel Coupled with Rabbit Anti-AFB₁ Anti-serum

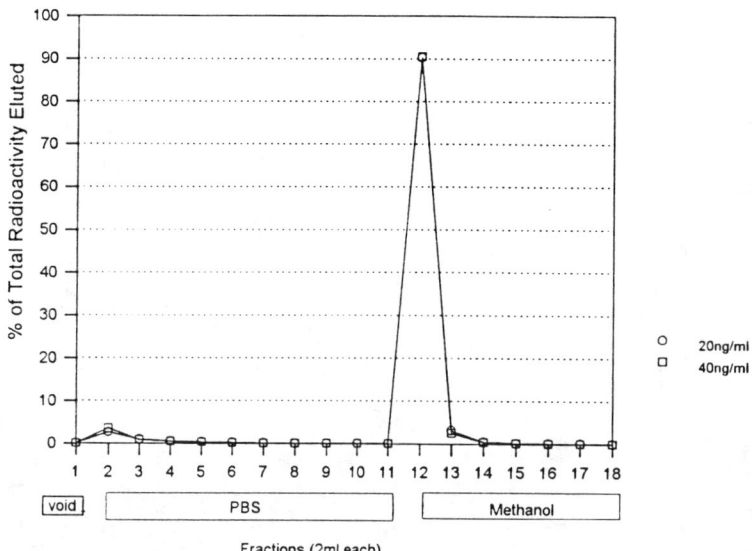

a. CNBr-Sepharose 4B Gel

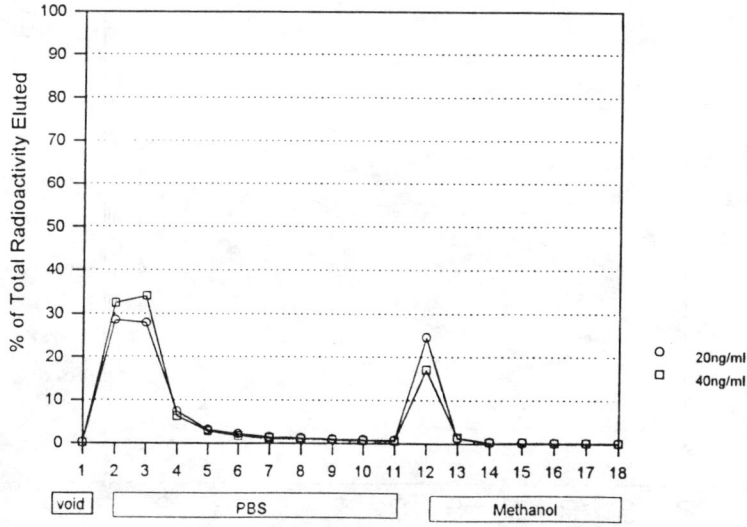

b. EAH-Sepharose 4B Gel

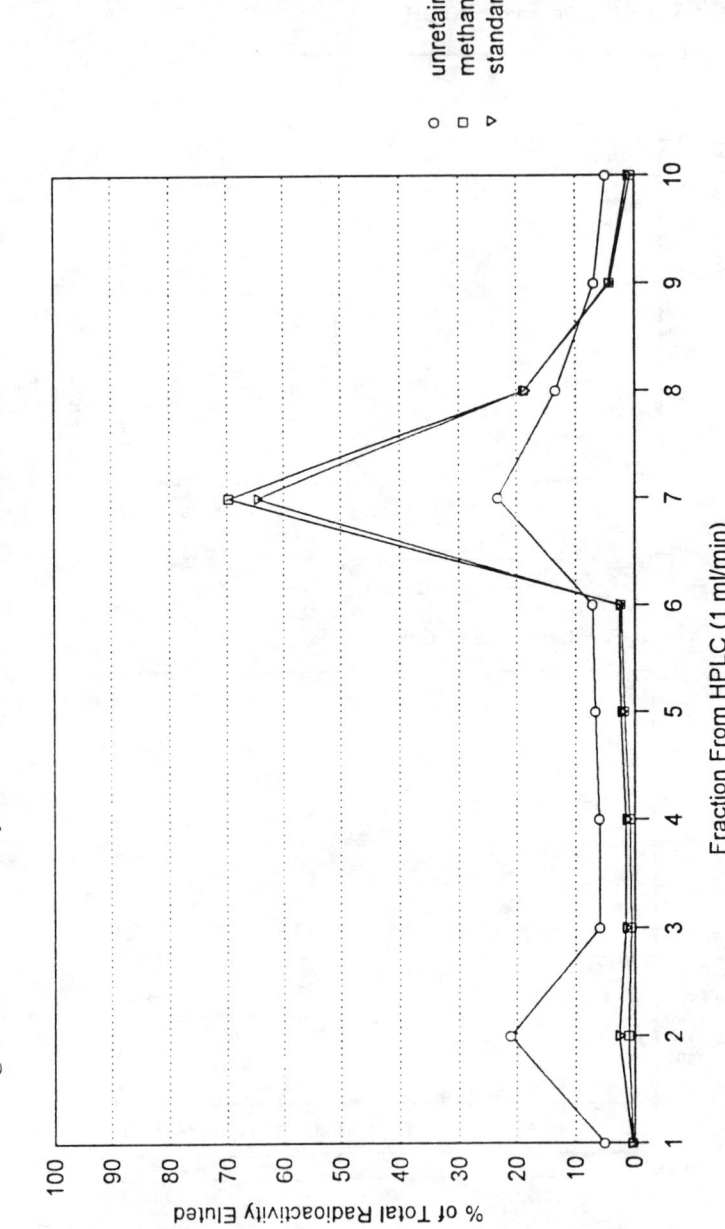

Figure 3.13 HPLC Analysis of Fractions Obtained from CNBr-Sepharose 4B Gel Immunoaffinity Columns

o   unretained fraction
□   methanol fraction
▽   standard ³H-AFB₁

When an immunoaffinity column was prepared from rabbit anti-AFB_1 serum coupled to EAH-Sepharose 4B gel, the elution profile of ^3H-AFB_1 was very different. It can be seen from Fig. 3.12b that a large percentage of the radioactivity appeared in the PBS fractions, indicating that the sample was not adsorbed onto the affinity gel and was easily eluted by just PBS. A small percentage of the radioactivity was retained and was subsequently eluted by methanol. This was probably due to a small amount of ligand being successfully coupled with the gel. However, this only gave a very small retention capacity for the affinity gel and such a gel was very unsatisfactory for the clean-up of AFB_1 samples.

The flow of solution through the immunoaffinity columns was only by the force of gravity and thus was fairly slow. The collection of a volume of 10 ml was not efficient and to evaporate 10 ml in a vacuum concentrator was inconvenient. The percentage recovery of radioactivity in the void (unretained) fraction, the first 4 ml of the PBS fraction and the first 4 ml of the methanol fraction are shown in Table 3.3. As about 93% of the total radioactivity could be recovered in the first 4 ml of the methanol fraction, it was decided that only 5 ml of PBS and methanol would be used in future analyses when eluting AFB1 from immunoaffinity columns.

Table 3.3 Radioactivity in fractions from immunoaffinity column, obtained after loading with 1 ml sample containing 20 ng or 40 ng of ^3H-AFB_1

CNBr-Sepharose 4B Gel

Fraction from affinity column	% of total radioactivity eluted	
Void (unretained)	0.08	0.11
PBS washing (first 4 ml)	3.68	4.35
Methanol washing (first 4 ml)	93.51	93.10

EAH-Sepharose 4B Gel

Fraction from affinity column	Radioactivity	
Void (unretained)	0.11	0.06
PBS washing (first 4 ml)	56.23	66.47
Methanol washing (first 4 ml)	25.54	18.51

In this experiment, eluates from the immunoaffinity columns were collected in 2 ml fractions. They were concentrated to about 0.5 ml and then the volume adjusted to 1 ml with PBS. This concentration procedure did not seem to affect the recovery of radioactivity or AFB_1 (see section 3.2.5.10).

For the same experiment using columns packed with immunoaffinity gel coupled with the rat monoclonal antibody, each column was eluted with only 5 ml of PBS and 5 ml of methanol after loading sample as this volume was to be sufficient. The elution profiles are shown in Fig. 3.14. Over 90% of the radioactivity was eluted in the methanol fractions.

3.2.5.7 Immunoaffinity column experiment of AFB₁-lysine

Most aflatoxins and related compounds exhibit a strong fluorescence when viewed under ultraviolet light. AFB_1 was found to have a maximum fluorescence emission at 425 nm (blue colour) whereas the maximum fluorescence emission for AFG_1 was found to be at 450 nm (green colour). In previous experiments, ^3H-AFB_1 was used in the investigation of AFB_1 in Sep-Pak C_{18} cartridges and immunoaffinity columns. It was necessary to confirm that lysine-AFB_1, the putative end product of AFB_1 albumin adduct digestion, would behave in a similar manner. Previously, the recovery of AFB_1 could be calculated from the associated radioactivity. Since tritiated AFB_1-lysine was not available, other physical and chemical properties of AFB_1-lysine must be employed. AFB_1-lysine was also found to be a fluorescent compound and thus its behaviour in immunoaffinity column was studied by determining the fluorescence of the different fractions collected.

The maximum excitation and emission wavelengths of lysine-AFB_1 were determined to be at 403 nm and 466 nm respectively. The fluorescence at these conditions was determined for all the fractions collected from the immunoaffinity column. It was found that under these conditions, PBS gave a fluorescence value of 14.5 (fixed scale 13). This was taken as the baseline value which was subtracted from the fluorescence readings of all other fractions. The fluorescence profile of the fractions are shown in Fig. 3.15. It can be seen that of all the fractions collected from the immunoaffinity column, only fraction 12 and 13, i.e. the first two methanol fractions, showed a significant fluorescence. It was evident that the sample of AFB_1-lysine, after being loaded onto the immunoaffinity column, was immobilised onto the gel. Even after being washed with 20 ml of PBS, it

Figure 3.14 Elution Characteristics of ^{3}H-AFB$_1$ from Immunoaffinity Columns Prepared from CNBr-Sepharose 4B Gel Coupled with Rat anti-AFB$_1$ Monoclonal Antibody

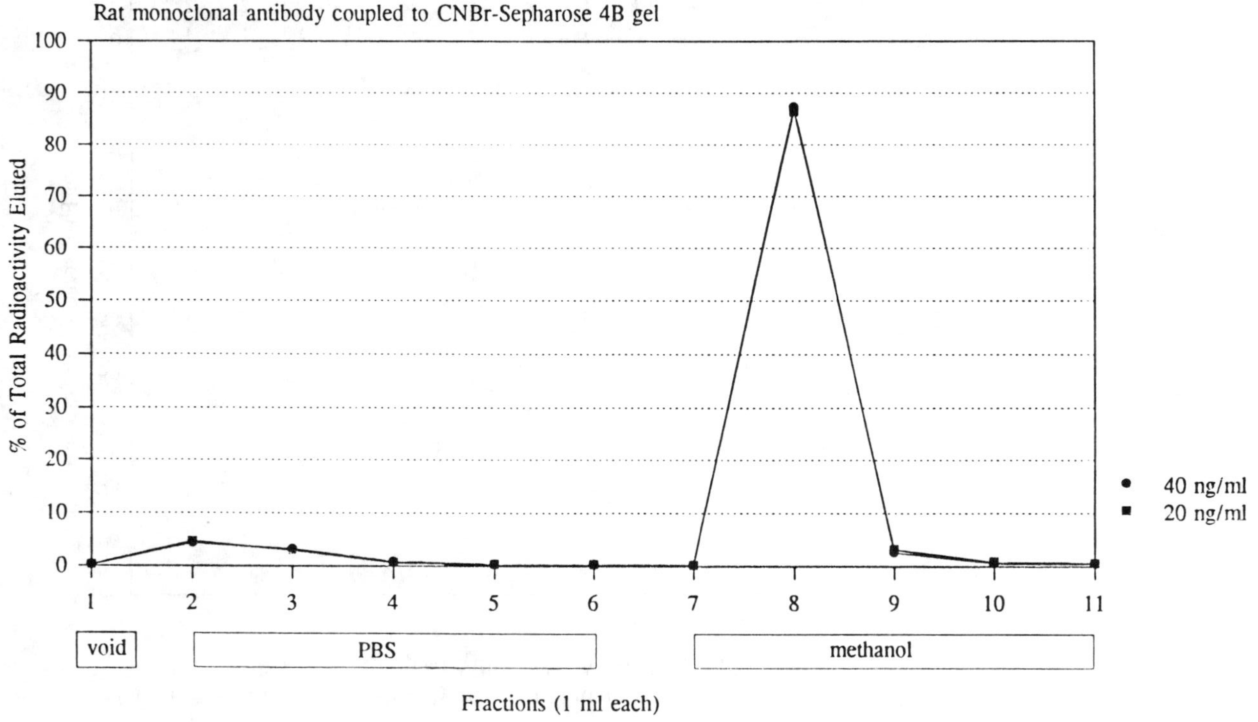

Rat monoclonal antibody coupled to CNBr-Sepharose 4B gel

Figure 3.15 Elution Characteristics of AFB$_1$-lysine from Immunoaffinity Columns Prepared from CNBr-Sepharose 4B Gel Coupled with Rabbit Anti-AFB$_1$ Anti-serum

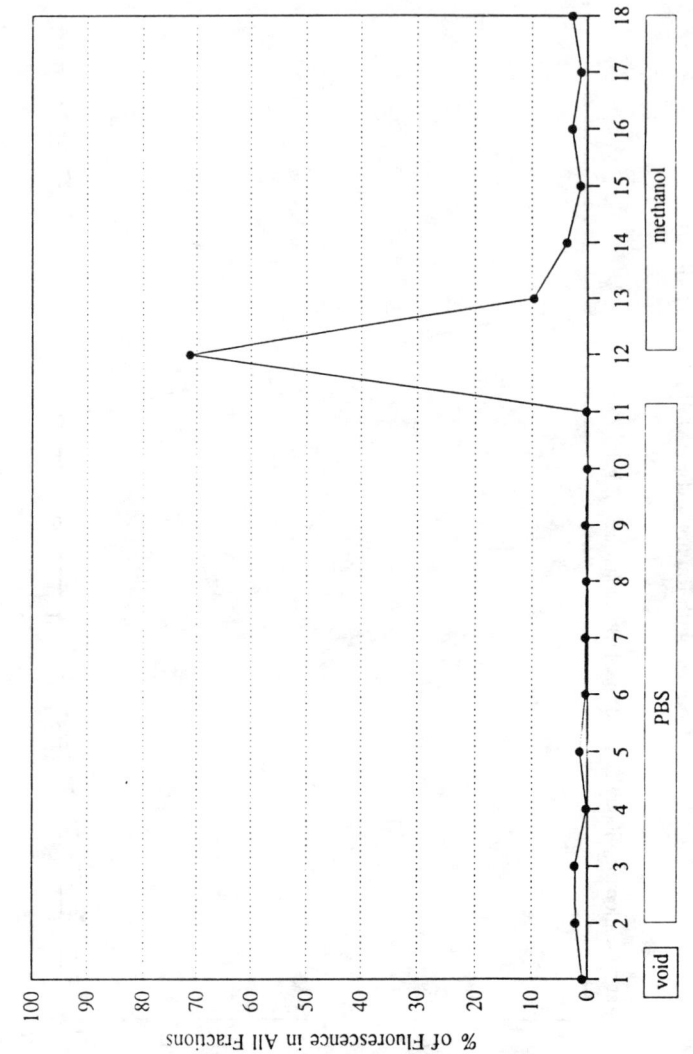

was not desorbed from the column. The ligand (anti-AFB_1 antibodies) coupled onto the gel thus showed a high affinity for AFB_1-lysine. The desorption of immobilised AFB_1-lysine was effected by washing with methanol. The recovery was 84.4% in the first 3 methanol fractions (Table 3.4). Since the recovery was high in this volume, it was decided that in future analyses, the column would be washed with 5 ml of PBS and 5 ml of methanol, to facilitate the concentration process.

Although this experiment was not repeated using a column packed with immunoaffinity gel prepared with the rat monoclonal antibody, since this monoclonal antibody was shown to have high specificity and sensitivity towards AFB_1-lysine (section 3.2.5.4), it was satisfactory to assume the same high retention of AFB_1-lysine by such an immunoaffinity column.

Table 3.4 Fluorescence in fractions collected from immunoaffinity column, obtained after loading with 1 ml sample containing 40 ng of AFB_1-lysine

Eluant	Fraction (2 ml each)	Fluorescence	Percentage	Remarks
Void	1	0.9	0.85	
PBS	2	2.2	2.07	4.43% eluted in
	3	2.3	2.17	first 6 ml PBS
	4	0.2	0.19	
	5	1.4	1.32	
	6	0.4	0.38	
	7	0.4	0.38	
	8	0.2	0.19	
	9	0.4	0.38	
	10	0.0	0.00	
	11	0.2	0.19	
Methanol	12	75.5	71.22	84.42% eluted
	13	10.2	9.62	in first 6 ml
	14	3.8	3.58	methanol
	15	1.2	1.13	
	16	2.8	2.64	
	17	1.1	1.04	
	18	2.8	2.64	

3.2.5.8 Digestion of serum albumin by proteinase K

The recoveries of serum albumin digestion and the subsequent precipitation step (to remove excess enzyme) of the 4 different regimens are shown in Table 3.5.

Table 3.5   Recovery of digested rat serum albumin modified by ^{3}H-AFB$_1$-lysine in different digestion regimens

Regimen	Radioactivity of digested material (DPM/ml)*	Recovery (%)**
A	7,423	7.2
B	70,528	68.9
C	69,170	67.6
D	69,550	67.9

Regimens
A   No Proteinase K
B   Proteinase K at 0 hr and 4 hr
C   Proteinase K at 0 hr, 2 hr and 4 hr
D   Proteinase K at 0 hr, 2 hr and 24 hr
*   Mean of duplicate readings
** Recovery calculated from the radioactivity of rat serum albumin solution at 102,373 DPM/ml

The modified rat serum albumin was found to have a level of modification of about 25 ng AFB$_1$/mg of albumin (section 3.2.5.2). The enzymatic action of proteinase K was a non-specific one and it would bring about proteolysis of any peptide linkage which it came across randomly. It is known that AFB$_1$ modifies serum albumin via the lysine residues. Therefore, during proteolysis by proteinase K, it could not be guaranteed that all the peptide linkages at the lysine residues would be broken up. Thus, not only lysine-AFB$_1$ would be released but also a variety of other modified or unmodified peptides. Also due to its non-specificity, proteinase K would hydrolyse other molecules of the enzyme, as well as serum albumin. The enzymatic action might terminate quite soon. Therefore, excess enzymes might be required to further the digestion process. But the duration of action depends on a number of factors including the type of enzyme, the digestion conditions e.g. pH and temperature, the amount and nature of the substrate present, etc. The requirement for the optimal performance of a digestion thus needed to be evaluated individually.

In this experiment, the substrate was about 1.5 mg of ^{3}H-AFB$_1$ modified serum albumin. After the digestion procedure, excess enzymes, whole digested serum albumin and some larger peptides would be precipitated by cold ethanol and freezing. The addition of a small amount of BSA would help precipitate these materials. The radioactivity in the end product represented released ^{3}H-AFB$_1$-lysine residues and other short peptides.

From Table 3.5, it can be seen that without any proteolytic enzymes (Regimen A), almost all ^{3}H-AFB$_1$-modified serum albumin was removed in the precipitation step. Only 7% of the original radioactivity of the starting material was recovered. Albumin is not soluble in ethanol and would be precipitated by cold ethanol. In the other 3 regimens, the recoveries were very similar, all at around 67–68%. It indicated that the amount of ^{3}H-AFB$_1$ in the post-digestion sample was similar. But at this stage, it was not possible to differentiate if the product of digestion was the same in these three samples. There might be more fully digested product i.e. AFB$_1$-lysine in one sample and in another more AFB$_1$-peptides. All that could be concluded was that the total amount of radioactive AFB$_1$, irrespective of the form it was contained, was about the same in the digestion end products of regimen B, C and D. Theoretically, with more enzyme added at regular intervals, the digestion of the substrate (serum albumin in this case) would be more complete. It might be expected that in regimen D, the recovery was higher than that in regimen B. This was not the case found in this experiment. This could be because the enzyme was in excess already or the digestion was complete already with the least amount of enzyme. This calls for further investigation.

3.2.5.9 Effect of ethanol in samples to be applied onto Sep-Pak C$_{18}$ cartridges

The percentage of recovery in the respective fractions of the three regimens is shown in Table 3.6. After digestion and removal of excess enzymes, there was still a lot of unwanted material in the reconstituted sample. e.g. large peptides and other water soluble materials. It was possible to remove these by a reverse phase Sep-Pak cartridge. ^{3}H-AFB$_1$-modified material e.g. lysine or peptides are water insoluble and would be retained by the cartridge. They could be recovered by eluting the Sep-Pak cartridge with methanol. The presence of organic solvent e.g. ethanol or methanol in the sample to be applied on the cartridge would affect the adsorption of ^{3}H-AFB$_1$-modified material onto the solid support.

In regimen A, the ethanol in the post digestion sample was removed in

Table 3.6   Recovery of radioactivity in different fractions from Sep-Pak C_{18} cartridges obtained after loading digested ^{3}H-AFB$_1$-modified rat serum albumin — effect of concentration of ethanol in samples

Protocol	Radioactivity recovered in fractions (% of total)		
	Void	PBS	Methanol
A	13.1 (1 ml)	11.1	75.8
B	80.8 (25 ml)	2.5	19.2
C	53.2 (50 ml)	2.4	44.5

a vacuum concentrator. When this sample was applied onto a Sep-Pak cartridge, 75.8% of the total recovered radioactivity was retained and was present in the methanol fraction. When comparing the results to that in regimen B, it can be seen clearly that the ethanol present prevented the adsorption of ^{3}H-AFB$_1$-modified material, most of which subsequently appeared in the 'void' fraction.

The small percentage of radioactive material adsorbed onto the cartridge was eluted by methanol. Clearly, dilution of the post-digestion sample to 25 ml was not able to negate the interfering action of ethanol present. Further dilution of the sample to 50 ml brought the recovery in the methanol fraction up to 44.5%, although this was not a good working regimen as the 'void' volume was excessively large and the recovery was still low. To ensure a good recovery in the methanol fraction, it was necessary to remove all ethanol in the sample to be applied onto a Sep-Pak C_{18} cartridge.

3.2.5.10   Recovery of radioactivity after drying in a vacuum concentrator

The effect of drying in a vacuum concentrator on the recovery of the radioactivity of ^{3}H-AFB$_1$ is shown in Table 3.7. Drying samples of radioactive AFB$_1$ in a vacuum concentrator seemed to reduce a small percentage of the radioactivity. Part of this loss could be accounted for by non-exchange tritium which evaporated with the solvent. Nevertheless, this percentage was less than 10% for a range of AFB$_1$ concentrations.

3.2.5.11   Recovery of the overall clean-up procedure for the analysis of serum albumin adducts of AFB1

The analysis of serum albumin AFB$_1$ adducts involved a number of clean

Table 3.7 Percentage recovery of radioactivity of a sample of ^{3}H-AFB$_1$ following drying in a vacuum concentrator

Sample	Volume of ^{3}H-AFB$_1$ spiked (μl)	Radioactive counts (DPM/ml)	Recovery compared to A (%)
A1	100	176912	—
A2	50	90410	—
A3	20	37718	—
A4	0	58	—
B1	100	160245	90.6
B2	50	84357	93.3
B3	20	36258	96.1
B4	0	79	—
C1	100	148807	84.1
C2	50	87517	96.8
C3	20	34894	92.5
C4	0	57	—

A   Counted directly
B   5 ml methanol, 0.5 ml PBS added for evaporation
C   5 ml PBS added for evaporation

up steps before the detection by ELISA or HPLC. It was necessary to determine the recovery of the individual steps, such that an overall recovery, as an indication of the sensitivity of the analytical procedure, could be obtained. From the detection method alone i.e. the ELISA or HPLC, a detection limit could be read directly from the detection results. The detection limit refers to the actual level measured by the detection method. It must be considered in the context of the percentage recovery of that particular method in order to obtain the 'real' level that needs to exist in the sample before detection is possible. For example, if in an analytical procedure, the detection limit of the detection method was 5 ng of the substance in question, it meant that during the detection, a sample containing 5 ng or more of the substance would be picked up as a 'positive' sample. However, it did not directly imply that if there was a study sample containing 5 ng of the substance, it would be detected as positive by the analytical procedure. If the recovery of the overall analytical procedure, i.e. all the different steps that a sample must be taken through, was 10%, then the 'real' level in the original study sample needed to be at least 50 ng or more in order to be detected. This would be known as the absolute detection limit. Therefore, the percentage recovery

is an important factor contributing to the sensitivity of an analytical procedure.

In this study of AFB_1 serum albumin adducts, a study sample needed
to be taken through the steps of albumin isolation, albumin digestion with
proteinase K, clean-up by a Sep-Pak C_{18} cartridge and clean-up by an
anti-AFB_1 immunoaffinity column before any AFB_1-albumin adducts
could be detected by either ELISA or HPLC. The percentage recovery at
each step, for each fraction, and the overall percentage recovery of the 4
different digestion regimens are shown in Table 3.8. In regimen A, where
no enzyme was present in the digestion process, the recovery of radioactivity following removal of insoluble proteins in ethanol was so low that
the amount of radioactivity was extremely small. Although this sample
was taken through the following steps, the percentage recovery calculated
were unreliable as the counts were not much more than the background
radioactivity. The results in regimen A were included for completeness

Table 3.8 Percentage recovery at each step for each fraction for
different study regimens

	Percentage recovery (%)			
	A*	B	C	D
Albumin digestion & removal of excess enzyme	7.25	68.9	67.7	67.9
Sep-Pak C_{18} cartridge				
void	24.6	9.4	8.9	10.7
PBS	28.7	8.0	6.9	9.5
methanol	**46.4**	**54.6**	**58.3**	**45.7**
total recovery	99.7	72.0	74.1	65.9
Immunoaffinity column				
void	26.0	3.0	2.4	3.1
PBS	33.0	12.0	11.8	12.4
methanol	**61.9**	**61.9**	**57.2**	**59.4**
total recovery	120.9	76.9	71.4	74.9
Overall recovery of clean UP steps	20.8	**23.3**	**22.5**	**18.4**

* Results for regimen A not reliable (see text)
Regimens
A   No proteinase K
B   Proteinase K at 0 hr & 4 hr
C   Proteinase K at 0 hr, 2 hr & 4 hr
D   Proteinase K at 0 hr, 2 hr, 4 hr & 24 hr

rather than as an indication of the efficiency of the digestion process. It should, therefore, not be taken into serious consideration. Regimens B, C and D all produced similar percentage recovery following the digestion process. In fact, the recoveries for the Sep-Pak cartridge clean up and the immunoaffinity column clean up did not differ by a wide margin among these three regimens. The overall recovery of the digestion and clean up steps of Regimen B, C and D were 23.3%, 22.5% and 18.4% respectively. The slightly lower value for regimen D was due to a lower percentage recovery at the Sep-Pak cartridge step. This was not anticipated. The total recovery of radioactivity from the Sep-Pak cartridge in regimen D was also lower than in regimens B and C. It was not known whether this was due to an artifact or the fact that the addition of too much enzyme added actually impaired the recovery. Other than this point, the recoveries in various fractions were very similar in these three regimens.

From Table 3.8, it can be seen that maximum recovery was obtained with regimen B. i.e. when proteinase K was added to the system at 0 hr and 4 hr and the incubation continued for a total of 28 hours. Further addition of enzymes did not increase the recovery further. Since maximum recovery was achieved in regimen B, there was no need to increase the amount of enzyme to be added. The recovery was maximized in regimen B when the starting material was 1.5 mg of serum albumin. The amount of enzyme required and how often it is necessary to add more enzyme into the digestion mixture will vary with the amount and nature of the starting material, the type of enzyme used and other incubation conditions. In this case, it was not known whether digestion was maximum or the enzyme was in excess. In any case, no improvement in the recovery could be achieved with more enzyme. Therefore, it has been decided to choose regimen B for further studies.

In this experiment, all the digestion regimens were incubated for a total of 28 hours. This was because enzyme was added at 24hr in regimen D and so another 4 hours were allowed. Since regimen B was chosen as the digestion regimen for future studies, it was decided for convenience purpose to allow a total of 24 hours for incubation. It was anticipated that beyond this length of time, further incubation would not improve digestion or recovery. Therefore, the chosen digestion regimen was:

Starting material 1.5 mg serum albumin;
1 mg proteinase K added at 0 hr & 4 hr;
Total incubation period 24 hours.

3.2.5.12   HPLC analysis of samples obtained after all clean-up procedures

It has been discussed previously that the end product of digestion of AFB_1-modified serum albumin was putatively AFB_1-lysine if digestion were complete (see section 3.1.3. and section 3.2.1.). In practice, it is expected that AFB_1-lysine will not be the only product of digestion. Instead, a range of AFB_1-peptides will be released. In a study by Wild *et al.* previous study, the recovery from a method involving albumin hydrolysis and detection by ELISA was 23%, compared to a recovery of only 5.5% if the detection method was HPLC with fluorescence detection (Wild *et al.*, 1990b). This was explained by the fact that in detection by HPLC and fluorescence detector, only one distinct entity, AFB_1-lysine was measured, whereas the anti-AFB_1 antibody used in ELISA was able to recognised a range of AFB_1-modified materials, although the inhibition produced may differ from the major adduct, AFB_1-lysine. This basic difference in the principle of detection of the two methods gave rise to the difference in the percentage recovery.

Detection by HPLC is no doubt a very precise method. It would be the method of choice when the amount of lysine-AFB_1 contained in a sample was known to be above the detection limit. Since a proportion of the AFB_1 adducted to serum albumin would end up in peptides following digestion, a falsely low reading would be produced if detection relied on HPLC/ fluorescence alone.

When AFB_1-modified serum albumin samples were studied using ELISA after having been taken through the many steps of digestion and clean up, they produced inhibition in ELISA which allowed estimation of AFB_1 equivalent that existed. These same samples were studied by HPLC by injecting 100 µl into the system.

The chromatograms produced for samples from regimens B, C and D are shown in Fig. 3.16. A standard sample of lysine-AFB_1 was detected by this system and was eluted at retention time 6.6 minutes. Converting from the radioactivity, in 1 ml of the sample from regimen B, there should be about 8 ng of AFB_1. If 100 µl was injected into the HPLC, there should be about 0.8 ng of AFB_1 applied. It was shown previously in this HPLC set up that the absolute detection limit was about 0.08 ng of AFB_1-lysine. Therefore, it was expected that if all the radioactivity in the sample from regimen B was in the form of AFB_1-lysine, there should be a very distinct peak, representing AFB_1-lysine being eluted at 6.6 minutes. This was not the

Figure 3.16　HPLC Chromatograms of Authentic AFB₁-lysine and Samples Ready for ELISA from Digestion Regimens B, C and D, Which Has Been Subject to the Clean-up Procedures

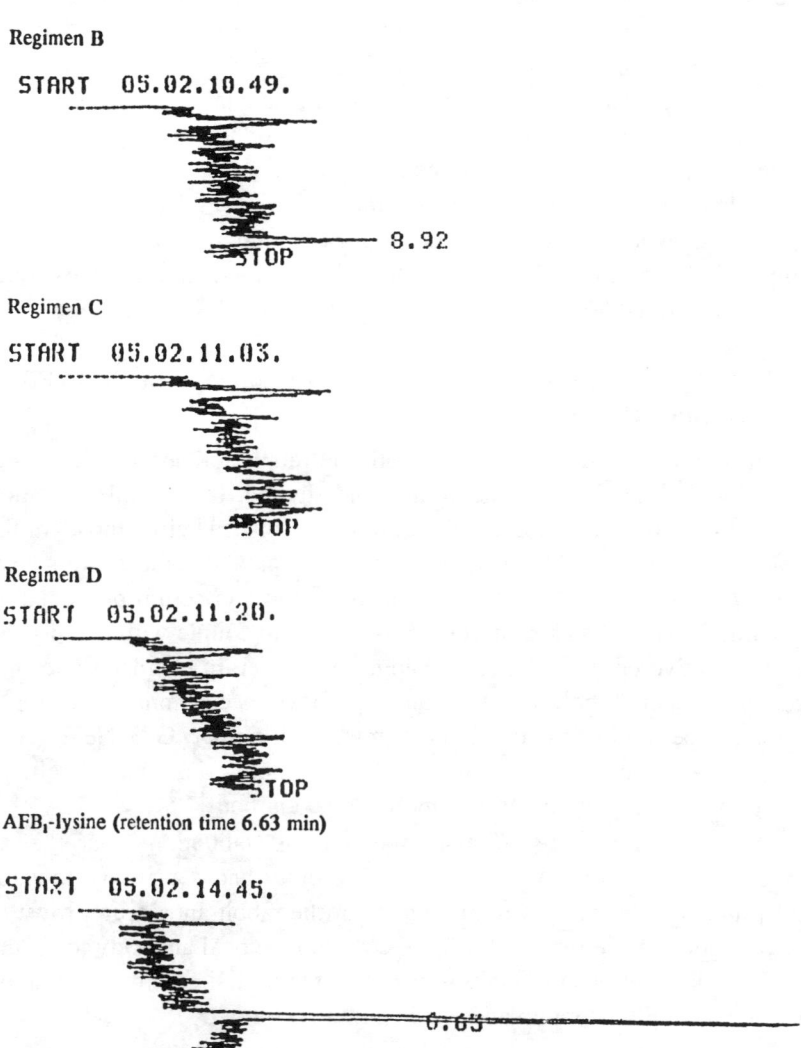

Regimen B

START　05.02.10.49.

8.92

Regimen C

START　05.02.11.03.

Regimen D

START　05.02.11.20.

AFB₁-lysine (retention time 6.63 min)

START　05.02.14.45.

6.63

case. Instead, no clearly visibly peaks were seen. Fluorescent materials were eluted at a range of retention times but there was no distinct peaks that could be integrated. These could be AFB_1-peptides. Similar chromatograms were obtained for samples from regimens C and D. It can be seen that though these samples produced inhibition in ELISA, indicating recognition by anti-AFB_1 antibodies, the results were negative in HPLC analyses. This disagreement can partly be explained by the principle outlined above, in that most of the digestion products in these regimens existed not as lysine-AFB_1 but some as peptides.

Perhaps it would be possible to combine these two detection methods after the digestion and clean up of serum albumin samples. Initially the sample could be screened by ELISA for inhibition. Positive samples could then be confirmed for AFB_1-lysine by HPLC.

3.2.5.13   The use of rabbit anti-AFB1 anti-serum and rat anti-AFB_1 monoclonal antibody

All through the validation process, both the rabbit anti-serum and the rat monoclonal antibody were mentioned and studied. In fact, all validation processes for using the rabbit anti-serum were finished before those for the monoclonal antibody. At that stage, it was then found that there might have been a change in the characteristics of the rabbit anti-serum produced by the animal as new batches of anti-serum failed to couple with affinity gel on consecutive occassions. This change in anti-serum characteristics has been encountered before when animals have been immunised for a prolonged period of time (personal communication, Dr. G.E. Neal). As a result, it was necessary to change over to a more constant and reliable source of supply of antibody — a monoclonal antibody.

It has been demonstrated by the various validations that the rat monoclonal antibody possesses high specificity and sensitivity towards AFB_1 and AFB_1-lysine, even more so than the rabbit anti-serum. Most of the validations were repeated using the rat monoclonal antibody to ensure that it could safely and reliably replace the rabbit anti-serum in our study regimen for AFB_1-albumin adducts in human serum.

3.2.6   *Summary*

Various methods of aflatoxin exposure assessment have been used. Measurement of AFB_1 levels in food does not provide any information on the biologically effective dose of this mycotoxin at the individual level, whereas the measurement of the AFB_1-DNA or protein adducts circulating in body fluids or tissues can serve as a marker for both AFB_1 exposure and in vivo metabolic activation. Immunological assays employing polyclonal antibody or monoclonal antibody are able to measure very low levels of AFB_1 and adducts.

In this study, a method was successfully developed and validated for the assay of AFB_1-albumin adducts in serum, employing both a rabbit anti-AFB_1 anti-serum and a rat anti-AFB1 monoclonal antibody. In the end, a rat monoclonal antibody was used for the study. The study regimen involved firstly the isolation of serum albumin which was digested by a protease proteinase K to release the major serum albumin adduct — AFB_1-lysine together with other AFB_1-peptides. This was followed by clean-up steps by a Sep-Pak C_{18} cartridge and a specific immunoaffinity column. The final sample was studied by ELISA and HPLC. The study by HPLC, due to its intrinsic properties, could only separate and quantify AFB_1-lysine as one entity. On the other hand, because the rat monoclonal antibody was capable of recognising AFB_1, AFB_1-lysine and a range of other AFB_1 metabolites, study by ELISA could give a representative estimation of exposure.

The optimal digestion process was determined to be a 24 hr digestion with proteinase K added at O hr and 4 hr. The capacity was over 40 ng of AFB_1 for both the Sep-Pak C_{18} cartridge and the immunoaffinity column. The overall process including the isolation of albumin from serum, digestion of albumin to release AFB_1-modified adducts and the clean-up process was validated using ^{3}H-AFB_1-modified animal serum by injecting them with ^{3}H-AFB_1. The overall percentage recovery of 23.3%, although low, was comparable to some similar studies (Wild et al., 1990b).

The rat monoclonal antibody was found to have high specificity and sensitivity towards both AFB_1, AFB_1-lysine and some other AFB_1 metabolites and adducts. It could be diluted 1:5,000 for use in the competitive ELISA assay developed in this study.

This regimen was used in the study of possible AFB_1 exposure in man.

3.3 Monitoring of AFB_1-albumin adducts in plasma of patients with liver disease and hepatocellular carcinoma

3.3.1 Introduction

There is considerable evidence indicating an association between aflatoxin exposure and hepatocellular carcinoma in man (see section 3.1.4.5). Epidemiology studies correlating the dietary levels of AFB_1 and the incidence of HCC have been carried out in China, Swaziland and Kenya, providing positive association and dosimetery data between high intakes of aflatoxins and high incidence rates of HCC. However, these data could not provide information on the biologically effective dose of aflatoxin at the individual level. i.e. the amount of activated agent that has actually reacted with critical cellular targets, including the nucleic acids and proteins, which may be influenced by intake, distribution, metabolic activation and excretion of aflatoxin. Thus there is a strong motivation to investigate further the circumstantial relationship between aflatoxin ingestion and HCC incidence by monitoring aflatoxin and its metabolites and adducts in human body fluids, in order to compile biochemical and molecular epidemiological data. The main goal of these studies is to identify individuals at high risk of HCC by obtaining evidence of high exposure to AFB_1, leading to pathobiological lesions in target cells, and/or increased oncogenic susceptibility due to host factors including chronic hepatitis B infection, consumption of alcohol or cigarettes and other possible procarcinogenic substances.

Monitoring of AFB_1 exposure or any other suspected carcinogen in man provides evidence of possible pathobiological lesions in target cells at an individual level and also a bridge between laboratory animal and human studies. However, since there may be a lag time, possibly of decades, between exposure and effects, biological exposure monitoring should ideally be parallelled with environmental monitoring.

To detect these extremely low levels of the carcinogen in human body fluids or tissues, the method used must be sensitive and specific. Possible modifying and confounding factors must also be taken into account when analysing the results of exposure monitoring which may affect their interpretation. For the association between AFB_1 and HCC, modifying factors include diet (especially the protein content), smoking habit, intake of alcohol and other drugs. These may play a role in the metabolic activation or detoxification of AFB_1 by affecting the various enzyme systems involved. When other confounding factors were removed, cigarette smoking was found to have a protective effect against HCC in Fujian Province of China where incidence of both HCC and dietary contamination by AFB_1 were high (Lin, Yang, Ye, Xu, Yang, Zhang, Wu & Nebert, 1991). A suggested possible mechanism was that cigarette smoking induced CYP1A2 and diverted the metabolism of AFB_1 to the less toxic AFM_1 and thus less of

AFB_1-8,9-epoxide was produced. Confounding factors which were known to be associated with HCC include hepatitis B infection and liver cirrhosis.

The southeast coast of China, including Hong Kong is considered to be an endemic area for HCC. The mortality rate of HCC could be up to 300 per 100,000/year for males in some parts of China. In Hong Kong, the rate is about 30 per 100,000/year for males. Shank and Wogan surveyed foodstuffs on the market in Hong Kong in the 70's and found evidence of contamination by AFB_1 (Shank & Wogan, 1972b). However, standards of living and the general storage of food and hygiene have much improved since then. In a case-control study conducted in Hong Kong where 107 HCC patients and 107 controls were studied, the relative risk of HCC was not related to the dietary intake of corn or beans, which were found to be the chief sources of AFB_1 contamination in Hong Kong. The relative risk was found to be increase by a factor of 2.2, though not significantly, for consumption of other grains, including wheat, barley and oats (Lam, Yu, Leung & Henderson, 1982).

The objective of the present study was to determine whether exposure to AFB_1 was an important factor associated with the high incidence of HCC in Hong Kong. An assay for AFB_1-albumin adducts in human serum employing an ELISA method was developed successfully (section 3.2) and was applied to the estimation of possible exposure to AFB1 among patients with HCC, other liver diseases and also patients without liver disease. As this was the first study of its kind in Hong Kong looking at human exposure to AFB_1 on an individual basis by monitoring AFB_1-albumin adducts in the serum, it was difficult to make a prediction of the probable levels of measurement, if the adduct was detectable. Both patients with and without liver diseases were recruited into this study for comparison as their involvement with the study was very little — only 10 ml whole blood to be taken at the same time of their other routine blood tests and some questions to be answered on their diet.

Nevertheless, since it is well established that cancer is a disease with a very long latent period, it is not to be expected that the presence of AFB_1 or its adducts in the blood samples would have any particular relevance in terms of the carcinogenic process in any individual patient. However, if the dietary patterns of the Hong Kong people have not changed dramatically during the past years, and especially for the liver disease/cancer patients, despite their illness, the data obtained may provide valuable information on probable HCC risk due to exposure to AFB_1 and its *in vivo* metabolic activation.

3.3.2 Material and methods

3.3.2.1 Subject

Subjects were recruited for 3 main categories:

> Group A: Subjects with no history or obvious evidence of liver disease
> Group B: Patients with various liver diseases
> Group C: Patients with hepatocellular carcinoma

All subjects were Chinese. Group B subjects were further divided into Group B1, B2 and B3. They were patients with chronic hepatitis B infection, alcoholics and other liver diseases (mostly Non A – Non B hepatitis), respectively. Group A subjects were either patients attending other clinics at the Li Ka Shing Specialist Clinics or patients and volunteers visiting the Clinical Pharmacology Studies Unit and Metabolic Investigation Unit at the Prince of Wales Hospital. They might suffer from other medical problems including hypertension and diabetes, but had no history or obvious evidence of liver disease. Details of their past medical history and current medications were noted. Subjects in Group B and Group C were patients of the Liver Clinic and the Joint Hepatoma Clinic at the Li Ka Shing Specialist Clinic, respectively. These patients all had detailed patient records and previous laboratory tests to confirm diagnoses and were referred by their physicians-in-charge. It was intended to recruit about 50 patients in each group. The final numbers recruited for Groups A, B and C were 51, 47 and 49, respectively.

A summary of the details of age, body weight and height of the subjects in each group are shown in Table 3.9 and the plasma biochemistry screen data are shown in Table 3.10. The study was explained in outline to each patient who was recruited for the study and informed consent was given by each subject. They were each questioned on their smoking and drinking habits and also on their diet, assisted by relatives when required.

3.3.2.2 Sample collections

10 ml venous blood sample was drawn from each subject into a heparinised tube either at the Li Ka Shing Specialist Clinics or The Clinical Pharmacology Studies Unit. The blood samples were kept on ice until returned to the laboratory within an hour. They were centrifuged at 1,400 xg for 10 minutes and the plasma separated for storage at $-70°C$ prior to analysis. A urine sample of 20 ml was also collected from each subject for reference.

Table 3.9 Details of Subjects in Different Groups

		Group A n = 51 Control	Group B1 n = 20 Chronic hepatitis B infection	Group B2 n = 18 Alcoholic	Group B3 n = 9 Other liver diseases	Group C n = 49 Hepatocellular carcinoma
Sex	M	40	18	17	4	42
	F	11	2	1	5	7
Age	Mean	50.9	53.4	56.5	59.6	52.2
	SD	9.9	10.2	9.3	10.5	13.2
	Range	16–68	36–68	44–75	39–73	19–79
Weight (kg)	Mean	64.9	58.9	53.4	56.8	58.0
	SD	10.8	10.2	7.8	13.6	9.9
	Range	40.0–90.0	35.5–75.0	35.7–66.0	36.7–84.8	42.5–84.0
Height (cm)	Mean	163.8	163.1	161.7	154.5	165.2
	SD	6.4	8.6	6.3	6.8	7.0
	Range	147–175	147–180	144–171	145–162	147–185

Table 3.10   Plasma Biochemistry Screen of Subjects in Different Study Groups

		Group A (n = 51)	Group B1 (n = 20)	Group B2 (n = 18)	Group B3 (n = 9)	Group C (n = 49)	Normal Range*
Na	Mean	139.4	140.1	137.7	138.5	136.7	137–142
(mmol l^{-1})	SD	2.5	2.5	4.0	2.9	4.0	
	Range	134–144	135–144	130–142	134–142	126–144	
K	Mean	4.1	3.9	3.8	4.0	4.1	3.5–5.1
(mmol l^{-1})	SD	0.6	0.5	0.5	0.9	0.5	
	Range	2.6–5.6	3.0–4.5	2.9–4.6	3.5–6.1	2.9–5.3	
Urea	Mean	6.3	6.6	4.9	5.9	5.9	3.4–8.9
(mmol l^{-1})	SD	1.4	1.9	1.6	2.5	1.8	
	Range	3.4–9.9	4.3–11.9	2.0–8.6	3.8–11.5	3.2–9.9	
Creatinine	Mean	96.6	94.2	87.7	93.5	85.8	64–96
(μmol l^{-1})	SD	31.4	17.1	8.2	41.3	16.4	
	Range	55–194	56–115	70–94	62–192	52–137	
Albumin	Mean	46.8	39.4	38.3	41.0	36.6	35–48
(g l^{-1})	SD	3.6	8.1	9.1	5.8	6.3	
	Range	38–57	20–48	22–50	32–48	23–50	
Total Bilirubin	Mean	11.5	24.8	18.9	18.4	22.4	0–15
(μmol l^{-1})	SD	7.2	19.5	17.8	18.0	18.8	
	Range	5–46	8–78	4–52	7–64	4–99	
Alkaline	Mean	74.5	159.0	104.5	94	171.8	40–136
Phosphatase	SD	22.7	108.3	45.6	33.3	114.7	
(IU l^{-1})	Range	36–166	59–444	68–210	58–167	56–564	
ALT	Mean	25.4	41.9	88.8	30.7	71.33	0–58
(IU l^{-1})	SD	23.5	40.8	110.8	19.1	61.0	
	Range	1–148	8–140	16–351	13–75	11–272	
α-foetoprotein	Mean	—	12.5	897.9	28.7	9861.8	< 10
(IU ml^{-1})	SD		11.9	3191	72.9	24036	
	Range		2–43	2–12800	2–223	3–132000	

* From the Department of Clinical Pathology, Prince of Wales Hospital, Shatin.

3.3.2.3   Assay for AFB_1-albumin adducts

Plasma samples (0.5 ml) were used in the assays for AFB_1-albumin adducts. Plasma albumin was isolated from each sample (section 3.2.3.7), digested with proteinase K (section 3.2.3.8) then subjected to clean-up procedures (section 3.2.3.2 and section 3.2.3.3) before analysing for AFB_1-albumin adducts by ELISA (section 3.2.3.1), using 6 replicates for each sample. Additional HPLC analyses would be done on positive samples (section 3.2.3.5). AFB_1-albumin adducts concentrations were expressed in AFB_1-lysine equivalents on a per mg of serum albumin basis.

3.3.2.4 Statistical analysis

Results were represented as mean standard deviation (SD) with the range. Descriptive statistics for each group and comparisons between groups were done by one way analysis of variance (ANOVA) with the computer statistics package SigmaStat (Version 1.01, 1993, Jandel Scientific, San Rafael, California, U.S.A.).

3.3.3 Results and discussion

The details of subjects in the study groups are shown in Table 3.9. The age, sex distribution and weight of the different groups were comparable. The mean age of subjects in each group was in the fifties but the range could be quite large. Male subjects in all Groups A, B and C outnumbered female subjects by a factor of 4 to 6. This ratio was expected for the incidence of HCC. Since none of the subjects was actually an in-patient of the hospital, their diet was essentially the same as the normal population except for some of the control subjects who might suffer from diabetes mellitus. Nevertheless, the appetite of the patients suffering from chronic illness might be impaired and the mean weights of subjects in Group B and Group C were lower than that of subjects in Group A. It was very difficult to obtain information on their diet from the patients. Rice is the staple food amongst the population in Hong Kong but not corn, peanuts and beans and a majority of the patients interviewed indicated intake of rice everyday.

The biochemistry screen of the subjects in different study groups is shown in Table 3.10. The mean results in each group were grossly normal except for elevated liver enzymes levels among patients with various liver diseases. The HCC group was also characterised by a much elevated serum α-foetoprotein of near 10,000 IU ml^{-1}.

From Fig. 3.9, it can be seen that the steep slope of the standard ELISA curves, representing the proportional region, lies between the percentage of inhibition of 20% to 80% and this is the most reliable portion of the standard curves to be used in the conversion to concentrations of the detected substances — AFB₁ and AFB₁-lysine. Using these standard curves, inhibition below 20% could still be detected but was not reliable. Therefore, a cut off point was taken at 20% inhibition. This corresponded to a concentration of approximately 0.03 ng ml^{-1} of AFB₁-lysine equivalent in the test samples. When converted to the actual amount of AFB₁-lysine loaded into the wells of ELISA plates, this was approximately 0.75 pg of AFB₁-lysine (volume loaded into each well was 50 μl of the 1:1

diluted original sample). This was the absolute detection limit of the assay which referred to the actual level measured and must be considered together with the percentage recovery in order to obtain the 'real' level required to be present in a sample for detection to be possible. The recovery of the whole assay process was found to be 23.3% (section 3.2.5.11), therefore, the detection limit would be approximately 3.2 pg AFB_1-lysine present in 1.5 mg albumin (starting material in validation). This was equivalent to approximately 2 pg AFB_1-lysine/mg albumin.

Under these assay conditions and detection limits, it was found that none of the 147 serum samples studied in the 3 study groups showed a percentage of inhibition higher that 20%. The distribution of the percentage of inhibition of the serum samples from subjects in these 3 study groups is shown in a box plot in Fig. 3.17 and there was no statistically significant difference between the 3 groups. Most of the results were near zero or just slightly negative and only a very small number of samples with values around 10% inhibition. A number of the samples showed a negative percentage of inhibition. This was due to the fact that the percentage of inhibition was calculated using a blank PBS solution as the level of zero inhibition. When a control human serum sample or a study human serum sample produced a slightly more intense colour on the ELISA plate, the calculated pecentage of inhibition would be negative. But the difference was very small and the largest negative value was only around −10%. Due to the low levels of inhibition by the study samples, it was not possible to convert them into AFB_1-lysine equivalent concentrations as they were below the proportional range of the standard ELISA curve. In other words, it could be said that all the samples presented for ELISA were of a concentration below 0.03 ng ml^{-1} of AFB_1-lysine equivalent or the serum samples of all the study subjects contained less than 2 pg AFB_1-lysine per mg of albumin, which was the detection limit of this assay. As expected, no identifiable peaks could be detected when these samples were injected into the HPLC system (section 3.2.3.5). The chromatograms resembled those shown in Fig 3.16 with no distinguishable peaks eluted at the retention time of AFB_1-lysine.

The objective of this study was to determine whether exposure to AFB1 was an important factor associated with the high incidence of HCC in Hong Kong by monitoring AFB_1-lysine from serum albumin. In trying to produce such retrospective or prospective epidemiological data, the laboratory assay used for analysis is required to possess several properties — sensitivity, specificity, noninvasive sampling, large sample capacity,

Figure 3.17   Box Plot Showing the Distribution of the Percentages of Inhibition
in ELSA Produced by Serum Samples of the Three Study Groups

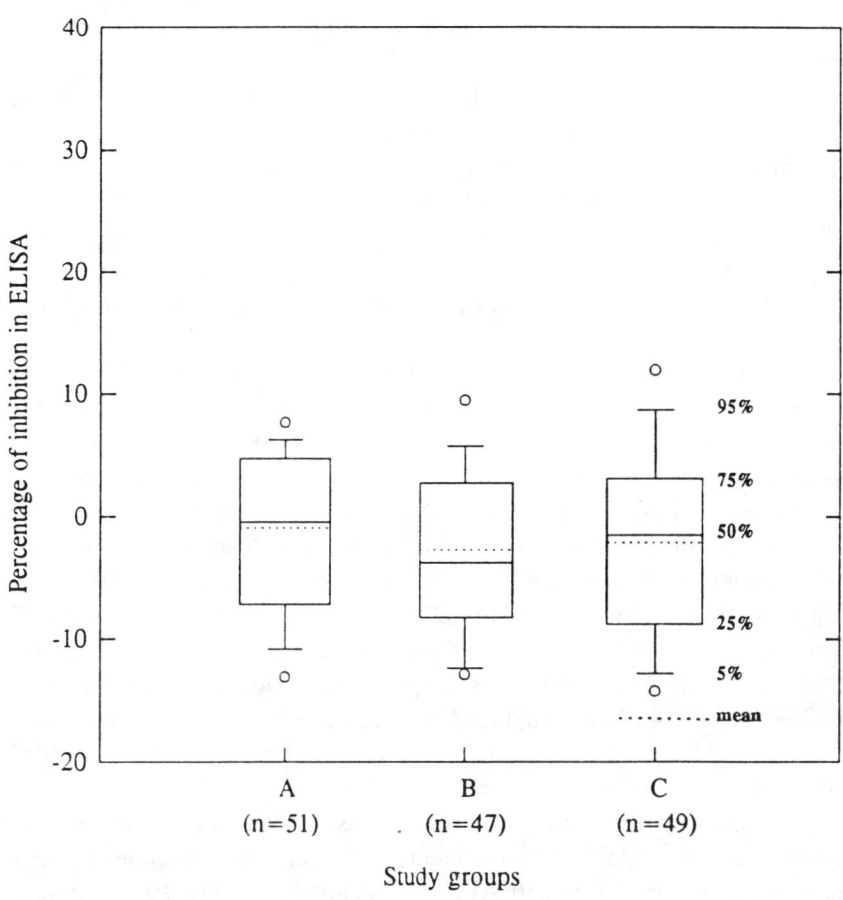

Group A — Control
Group B — Liver diseases
Group C — Hepatocellular carcinoma

inexpensive and easy to perform (Wild *et al.*, 1990b). Analysis of AFB₁-
albumin adducts has been considered to be a most promising approach in
the study in this area, but an unreasonably high number of false positives
were found when an ELISA was done directly on serum albumin without
previous hydrolysis or digestion (Wild *et al.*, 1990b). These false positives

were from subjects whose serum albumin showed yellow green colour, suggesting a high level of bound bilirubin which may be interfering in ELISA. Therefore, direct ELISA has the inherent property of non-specificity and could not be used in serum samples from patients with liver diseases, who very often have elevated bilirubin levels. It has also been found that recognition by specific anti-AFB$_1$ antibodies of the isolated AFB$_1$-lysine adduct was more than 30-fold greater than when the adduct is present in the intact albumin molecule (Wild *et al.*, 1990b). This could be due to the steric arrangement of the adduct when it is still attached to albumin whereby the specific antibody could not get to the epitope that it recognises. Thus, ELISA for AFB$_1$-lysine after hydrolysis or digestion is a superior study method to direct ELISA on serum albumin in terms of both specificity and sensitivity.

Serum samples from study subjects were required for the AFB$_1$-lysine ELISA assay used in this study. Blood-taking is an invasive procedure but most of these subjects were due for some routine blood tests when they visited the clinics. Therefore, they were not subjected to an extra invasive procedure. A large number of samples can be processed on the same ELISA plate but usually, a number of replicate wells are used. The entire experimental procedure of this study, starting from albumin isolation, to digestion by proteinase K, clean-up by Sep-Pak cartridge and immunoaffinity column, then finally to detection by ELISA, is a very long and 'labour intensive' process. In particular, the loading of samples onto ELISA wells requires a high degree of concentration and clear documentation to avoid mix-up. Nevertheless, it does not require very expensive equipment or instrumentation except an ELISA plate reader.

In summary, this study employed a sensitive and specific method for the monitoring of AFB$_1$-lysine adducts in human serum samples through their recognition by a rat anti-AFB$_1$ monoclonal antibody developed specially for this study in an ELISA assay. The detection limit of this assay was found to be approximately 2 pg AFB$_1$-lysine per mg of albumin. Nevertheless, even with this very high sensitivity, the assay failed to detect significant amounts of the adduct amongst the 147 serum samples collected for this study. These serum samples came from three groups of patients: a group of control patients who did not have any history or evidence of liver disease, a group of patients with various liver diseases including chronic hepatitis B infection and alcoholic liver disease and finally a group of patients diagnosed to suffer from HCC.

There could be several reasons for the non-detection of AFB$_1$-albumin adducts in the serum of the subjects in this study. One of the most easily explained reasons would be a low sensitivity of the assay used, thereby producing a large number of false negatives. This could result from a low level of recognition of AFB_1-lysine and related albumin adducts by the rat monoclonal antibody used and/or a low percentage of recovery of the assay process such that a large proportion of the adducts was lost during the process. Looking at the validations carried out on the assay process, these explanations might not be substantiated. The monoclonal antibody was found to be very specific and sensitive towards AFB_1-lysine. In the ELISA standard curves, the proportion part of the curve has a very steep slope. This signifies high specificity of the monoclonal antibody against the substrate, AFB_1-lysine. The dilution used for the assay was 1:5,000 and using this dilution in ELISA, levels down to 0.75 pg of AFB_1-lysine could be detected. Although the overall recovery of the preparation and clean-up process was 23.3%, it is comparable to that of a similar study (Wild *et al.*, 1990b) and in fact the detection limit was approximately 2 pg AFB_1-lysine per mg of albumin. In the study of Wild et al., 17 out of 19 serum samples from Gambia and 5 out of 38 serum samples from Thailand were shown to contain measurable amounts of AFB_1-lysine, but not in any of 14 serum samples from France. The detection limit of our assay method was even lower than that of Wild *et al.*. Thus the non-detection of AFB_1-lysine in our Hong Kong serum samples was likely to be a real phenonmenon and not a false negative result due to the assay having low sensitivity and specificity.

It follows that the actual amounts of AFB_1-albumin adducts that exist in the serum of our subjects were of an extremely low level, if they existed at all. Very little work has been carried out on the aflatoxins in Hong Kong since Shank and Wogan conducted surveys on the contamination of foodstuffs available on the Hong Kong market in the 70's (Shank & Wogan, 1972b). The general standards of living and hygiene and the for food storage have much improved since then, but part of the population still live in poor conditions with some still in rural areas. The Harmful Substances in Food Regulations of the Public Health and Municipal Service Ordinance in Hong Kong stipulate that the amount of AFB_1 in foodstuffs in Hong Kong should not exceed 15 ppb (Hong Kong Government, 1990). Enquiries were made at the Hygiene Division of the Department of Health, the department responsible for the enforcement of this regulation, regarding the actual frequency and results of test purchasea and the analysis of AFB_1 in foodstuffs from the general market in Hong Kong.

They replied that adherence to these regulations was voluntary from the manufacturer's and importer's part. Test purchases and analyses carried out by the department were done infrequently and the normal work schedule was impaired lately by the problem of organophosphate pesticides contamination of vegetables, which was very time consuming. Also, they would not disclose the results of previous analyses claiming to want 'to avoid misintepretation'. Therefore, although a regulation exists to control the level of AFB_1 that can exist in foodstuffs on the market in Hong Kong, it might not be fully enforced. If the subjects recruited for our study were representative of the whole population in Hong Kong, then it would be truly fortunate that according to the findings of this study, exposure to AFB_1 was not found to be a health hazard in the local scene.

Several studies have tried to correlate the dietary intake of AFB_1 with serum albumin adducts (Gan *et al.*, 1988; Sabbioni *et al.*, 1990; Wild *et al.*, 1990a) and a highly significant association has been shown. A functional relationship describing adduct levels under conditions of chronic exposure to xenobiotics which form covalent bonds to serum albumin has been derived (Sabbioni *et al.*, 1987). The two important parameters are the dose-adduct relationship for single doses and the chronic average daily dose. The former parameter was determined using a rat model (Sabbioni *et al.*, 1987) and Gan et al. determined that the rat is an appropriate surrogate for humans with respect to this parameter (Gan *et al.*, 1988). When studying subjects from Gangxi Province, China, Gan *et al.* constructed a regression line between the level of AFB_1-albumin adduct and daily AFB_1 intake with a slope of 1.05 ng adduct (per g albumin) per 1 µg AFB_1 intake/day (Gan *et al.*, 1988). Using this as the basis of conversion, the detection limit of 2 pg AFB_1-lysine equivalents per mg of serum albumin in our assay would indicate an ingestion level of about 1.9 ng AFB_1 per day on the average. A correction factor of 3–5 was also proposed to take into account underestimation of the amount of AFB_1 ingested. The subjects that we studied from Hong Kong thus should have a daily ingestion of at least below approximately 2 ng AFB_1.

The other constraint of our study was that assumptions were made that the diet of the study subjects was not modified significantly as compared to the normal population. Nevertheless, the majority of these subjects were patients attending the Li Ka Shing Specialist Clinics with various disorders, including hypertension, diabetes and liver diseases. There is a tendency for Chinese patients to take special care of their diet irrespective of what kind of disease they suffer from and so they might be taking 'better quality food' as compared to the general population. Also, there might be subtle changes in their diet over the years if their illnesses were chronic. The half-life of albumin in man is about 20–30 days and so the monitoring of AFB_1-albumin adducts, including AFB_1-lysine, can reflect dietary exposure to AFB_1 during the past few months at the most. Possible exposure months or years before would not be revealed by this assay method.

Monitoring of AFB_1-DNA adducts measures even more recent AFB_1 exposure as the major DNA adduct AFB_1-N ^{7}-Gua adduct is rapidly excised from DNA and excreted in the urine with a half-life of about 12 hours. The demonstration of actual mutational hotspot in genetic material would be a more long-lasting and definite proof of carcinogenesis (Bressac, Kew, Wands & Ozturk, 1991; Hsu, Metcalf, Sun, Welsh, Wang & Harris, 1991). The p53 gene is a putative tumour-suppressor gene and mutational hot spot in this gene has been reported in carcinoma of human lung, colon, oesophagus, breast and also liver. It was found that mutations of p53 in HCCs are preferentially $G \rightarrow T$ or $G \rightarrow C$ substitutions at condon 249. These HCC samples came from southern Africa and Qidong, China, where dietary exposure to AFB_1 was evident; therefore these findings were of much interest as AFB_1 is known to bind preferentially to G residues of genetic material and induces $G \rightarrow T$ substitutions almost exclusively.

Our study revealed no circulating AFB_1-albumin adduct detectable by our assay. It was planned to further this study by monitoring AFB_1-DNA adducts freed from isolated heptic DNA and immunocytochemical studies as well if there was evidence that exposure to AFB_1 was a sizable problem in Hong Kong. Since the results of the AFB_1-albumin adduct study were mostly negative, this was not pursued further. Perhaps a study of the mutational hotspot of HCC from Hong Kong would be of more value. However, these studies all involve the difficulty of obtaining liver tissues, tumour and non-tumour, from study subjects. This would have to rely on biopsy materials and resected tissues from suitable patients. HCC patients who cannot undergo surgery or chemotherapy would ultimately be incurable. Organ donation from patients of Chinese origin is especially difficult due to cultural beliefs and thus poses further hindrance to studies requiring human tissues.

CHAPTER 4

Summary and Ideas for Further Studies

The theme of this PhD thesis is on the metabolic activation of drugs and carcinogens in relation to toxicity and carcinogenesis. The two xenobiotics studied in this project were paracetamol and aflatoxin B1. For the first part of the project, we hoped to show whether patients with hepatocellular carcinoma (HCC), who also have evidence of increased metabolic activation of paracetamol, have normal or prolonged plasma paracetamol half-lives and also confirm that there is a close relationship between plasma paracetamol half life, the AUC and the urinary recovery of unchanged paracetamol. A study was done to assess the full pharmacokinetics of paracetamol in these patients and the differences, if any, from healthy subjects and patients with other liver diseases. The results were used to help explain the mechanism and significance of the finding of increased metabolic activation of paracetamol in patients with HCC. The other xenobiotic whose metabolic activation was studied in this project was the mycotoxin aflatoxin B_1. For this part of the project, a study was carried out to monitor the levels of the major albumin adduct of aflatoxin B1 in the serum of healthy individuals and patients with HCC and other liver disease.

The results of the comparative pharmacokinetic study of paracetamol among different groups of patients showed that the metabolic activation of paracetamol was genuinely enhanced among patients with HCC and a small proportion of patients with chronic liver diseases, and not due to an impairment of other metabolic pathways. It was postulated that metabolic activation by microsomal enzymes might be involved in the formation of carcinogenic substances from xenobiotics with some implications in the pathogenesis of HCC. Although it was shown clearly that the oxidative pathway of paracetamol was enhanced amongst these patients, it was not known which specific metabolising enzymes were involved. It was known that cytochrome P450 enzymes, most probably CYP2E1 and CYP1A2, are involved in the metabolic activation of paracetamol, however, an enhancement of their activity has not been demonstrated amongst patients with HCC. It is also not known whether the activity of other families of cytochrome P450 enzymes are enhanced. To find out the identity of the cytochrome P450 enzyme(s) which is causing the enhanced metabolic activation of paracetamol in HCC patients, a study on the enzyme content of liver tissues from these patients is needed. The relative expression of various microsomal enzymes can be studied by separation by gel electrophoresis with Western blots and the rate of metabolism of known specific substrates to assess individual subject's capacity for the metabolic activation of paracetamol.

Although our study on the metabolic activation of AFB_1-albumin adduct showed that even at high sensitivity of detection, we failed to detect significant amount of the adducts in all the plasma samples studied. This follows that the actual amounts of AFB1-albumin adducts that exist in the serum of our subjects were of an extremely low level, if they existed at all. It was planned to further this study by monitoring AFB_1-DNA adducts freed from isolated hepatic DNA and immunocytochemical studies as well if there was evidence that exposure to AFB1 was of a sizable problem in Hong Kong. Since the results of the AFB1-albumin adduct study was mostly negative, this was not further pursued. Perhaps a study of the mutational hotspot of HCC, a more long-lasting and definite proof of carcinogenesis, would be of more value. Mutation of the p53 gene, a putative tumour-supressor gene, has been reported in carcinoma of human lung, colon, oesophagus, breast and also liver. It was found that mutations of p53 in HCCs are preferentially $G \rightarrow T$ or $G \rightarrow C$ substitutions at codon 249 (Bressac *et al.*, 1991; Hsu *et al.*, 1991) and these findings are of much interest as AFB1 is also known to induce $G \rightarrow T$ substitutions in genetic material.

AFB_1-lysine is one of the end products of the in vivo metabolic activation of AFB_1. Another way of assessing the status of metabolic activation of AFB_1 in individuals is to study the specific cytochrome P450 enzymes responsible for this process. It has been shown that multiple forms of cytochrome P450 are involved in the metabolic activation of

AFB$_1$ (Forrester *et al.*, 1990), which are also highly sensitive to environmental factors such as diet and cigarette smoking and are subject to considerable inter-individual variations. Identification and quantification of their relative expression by Western blots and the rate of metabolism of known specific substrates (drugs and other xenobiotics) (Forrester, Henderson, Glancey, Back, Park, Ball, Kitteringham, McLaren, Miles, Skett & Wolf, 1992) would be another method of assessing an individual's capacity for the metabolic activation of AFB$_1$ *in vivo*.

APPENDICES

Appendix 2.1   Chemical and pharmacokinetic data of paracetamol

HNCOCH$_3$

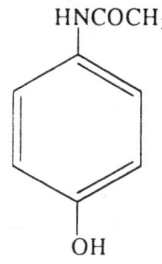

OH

Paracetamol [acetaminophen, N-acetyl-p-aminophenol, 4-hydroxyacetanilide, N-(4-hydroxyphenyl) acetamide] is an antipyretic and analgesic agent

Description: White odourless crystalline powder with bitter taste

Molecular weight: 151.2

Melting point: 168 - 172°C

pKa: 9.5

Soluble in: 70 parts water, 7 parts alcohol, 13 parts acetone, 40 parts glycerol, 9 parts propylene glycol, 50 parts chloroform and 10 parts methyl alcohol

Insoluble in: Ether, pentane and benzene

Oral bioavailability 70 -80%

Plasma clearance   5.0 $\pm$ 1.4 ml min^{-1} kg^{-1}

V$_d$ 0.95 $\pm$ 0.12 l kg^{-1}

t$_{1/2}$ 2.0 $\pm$ 0.4 hr

Protein binding   neglibible at < 60 μg ml^{-1}

Appendix 2.2 Individual Plasma Paracetamol Concentrations in 14 Healthy Subjects Following Ingestion of a 20 mg kg^{-1} Body Weight Dose

Plasma Paracetamol Concentration (μg ml^{-1})

TIME (hr)	CWH	WR	WKKW	KWSC	CSYC	LHY	CWSD	NPSD	LCKJ	WP	WH	YAS	SPY	KKH
0	0	0	0	0	0	0	0	0	0	0	0	0	0	0
0.5	21.16	13.33	16.53	17.42	23.55	19.12	15.94	28.88	28.71	15.15	31.23	10.17	18.79	33.83
1	16.89	17.66	13.97	16.85	18.98	19.44	19.75	17.04	28.81	18.59	18.16	15.53	20.62	26.64
1.5	18.98	13.46	9.90	17.55	14.83	15.33	16.66	14.51	23.55	16.43	15.26	16.77	21.18	17.71
2	14.65	12.15	7.75	14.93	12.57	13.16	14.29	12.86	18.40	14.54	13.33	14.59	19.07	16.86
3	10.63	10.26	5.95	11.43	9.04	10.85	11.89	10.68	15.15	10.63	9.51	12.70	14.76	13.41
4	7.96	7.96	4.21	7.68	6.83	8.21	9.01	8.24	11.67	9.03	7.76	9.42	10.95	10.61
5	6.16	6.35	2.90	5.82	5.42	6.96	7.24	6.08	7.93	6.17	5.15	7.02	8.27	7.50
6	4.75	4.90	1.85	4.48	4.25	5.40	5.43	3.82	5.89	4.98	3.96	5.27	6.40	6.34
7	3.74	4.31	1.33	3.66	3.43	4.12	4.26	3.27	3.95	3.53	2.99	4.52	4.80	5.22
8	2.85	3.49	0.91	2.62	2.46	3.21	3.14	2.88	3.12	2.66	2.40	3.57	3.83	4.25
9	2.23	2.47	0.71	1.70	1.89	2.17	2.48	2.12	2.25	1.99	1.71	2.91	2.84	3.17
10	1.82	1.97	0.65	1.45	2.66	1.44	2.09	1.74	1.59	1.51	2.65	2.31	2.11	2.63
11	1.57	1.59	0.42	1.14	1.14	1.83	1.56	1.46	1.19	1.21	0.89	1.79	1.67	2.18
12	1.25	1.13	0.33	0.89	0.98	1.54	1.30	1.24	0.97	0.94	0.74	1.48	1.29	1.77
24	0.22	0.23	0.09	0.22	0.28	0.33	0.17	0.15	0.32	0.22	0.23	0.28	0.29	0.36

Appendix 2.3 Individual Plasma Paracetamol Glucuronide Concentrations in 14 Healthy Subjects Following Ingestion of a 20 mg kg^{-1} Body Weight Dose

TIME (hr)	Plasma Paracetamol Glucuronide Concentration (μg ml^{-1}) — Subject													
	CWH	WR	WKKW	KWSC	CSYC	LHY	CWSD	NPSD	LCKJ	WP	WH	YAS	SPY	KKH
0	0.00	0.00	0.00	0.00	0.00	0.00	0.00	0.00	0.00	0.00	0.00	0.00	0.00	0.00
0.5	3.32	1.10	2.16	1.15	1.46	1.23	1.52	3.90	2.65	1.78	2.88	0.45	3.11	2.01
1	6.62	3.18	6.68	4.19	5.63	3.34	5.61	6.34	6.37	5.69	6.04	3.71	8.29	6.71
1.5	10.39	3.91	10.27	5.92	7.16	4.19	7.37	7.17	7.63	9.39	8.45	5.58	11.23	8.18
2	11.24	4.90	12.23	7.19	7.45	4.89	9.80	8.89	8.05	10.04	8.73	6.34	13.64	9.50
3	11.79	5.92	12.15	8.25	7.36	5.65	11.38	8.66	8.67	10.54	9.40	7.56	15.10	10.15
4	11.08	6.30	11.88	8.02	6.31	5.59	12.57	8.74	8.76	10.63	9.09	7.40	14.40	9.62
5	9.78	6.17	9.42	6.90	5.52	5.49	10.95	7.50	7.94	9.14	8.11	6.63	12.62	8.32
6	8.86	5.60	7.42	5.70	4.96	4.87	9.37	5.64	6.07	7.46	6.82	5.67	10.89	7.72
7	7.88	4.77	4.79	4.35	4.16	3.73	7.55	4.60	4.53	6.07	5.69	4.92	8.69	6.43
8	6.50	3.99	4.07	2.62	3.36	3.03	6.39	3.54	3.55	4.66	4.79	4.14	7.31	5.39
9	4.44	3.19	3.10	2.94	2.65	2.29	5.36	2.65	2.78	3.83	3.67	3.64	5.96	4.18
10	4.60	2.59	2.63	2.18	2.54	2.10	4.44	2.44	2.05	3.24	9.51	3.15	4.86	3.86
11	3.31	1.98	1.74	1.86	1.54	1.60	3.56	1.88	1.73	2.53	2.37	2.53	4.15	3.31
12	2.83	1.50	1.18	1.44	1.29	1.38	3.02	1.51	1.31	1.91	1.99	2.14	3.22	2.71
24	0.47	0.28	0.18	0.27	0.15	0.26	0.30	0.27	0.22	0.36	0.36	0.34	0.51	0.54

Appendix 2.4 Individual Plasma Paracetamol Sulphate Concentrations in 14 Healthy Subjects Following Ingestion of a 20 mg kg^{-1} Body Weight Dose

Plasma Paracetamol Sulphate Concentration (μg ml^{-1})

Subject

TIME (hr)	CWH	WR	WKKW	KWSC	CSYC	LHY	CWSD	NPSD	LCKJ	WP	WH	YAS	SPY	KKH
0	0.00	0.00	0.00	0.00	0.00	0.00	0.00	0.00	0.00	0.00	0.00	0.00	0.00	0.00
0.5	2.61	1.69	2.49	2.36	3.14	3.05	1.32	5.00	4.38	2.75	4.19	1.17	2.91	3.53
1	3.84	2.85	3.54	3.90	5.72	5.31	2.23	5.49	6.75	4.71	5.29	4.26	4.57	6.83
1.5	4.43	2.79	3.88	4.25	6.22	5.35	2.63	5.52	7.15	6.10	5.78	5.20	4.91	6.89
2	4.28	2.79	3.71	4.23	6.21	5.34	3.12	5.39	7.09	5.87	5.45	4.80	5.28	6.87
3	3.55	2.63	3.42	3.88	5.69	4.91	2.89	4.74	6.68	6.05	5.27	4.77	5.07	6.36
4	3.08	2.22	3.02	2.96	4.95	4.07	2.84	4.07	5.94	5.92	4.40	3.81	4.17	5.57
5	2.56	1.92	2.46	2.66	4.19	3.60	2.59	3.20	5.15	5.32	3.63	3.10	3.53	4.63
6	2.37	1.55	1.80	2.14	3.94	3.03	2.26	2.48	4.91	4.54	3.00	2.60	2.91	3.91
7	1.83	1.49	1.36	1.73	3.53	2.45	1.97	2.06	3.93	3.73	2.30	2.33	2.34	3.28
8	1.47	1.19	1.32	0.85	2.85	1.97	1.68	1.66	3.31	2.95	1.90	1.91	2.00	2.63
9	1.17	0.90	0.77	0.93	2.22	1.29	1.39	1.22	2.59	2.52	1.50	1.66	1.49	2.23
10	1.00	0.72	0.67	0.69	1.64	1.70	1.15	1.10	2.00	2.13	5.48	1.34	1.20	1.81
11	0.79	0.63	0.48	0.66	1.39	1.05	0.90	0.83	1.58	1.55	0.95	1.03	0.92	1.59
12	0.68	0.45	0.34	0.53	1.18	0.94	0.86	0.75	1.24	1.41	0.72	0.93	0.75	1.29
24	0.14	0.09	0.06	0.14	0.21	0.20	0.10	0.14	0.28	0.30	0.24	0.17	0.09	0.25

Appendix 2.5 Individual Plasma Paracetamol Cysteine Concentrations in 14 Healthy Subjects Following Ingestion of a 20 mg kg^{-1} Body Weight Dose

Plasma Paracetamol Cysteine Concentration (μg ml^{-1})

TIME (hr)	CWH	WR	WKKW	KWSC	CSYC	LHY	CWSD	NPSD	LCKJ	WP	WH	YAS	SPY	KKH
0	0.00	0.00	0.00	0.00	0.00	0.00	0.00	0.00	0.00	0.00	0.00	0.00	0.00	0.00
0.5	0.00	0.00	0.08	0.00	0.00	0.00	0.00	0.02	0.00	0.00	0.00	0.00	0.00	0.00
1	0.04	0.03	0.18	0.06	0.02	0.03	0.03	0.07	0.00	0.10	0.06	0.00	0.00	0.00
1.5	0.08	0.04	0.18	0.09	0.03	0.06	0.09	0.04	0.00	0.17	0.13	0.08	0.00	0.15
2	0.11	0.07	0.16	0.11	0.09	0.09	0.00	0.11	0.14	0.12	0.08	0.09	0.06	0.20
3	0.16	0.11	0.21	0.19	0.08	0.12	0.14	0.12	0.17	0.21	0.08	0.15	0.00	0.28
4	0.19	0.12	0.18	0.22	0.11	0.16	0.14	0.12	0.22	0.26	0.15	0.20	0.17	0.38
5	0.21	0.14	0.18	0.19	0.13	0.16	0.17	0.12	0.18	0.23	0.15	0.20	0.15	0.37
6	0.19	0.17	0.16	0.19	0.08	0.13	0.16	0.12	0.14	0.17	0.13	0.19	0.15	0.30
7	0.17	0.12	0.17	0.19	0.07	0.11	0.13	0.07	0.00	0.16	0.09	0.16	0.00	0.32
8	0.14	0.11	0.18	0.13	0.08	0.10	0.12	0.06	0.09	0.17	0.08	0.16	0.00	0.28
9	0.12	0.00	0.13	0.17	0.03	0.06	0.10	0.00	0.11	0.17	0.07	0.15	0.11	0.28
10	0.11	0.00	0.14	0.15	0.09	0.04	0.12	0.06	0.08	0.14	0.20	0.15	0.00	0.25
11	0.10	0.00	0.11	0.13	0.02	0.08	0.05	0.06	0.06	0.05	0.08	0.12	0.06	0.24
12	0.04	0.00	0.08	0.10	0.02	0.08	0.05	0.06	0.00	0.10	0.05	0.10	0.09	0.20
24	0.00	0.00	0.06	0.00	0.00	0.00	0.00	0.06	0.00	0.00	0.00	0.00	0.00	0.03

Subject

Appendix 2.6 Urinary Recovery of Paracetamol Glucuronide in Each Sample Following Ingestion of a 20 mg kg^{-1} Body Weight Dose

Time after dosing (hr)	Urinary Recovery of Paracetamol Glucuronide (mg) Subject															
	CWH	WR	WKKW	KWSC	CSYC	LHY	CWSD	NPSD	LCKJ	WP	WH	YAS	SPY	KKH
Predose	0	0	0	0	0	0	0	0	0	0	0	0	0	0
0-4	282.61	123.91	309.24	134.43	168.06	92.70	492.19	296.03	209.56	286.13	285.26	119.71	212.59	179.45
4-8	105.39	115.45	298.66	252.23	103.19	119.45	309.57	216.43	215.69	226.76	284.60	262.47	378.39	179.12
8-12	112.82	65.27	81.39	73.36	52.66	68.99	163.59	87.50	79.82	96.12	104.94	167.66	154.21	93.48
12-24	111.66	25.10	41.60	44.37	27.75	31.73	134.52	58.28	36.74	61.99	51.28	91.99	98.91	85.17

Appendix 2.7 Urinary Recovery of Paracetamol Sulphate in Each Sample Following Ingestion of a 20 mg kg^{-1} Body Weight Dose

Time after dosing (hr)	Urinary Recovery of Paracetamol Sulphate (mg) Subject													
	CWH	WR	WKKW	KWSC	CSYC	LHY	CWSD	NPSD	LCKJ	WP	WH	YAS	SPY	KKH
Predose	0	0	0	0	0	0	0	0	0	0	0	0	0	0
0-4	127.42	91.33	131.58	101.61	176.38	129.66	161.52	230.21	221.21	199.12	215.12	135.94	107.34	162.46
4-8	33.60	49.16	96.25	114.99	102.47	115.75	94.33	118.63	190.00	152.81	148.30	166.75	136.58	122.89
8-12	33.70	25.72	27.00	30.02	57.95	58.78	54.63	52.44	87.12	71.34	52.35	100.06	50.35	61.99
12-24	36.52	11.58	16.76	21.15	32.61	31.88	47.73	37.69	48.56	55.76	30.81	56.70	34.38	56.57

Appendix 2.8 Urinary Recovery of Paracetamol Cysteine in Each Sample Following Ingestion of a 20 mg kg^{-1} Body Weight Dose

Time after dosing (hr)	Urinary Recovery of Paracetamol Cysteine (mg) Subject													
	CWH	WR	WKKW	KWSC	CSYC	LHY	CWSD	NPSD	LCKJ	WP	WH	YAS	SPY	KKH
Predose	0	0	0	0	0	0	0	0	0	0	0	0	0	0
0-4	7.70	6.30	8.58	5.16	4.46	5.93	10.47	6.19	9.19	11.54	10.39	4.70	1.99	7.57
4-8	5.31	9.63	10.88	18.97	6.30	11.07	7.70	7.33	10.13	13.10	11.19	17.15	9.40	16.18
8-12	8.27	8.92	5.24	10.82	3.82	7.60	7.23	4.92	5.28	9.07	5.83	20.36	5.86	12.18
12-24	12.78	4.24	2.21	9.86	2.63	7.85	8.45	6.00	4.88	11.27	4.40	15.18	4.51	16.78

Appendix 2.9 Urinary Recovery of Paracetamol in Each Sample Following Ingestion of a 20 mg kg^{-1} Body Weight Dose

Time after dosing (hr)	Urinary Recovery of Paracetamol (mg)														
	Subject														
	CWH	WR	WKKW	KWSC	CSYC	LHY	CWSD	NPSD	LCKJ	WP	WH	YAS	SPY	KKH
Predose	0	0	0	0	0	0	0	0	0	0	0	0	0	0
0-4	33.08	18.87	17.12	30.13	27.78	34.07	53.94	30.15	23.01	27.35	53.51	32.15	37.13	51.54
4-8	4.27	6.28	10.84	16.38	5.59	15.73	12.17	13.46	16.39	13.70	21.26	27.67	19.47	18.30
8-12	5.35	3.47	2.94	4.55	4.50	11.76	7.04	6.25	7.78	5.21	5.56	12.99	9.01	14.12
12-24	6.95	2.74	3.32	3.07	4.98	7.74	7.06	7.02	2.83	6.11	4.90	11.66	5.84	7.96

Appendix 2.10 Urinary Recovery of Paracetamol Mercapturate in Each Sample Following Ingestion of a 20 mg kg^{-1} Body Weight Dose

Time after dosing (hr)	Urinary Recovery of Paracetamol Mercapturate(mg) Subject													
	CWH	WR	WKKW	KWSC	CSYC	LHY	CWSD	NPSD	LCKJ	WP	WH	YAS	SPY	KKH
Predose	0	0	0	0	0	0	0	0	0	0	0	0	0	0
0-4	8.86	5.06	7.09	2.18	3.62	3.31	9.80	5.49	6.67	10.70	3.13	4.55	4.95	8.41
4-8	2.51	6.30	10.84	9.10	4.87	5.84	8.30	5.78	9.21	10.64	4.49	19.20	13.18	13.92
8-12	7.61	3.68	4.62	4.21	3.05	3.84	7.09	3.74	5.28	5.93	4.67	19.60	8.13	9.95
12-24	11.44	3.46	3.65	5.95	2.82	4.64	6.34	3.53	2.45	3.99	1.03	15.01	7.05	13.72

Appendix 2.11 Metabolic Clearance of Paracetamol and Its Glucuronide, Sulphate, Cysteine and Mercapturate Conjugate in 14 Healthy Subjects Following Ingestion of a 20 mg kg^{-1} Body Weight Dose

Model 1

Subject	Metabolic Clearance of Paracetamol and Metabolites						
	T	G	S	C	P	M	M+C
CWH	3.62	2.32	0.87	0.13	0.19	0.12	0.24
WR	3.93	2.21	1.19	0.20	0.21	0.12	0.32
WKKW	6.89	4.62	1.72	0.17	0.22	0.17	0.34
KWSC	3.88	2.19	1.16	0.20	0.24	0.09	0.29
CSYC	3.93	1.74	1.82	0.09	0.21	0.07	0.16
LHY	3.49	1.42	1.53	0.15	0.32	0.08	0.23
CWSD	3.54	2.42	0.79	0.08	0.18	0.07	0.14
NPSD	3.71	2.04	1.36	0.08	0.18	0.06	0.13
LCKY	2.81	1.28	1.29	0.07	0.12	0.06	0.13
WP	3.84	2.02	1.44	0.14	0.16	0.09	0.23
WH	4.42	2.46	1.52	0.11	0.29	0.05	0.15
YAS	3.51	1.73	1.24	0.16	0.23	0.16	0.31
SPY	2.96	1.92	0.75	0.05	0.16	0.08	0.13
KKH	2.70	1.28	0.96	0.13	0.22	0.11	0.24
Mean	3.80	2.12	1.26	0.12	0.21	0.09	0.22
SD	1.01	0.82	0.33	0.05	0.05	0.04	0.08

T = Total clearance
G = Metabolic clearance to the glucuronide conjugate
S = Metabolic clearance to the sulphate conjugate
C = Metabolic clearance to the cysteine conjugate
P = Metabolic clearance to unchanged paracetamol
M = Metabolic clearance to the mercapturate conjugate
M+C = Sum of the metabolic clearances to the cysteine and mercapturate conjugate

Appendix 2.12   Metabolic Clearance of Paracetamol and Its Glucuronide, Sulphate, Cysteine and Mercapturate Conjugate in 14 Healthy Subjects Following Ingestion of a 20 mg kg^{-1} Body Weight Dose

Model 2

Subject	Metabolic Clearance of Paracetamol and Metabolites						
	T	G	S	C	P	M	M+C
CWH	3.77	2.41	0.91	0.13	0.20	0.12	0.25
WR	4.15	2.33	1.26	0.21	0.22	0.13	0.34
WKKW	7.18	4.82	1.79	0.18	0.23	0.17	0.35
KWSC	4.11	2.32	1.23	0.21	0.25	0.10	0.31
CSYC	4.11	1.82	1.91	0.09	0.22	0.07	0.16
LHY	3.51	1.43	1.54	0.15	0.32	0.08	0.23
CWSD	3.63	2.49	0.81	0.08	0.18	0.07	0.15
NPSD	3.85	2.12	1.41	0.08	0.18	0.06	0.14
LCKY	2.97	1.35	1.36	0.07	0.13	0.06	0.13
WP	4.06	2.13	1.52	0.14	0.17	0.10	0.24
WH	4.70	2.62	1.61	0.12	0.31	0.05	0.16
YAS	3.71	1.83	1.31	0.16	0.24	0.17	0.33
SPY	3.14	2.04	0.80	0.05	0.17	0.08	0.13
KKH	2.83	1.34	1.01	0.13	0.23	0.12	0.25
Mean	3.98	2.22	1.32	0.13	0.22	0.10	0.23
SD	1.05	0.86	0.35	0.05	0.05	0.04	0.08

T = Total clearance
G = Metabolic clearance to the glucuronide conjugate
S = Metabolic clearance to the sulphate conjugate
C = Metabolic clearance to the cysteine conjugate
P = Metabolic clearance to unchanged paracetamol
M = Metabolic clearance to the mercapturate conjugate
M+C = Sum of the metabolic clearances to the cysteine and mercapturate conjugate

Appendix 2.13 Metabolic Clearance of Paracetamol and Its Glucuronide, Sulphate, Cysteine and Mercapturate Conjugate in 14 Healthy Subjects Following Ingestion of a 20 mg kg^{-1} Body Weight Dose

Model 3

Subject	Metabolic Clearance of Paracetamol and Metabolites						
	T	G	S	C	P	M	M+C
CWH	3.33	2.13	0.80	0.12	0.17	0.11	0.22
WR	3.40	1.91	1.03	0.17	0.18	0.11	0.28
WKKW	6.49	4.35	1.62	0.16	0.20	0.16	0.32
KWSC	3.49	1.97	1.05	0.18	0.21	0.08	0.26
CSYC	3.62	1.60	1.68	0.08	0.20	0.07	0.14
LHY	3.19	1.30	1.40	0.14	0.29	0.07	0.21
CWSD	3.21	2.20	0.72	0.07	0.16	0.06	0.13
NPSD	3.39	1.86	1.24	0.07	0.16	0.05	0.12
LCKY	2.56	1.17	1.18	0.06	0.11	0.05	0.11
WP	3.47	1.82	1.30	0.12	0.14	0.09	0.21
WH	3.95	2.20	1.35	0.10	0.26	0.04	0.14
YAS	3.16	1.56	1.12	0.14	0.21	0.14	0.28
SPY	2.64	1.71	0.67	0.04	0.15	0.07	0.11
KKH	2.45	1.16	0.87	0.11	0.20	0.10	0.21
Mean	3.45	1.93	1.14	0.11	0.19	0.09	0.20
SD	0.97	0.78	0.31	0.04	0.05	0.03	0.07

T = Total clearance
G = Metabolic clearance to the glucuronide conjugate
S = Metabolic clearance to the sulphate conjugate
C = Metabolic clearance to the cysteine conjugate
P = Metabolic clearance to unchanged paracetamol
M = Metabolic clearance to the mercapturate conjugate
M+C = Sum of the metabolic clearances to the cysteine and mercapturate conjugate

Appendix 2.14 Metabolic Clearance of Paracetamol and Its Glucuronide, Sulphate, Cysteine and Mercapturate Conjugate in 14 Healthy Subjects Following Ingestion of a 20 mg kg^{-1} Body Weight Dose

Model 4

Subject	Metabolic Clearance of Paracetamol and Metabolites						
	T	G	S	C	P	M	M+C
CWH	3.85	2.46	0.93	0.14	0.20	0.12	0.26
WR	4.17	2.35	1.27	0.21	0.22	0.13	0.34
WKKW	7.25	4.86	1.81	0.18	0.23	0.17	0.35
KWSC	4.13	2.33	1.24	0.21	0.25	0.10	0.31
CSYC	4.29	1.90	1.99	0.09	0.23	0.08	0.17
LHY	3.78	1.54	1.65	0.16	0.34	0.09	0.25
CWSD	3.71	2.55	0.83	0.08	0.19	0.07	0.15
NPSD	3.91	2.15	1.43	0.08	0.19	0.06	0.14
LCKY	3.01	1.37	1.38	0.07	0.13	0.06	0.13
WP	4.08	2.14	1.53	0.14	0.17	0.10	0.24
WH	4.78	2.66	1.64	0.12	0.31	0.05	0.17
YAS	3.75	1.85	1.32	0.17	0.24	0.17	0.33
SPY	3.15	2.05	0.80	0.05	0.17	0.08	0.13
KKH	2.89	1.37	1.03	0.13	0.23	0.12	0.25
Mean	4.05	2.26	1.35	0.13	0.22	0.10	0.23
SD	1.05	0.86	0.36	0.05	0.06	0.04	0.08

T = Total clearance
G = Metabolic clearance to the glucuronide conjugate
S = Metabolic clearance to the sulphate conjugate
C = Metabolic clearance to the cysteine conjugate
P = Metabolic clearance to unchanged paracetamol
M = Metabolic clearance to the mercapturate conjugate
M+C = Sum of the metabolic clearances to the cysteine and mercapturate conjugate

Appendix 2.15 Metabolic Clearance of Paracetamol and Its Glucuronide, Sulphate, Cysteine and Mercapturate Conjugate in 14 Healthy Subjects Following Ingestion of a 20 mg kg^{-1} Body Weight Dose

Model 5

Subject	Metabolic Clearance of Paracetamol and Metabolites						
	T	G	S	C	P	M	M+C
CWH	3.92	2.51	0.95	0.14	0.20	0.12	0.26
WR	4.03	2.27	1.22	0.20	0.22	0.13	0.33
WKKW	7.39	4.95	1.84	0.18	0.23	0.18	0.36
KWSC	4.09	2.31	1.23	0.21	0.25	0.10	0.30
CSYC	4.41	1.95	2.05	0.10	0.24	0.08	0.18
LHY	3.83	1.56	1.67	0.16	0.35	0.09	0.25
CWSD	3.76	2.58	0.84	0.08	0.19	0.07	0.15
NPSD	4.51	2.48	1.65	0.09	0.21	0.07	0.16
LCKY	3.02	1.37	1.39	0.08	0.13	0.06	0.13
WP	4.11	2.16	1.54	0.15	0.17	0.10	0.25
WH	4.13	2.30	1.41	0.10	0.27	0.04	0.14
YAS	3.83	1.89	1.35	0.17	0.25	0.17	0.34
SPY	3.15	2.04	0.80	0.05	0.17	0.08	0.13
KKH	2.89	1.37	1.03	0.14	0.24	0.12	0.25
Mean	4.08	2.27	1.35	0.13	0.22	0.10	0.23
SD	1.07	0.87	0.37	0.05	0.05	0.04	0.08

T = Total clearance
G = Metabolic clearance to the glucuronide conjugate
S = Metabolic clearance to the sulphate conjugate
C = Metabolic clearance to the cysteine conjugate
P = Metabolic clearance to unchanged paracetamol
M = Metabolic clearance to the mercapturate conjugate
M+C = Sum of the metabolic clearances to the cysteine and mercapturate conjugate

Appendix 2.16   Comparison between Model 4 and Model 5 for
Modified Bland-Altman Plot

1. Clearance

Subject	$Cl_{Model\ 4}$ (ml min^{-1} kg^{-1})	$Cl_{Model\ 5}$ (ml min^{-1} kg^{-1})	δ	mean	% of δ as mean	mean δ - 2SD	mean δ + 2SD
CWH	3.85	3.92	-0.07	3.89	1.78	-0.51	0.47
WR	4.17	4.03	0.14	4.10	3.46		
WKKW	7.25	7.39	-0.14	7.32	1.93		
KWSC	4.13	4.09	0.04	4.11	0.90		
CSYC	4.29	4.41	-0.12	4.35	2.71		
LHY	3.78	3.83	-0.05	3.80	1.24		
CWSD	3.71	3.76	-0.05	3.74	1.31		
NPSD	3.91	4.51	-0.60	4.21	14.14		
LCKY	3.01	3.02	-0.01	3.02	0.23		
WP	4.08	4.11	-0.03	4.10	0.76		
WH	4.78	4.13	0.65	4.45	14.69		
YAS	3.75	3.83	-0.08	3.79	2.22		
SPY	3.15	3.15	0.01	3.15	0.19		
KKH	2.89	2.89	0.00	2.89	0.07		
Mean			-0.02		3.26		
SD			0.25		4.65		

$\delta = Cl_{Model\ 4} - Cl_{Model\ 5}$

Appendix 2.17   Comparison between Model 4 and Model 5 for
Modified Bland-Altman Plot

2. $t_{1/2}$

Subject	$t_{1/2}$ Model 4 (hr)	$t_{1/2}$ Model 5 (hr)	δ	mean	% of δ as mean	mean δ - 2SD	mean δ + 2SD
CWH	2.60	2.64	-0.04	2.62	1.47	-0.26	0.28
WR	2.88	3.15	-0.27	3.02	8.79		
WKKW	1.86	1.83	0.03	1.85	1.63		
KWSC	2.45	2.63	-0.17	2.54	6.76		
CSYC	2.22	2.06	0.15	2.14	7.18		
LHY	2.89	2.84	0.05	2.86	1.73		
CWSD	2.78	2.72	0.06	2.75	2.21		
NPSD	2.50	2.59	-0.10	2.55	3.75		
LCKY	2.22	2.20	0.02	2.21	0.89		
WP	2.58	2.45	0.13	2.52	5.25		
WH	2.30	2.28	0.02	2.29	0.85		
YAS	3.05	2.74	0.31	2.89	10.62		
SPY	2.62	2.58	0.03	2.60	1.34		
KKH	2.96	3.01	-0.05	2.99	1.76		
Mean			0.01		3.87		
SD			0.13		3.14		

δ = $t_{1/2}$ Model 4 - $t_{1/2}$ Model 5

Appendix 2.18   Comparison between Model 4 and Model 5 for
Modified Bland-Altman Plot

3. AUC

Subject	$AUC_{Model\ 4}$ ($\mu g\ ml^{-1}$ hr)	$AUC_{Model\ 5}$ ($\mu g\ ml^{-1}$ hr)	δ	mean	% of δ as mean	mean δ - 2SD	mean δ + 2SD
CWH	86.5	85.0	1.5	85.8	1.8	-8.3	9.2
WR	79.9	82.7	-2.8	81.3	3.5		
WKKW	46.0	45.1	0.9	45.6	1.9		
KWSC	80.7	81.4	-0.7	81.1	0.9		
CSYC	77.7	75.6	2.1	76.7	2.7		
LHY	88.2	87.1	1.1	87.7	1.2		
CWSD	89.8	88.6	1.2	89.2	1.3		
NPSD	85.2	74.0	11.3	79.6	14.1		
LCKY	110.7	110.4	0.3	110.5	0.2		
WP	81.7	81.1	0.6	81.4	0.7		
WH	69.7	80.8	-11.0	75.3	14.7		
YAS	88.9	87.0	1.9	88.0	2.2		
SPY	105.7	106.0	-0.2	105.9	0.2		
KKH	115.5	115.4	0.1	115.5	0.1		
Mean			0.4		3.3		
SD			4.4		4.6		

$\delta = AUC_{Model\ 4} - AUC_{Model\ 5}$

Appendix 2.19 Comparison between Model 1 and Model 2 for
Modified Bland-Altman Plot

1. Clearance

Subject	$Cl_{Model\ 1}$ (ml min^{-1} kg^{-1})	$Cl_{Model\ 2}$ (ml min^{-1} kg^{-1})	δ	mean	% of δ as mean	mean δ - 2SD	mean δ + 2SD
CWH	3.62	3.77	-0.15	3.70	4.14	-0.32	-0.04
WR	3.93	4.15	-0.22	4.04	5.55		
WKKW	6.89	7.18	-0.29	7.04	4.12		
KWSC	3.88	4.11	-0.23	3.99	5.66		
CSYC	3.93	4.11	-0.19	4.02	4.63		
LHY	3.49	3.51	-0.02	3.50	0.60		
CWSD	3.54	3.63	-0.10	3.58	2.73		
NPSD	3.71	3.85	-0.14	3.78	3.79		
LCKY	2.81	2.97	-0.16	2.89	5.61		
WP	3.84	4.06	-0.22	3.95	5.57		
WH	4.42	4.70	-0.28	4.56	6.20		
YAS	3.51	3.71	-0.20	3.61	5.57		
SPY	2.96	3.14	-0.19	3.05	6.13		
KKH	2.70	2.38	-0.13	2.77	4.59		
Mean			-0.18		4.63		
SD			0.07		1.47		

$\delta = Cl_{Model\ 1} - Cl_{Model\ 2}$

Appendix 2.20 Comparison between Model 1 and Model 2 for
Modified Bland-Altman Plot

2. $t_{1/2}$

Subject	$t_{1/2}$ Model 1 (hr)	$t_{1/2}$ Model 2 (hr)	δ	mean	% of δ as mean	mean δ - 2SD	mean δ + 2SD
CWH	4.39	3.60	0.79	4.00	19.76	-0.92	4.58
WR	4.49	3.11	1.38	3.80	36.30		
WKKW	5.75	2.75	3.01	4.25	70.76		
KWSC	5.34	2.83	2.51	4.09	61.42		
CSYC	6.89	4.58	2.30	5.74	40.16		
LHY	5.25	5.91	-0.66	5.58	11.77		
CWSD	3.77	3.84	-0.07	3.81	1.86		
NPSD	3.95	3.97	-0.02	3.96	0.51		
LCKY	7.54	3.41	4.13	5.47	75.52		
WP	5.15	2.86	2.28	4.00	56.99		
WH	6.92	3.34	3.58	5.13	69.76		
YAS	4.83	3.45	1.38	4.14	33.23		
SPY	5.64	2.77	2.87	4.21	68.16		
KKH	5.22	3.10	2.12	4.16	51.00		
Mean			1.83		42.66		
SD			1.38		25.26		

$\delta = t_{1/2}$ Model 1 - $t_{1/2}$ Model 2

Appendix 2.21   Comparison between Model 1 and Model 2 for
Modified Bland-Altman Plot

3. AUC

Subject	$AUC_{Model\ 1}$ (μg ml^{-1} hr)	$AUC_{Model\ 2}$ (μg ml^{-1} hr)	δ	mean	% of δ as mean	mean δ - 2SD	mean δ + 2SD
CWH	92.1	88.3	3.7	90.2	4.1	0.9	7.4
WR	84.9	80.3	4.6	82.6	5.5		
WKKW	48.4	46.4	2.0	47.4	4.1		
KWSC	85.9	81.2	4.7	83.5	5.6		
CSYC	84.9	81.1	3.9	83.0	4.7		
LHY	95.5	94.9	0.6	95.2	0.6		
CWSD	94.3	91.8	2.5	93.0	2.7		
NPSD	90.0	86.6	3.3	88.3	3.8		
LCKY	118.8	112.3	6.5	115.6	5.6		
WP	86.8	82.1	4.7	84.4	5.6		
WH	75.4	70.9	4.5	73.1	6.2		
YAS	94.9	89.8	5.1	92.4	5.6		
SPY	112.7	106.0	6.7	109.4	6.1		
KKH	123.4	117.9	5.6	120.6	4.6		
Mean			4.2		4.6		
SD			1.6		1.5		

$\delta = AUC_{Model\ 1} - AUC_{Model\ 2}$

Appendix 2.22   Comparison between Model 1 and Model 3 for
Modified Bland-Altman Plot

1. Clearance

Subject	$Cl_{Model\ 1}$ (ml min^{-1} kg^{-1})	$Cl_{Model\ 3}$ (ml min^{-1} kg^{-1})	δ	mean	% of δ as mean	mean δ - 2SD	mean δ + 2SD
CWH	3.62	3.33	0.29	3.47	8.46	0.20	0.50
WR	3.93	3.40	0.53	3.67	14.35		
WKKW	6.89	6.49	0.40	6.69	5.95		
KWSC	3.88	3.49	0.39	3.69	10.64		
CSYC	3.93	3.62	0.31	3.77	8.22		
LHY	3.49	3.19	0.30	3.3+	8.98		
CWSD	3.54	3.21	0.32	3.37	9.51		
NPSD	3.71	3.39	0.32	3.55	8.94		
LCKY	2.81	2.56	0.24	2.68	9.09		
WP	3.84	3.47	0.37	3.66	10.12		
WH	4.42	3.95	0.47	4.19	11.20		
YAS	3.51	3.16	0.35	3.34	10.46		
SPY	2.96	2.64	0.32	2.80	11.52		
KKH	2.70	2.45	0.25	2.57	9.83		
Mean			0.35		9.80		
SD			0.08		1.85		

$\delta = Cl_{Model\ 1} - Cl_{Model\ 3}$

Appendix 2.23 Comparison between Model 1 and Model 3 for Modified Bland-Altman Plot

2. $t_{1/2}$

Subject	$t_{1/2}$ Model 1 (hr)	$t_{1/2}$ Model 3 (hr)	δ	mean	% of δ as mean	mean δ - 2SD	mean δ + 2SD
CWH	4.39	4.59	-0.20	4.49	4.43	-0.71	2.76
WR	4.49	4.06	0.44	4.28	10.17		
WKKW	5.75	4.87	0.89	5.31	16.67		
KWSC	5.34	4.17	1.18	4.76	24.72		
CSYC	6.89	4.87	2.02	5.88	34.28		
LHY	5.25	4.58	0.68	4.91	13.75		
CWSD	3.77	3.79	-0.02	3.78	0.62		
NPSD	3.94	3.56	0.39	3.75	10.38		
LCKY	7.54	4.58	2.95	6.06	48.76		
WP	5.14	4.09	1.06	4.62	22.86		
WH	6.92	4.49	2.43	5.70	42.57		
YAS	4.83	4.27	0.56	4.55	12.22		
SPY	5.64	4.38	1.26	5.01	25.21		
KKH	5.22	4.48	0.74	4.85	15.32		
Mean			1.03		20.14		
SD			0.87		13.46		

$\delta = t_{1/2}$ Model 1 - $t_{1/2}$ Model 3

Appendix 2.24 Comparison between Model 1 and Model 3 for
Modified Bland-Altman Plot

3. AUC

Subject	$AUC_{Model\ 1}$ (μg ml^{-1} hr)	$AUC_{Model\ 3}$ (μg ml^{-1} hr)	δ	mean	% of δ as mean	mean δ - 2SD	mean δ + 2SD
CWH	92.1	100.2	-8.1	96.1	8.5	-14.9	-4.3
WR	84.9	98.0	-13.1	91.4	14.3		
WKKW	48.4	51.3	-3.0	49.9	5.9		
KWSC	85.9	95.5	-9.6	90.7	10.6		
CSYC	84.9	92.2	-7.3	88.6	8.2		
LHY	95.5	104.5	-9.0	100.0	9.0		
CWSD	94.3	103.7	-9.4	99.0	9.5		
NPSD	90.0	98.4	-8.4	94.2	9.0		
LCKY	118.8	130.1	-11.3	124.5	9.1		
WP	86.8	96.0	-9.2	91.4	10.1		
WH	75.4	84.3	-8.9	79.9	11.2		
YAS	94.9	105.4	-10.5	100.2	10.5		
SPY	112.7	126.5	-13.8	119.6	11.5		
KKH	123.4	136.1	-12.7	129.8	9.8		
Mean			-9.6		9.8		
SD			2.6		1.8		

δ = $AUC_{Model\ 1}$ - $AUC_{Model\ 3}$

Appendix 2.25 Comparison between Model 2 and Model 4 for
Modified Bland-Altman Plot

1. Clearance

Subject	$Cl_{Model\ 2}$ (ml min^{-1} kg^{-1})	$Cl_{Model\ 4}$ (ml min^{-1} kg^{-1})	δ	mean	% of δ as mean	mean δ - 2SD	mean δ + 2SD
CWH	3.77	3.85	-0.08	3.81	2.05	-0.21	0.06
WR	4.15	4.17	-0.02	4.16	0.48		
WKKW	7.18	7.25	-0.07	7.21	0.92		
KWSC	4.11	4.13	-0.02	4.12	0.58		
CSYC	4.11	4.29	-0.18	4.20	4.24		
LHY	3.51	3.78	-0.27	3.65	7.35		
CWSD	3.63	3.71	-0.08	3.67	2.18		
NPSD	3.85	3.91	-0.06	3.88	1.60		
LCKY	2.97	3.01	-0.04	2.99	1.47		
WP	4.06	4.08	-0.02	4.07	0.47		
WH	4.70	4.78	-0.08	4.74	1.60		
YAS	3.71	3.75	-0.04	3.73	0.97		
SPY	3.14	3.15	-0.01	3.15	0.25		
KKH	2.83	2.89	-0.06	2.86	1.86		
Mean			-0.07		1.86		
SD			0.07		1.81		

$\delta = Cl_{Model\ 2} - Cl_{Model\ 4}$

Appendix 2.26 Comparison between Model 2 and Model 4 for
Modified Bland-Altman Plot

2. $t_{1/2}$

Subject	$t_{1/2}$ Model 2 (hr)	$t_{1/2}$ Model 4 (hr)	δ	mean	% of δ as mean	mean δ - 2SD	mean δ + 2SD
CWH	3.60	2.60	1.00	3.10	32.24	-0.68	2.62
WR	3.11	2.88	0.23	3.00	7.65		
WKKW	2.75	1.86	0.88	2.31	38.30		
KWSC	2.83	2.45	0.38	2.64	14.29		
CSYC	4.58	2.22	2.37	3.40	69.64		
LHY	5.91	2.89	3.02	4.40	68.64		
CWSD	3.84	2.78	1.06	3.31	32.14		
NPSD	3.97	2.50	1.47	3.23	45.37		
LCKY	3.41	2.22	1.18	2.81	41.98		
WP	2.86	2.58	0.28	2.72	10.26		
WH	3.34	2.30	1.04	2.82	36.91		
YAS	3.45	3.05	0.41	3.25	12.48		
SPY	2.77	2.62	0.16	2.70	5.82		
KKH	3.10	2.96	0.14	3.03	4.60		
Mean			0.97		30.02		
SD			0.82		21.12		

$\delta = t_{1/2}$ Model 2 - $t_{1/2}$ Model 4

Appendix 2.27 Comparison between Model 2 and Model 4 for
Modified Bland-Altman Plot

3. AUC

Subject	$AUC_{Model\ 2}$ (μg ml^{-1} hr)	$AUC_{Model\ 4}$ (μg ml^{-1} hr)	δ	mean	% of δ as mean	mean δ - 2SD	mean δ + 2SD
CWH	88.3	86.5	1.8	87.4	2.1	-1.6	5.0
WR	80.3	79.9	0.4	80.1	0.5		
WKKW	46.4	46.0	0.4	46.2	0.9		
KWSC	81.2	80.7	0.5	80.9	0.6		
CSYC	81.1	77.7	3.3	79.4	4.2		
LHY	94.9	88.2	6.7	91.5	7.3		
CWSD	91.8	89.8	2.0	90.8	2.2		
NPSD	86.6	85.2	1.4	85.9	1.6		
LCKY	112.3	110.7	1.7	111.5	1.5		
WP	82.1	81.7	0.4	81.9	0.5		
WH	70.9	69.7	1.1	70.3	1.6		
YAS	89.8	88.9	0.9	89.4	1.0		
SPY	106.0	105.7	0.3	105.9	0.3		
KKH	117.9	115.5	2.4	116.7	2.0		
Mean			1.7		1.9		
SD			1.6		1.8		

$\delta = AUC_{Model\ 2} - AUC_{Model\ 4}$

Appendix 2.28   Individual Plasma Paracetamol Concentrations Following
Ingestion of a 20 mg kg^{-1} Body Weight Dose — Group A

Time (hr)	Plasma Paracetamol Concentration (μg ml^{-1})						
	Group A Subject						
	1	2	3	4	5	6	7
0	0	0	0	0	0	0	0
0.5	15.52	19.72	19.28	23.59	25.14	20.37	26.87
1	14.51	15.28	21.23	19.69	29.21	24.26	17.42
1.5	12.21	-	-	16.38	123.00	19.45	13.90
2	13.67	12.22	15.05	12.85	19.39	16.28	12.07
3	9.56	8.13	10.15	9.24	13.66	11.43	8.73
4	6.76	5.24	7.89	5.76	10.35	8.31	6.51
5	4.76	4.17	5.24	3.79	7.06	5.86	4.91
6	3.38	2.91	3.73	2.66	5.83	4.14	3.47
7	2.63	1.94	2.72	1.96	4.43	3.01	2.58
8	1.87	1.48	1.97	1.45	3.59	2.56	1.79
24	0.09	0.14	0.10	0.15	0.17	0.16	0.17

Appendix 2.29   Individual Plasma Paracetamol Concentrations Following
Ingestion of a 20 mg kg^{-1} Body Weight Dose — Group B

Time (hr)	Plasma Paracetamol Concentration (ug m-1)							
	Group B Subject							
	1	2	3	4	5	6	7	8
0	0	0	0	0	0	0	0	0
0.5	12.57	26.92	15.39	13.41	30.24	20.38	18.39	8.90
1	12.49	20.34	13.23	31.38	19.86	24.39	19.53	14.69
1.5	9.57	17.14	11.15	17.91	16.02	23.65	-	11.51
2	7.52	15.89	9.57	11.01	13.72	20.93	15.26	11.56
3	5.29	13.98	7.59	6.43	10.09	16.34	12.25	8.11
4	3.49	11.24	5.78	3.80	7.97	13.33	9.82	5.26
5	2.24	9.21	4.51	2.38	6.02	10.72	6.80	3.58
6	1.31	7.92	3.99	1.39	4.08	8.54	5.23	2.61
7	0.98	6.87	2.89	1.29	2.93	7.05	4.57	1.80
8	0.75	5.15	2.32	0.68	2.89	6.06	3.51	1.40
24	ND	ND	0.09	ND	ND	0.35	0.15	0.15

Appendix 2.30   Individual Plasma Paracetamol Concentrations Following
Ingestion of a 20 mg kg^{-1} Body Weight Dose — Group C

Time (hr)	Individual Plasma Paracetamol Concentration (μg ml^{-1})								
	Group C Subject								
	1	2	3	4	5	6	7	8	9
0	0	0	0	0	0	0	0	0	0
0.5	15.10	21.59	15.43	15.77	19.84	21.31	3.68	13.54	15.29
1	22.93	20.18	15.59	17.55	23.51	21.22	17.73	21.88	29.15
1.5	19.84	15.73	12.78	27.15	12.18	19.17	15.38	18.24	20.07
2	18.20	13.89	10.80	17.47	9.31	18.08	11.00	17.57	20.71
3	15.88	9.99	8.20	12.41	6.80	13.34	6.25	14.58	22.37
4	13.53	7.03	6.50	8.66	4.96	12.85	5.02	13.02	18.34
5	11.54	5.29	4.40	5.98	3.72	10.53	2.63	10.87	18.01
6	9.67	4.01	3.34	4.41	2.83	9.48	1.88	8.01	13.59
7	8.52	3.16	2.58	3.39	2.22	8.76	1.31	6.27	11.85
8	7.85	2.52	1.86	2.61	1.84	9.00	1.22	6.11	11.57
24	0.56	0.13	0.09	0.04	0.08	1.63	0.04	0.35	3.03

Appendix 2.31   Individual Plasma Paracetamol Concentrations Following
Ingestion of a 20 mg kg^{-1} Body Weight Dose — Group D

Time (hr)	Plasma Paracetamol Concentration (μg ml^{-1})							
	Group D Subject							
	1	2	3	4	5	6	7	8
0	0	0	0	0	0	0	0	0
0.5	22.49	18.88	20.23	19.82	28.27	23.89	6.65	25.03
1	15.26	19.73	18.61	29.30	30.81	17.98	12.85	18.12
1.5	11.35	17.60	13.08	31.05	29.22	14.59	16.29	15.04
2	9.30	15.70	10.90	21.07	27.35	12.56	14.86	13.27
3	6.01	13.02	8.07	16.56	19.46	9.74	11.53	10.36
4	4.62	10.18	5.11	12.80	13.89	7.93	9.87	8.69
5	3.39	8.11	4.03	10.80	11.01	6.12	8.00	6.68
6	2.70	6.55	3.02	9.37	6.59	4.29	6.22	5.47
7	1.99	5.28	2.35	8.38	6.13	3.69	5.01	4.41
8	1.62	4.25	1.79	7.23	4.07	2.73	4.01	3.56
24	0.40	2.22	0.11	1.41	0.17	0.07	0.08	0.20

Appendix 2.32   Individual Plasma Paracetamol Concentrations Following Ingestion of a 20 mg kg^{-1} Body Weight Dose — Group R

Time (hr)	Plasma Paracetamol Concentration (μg ml^{-1}) Group R Subject						
	1	2	3	4	5	6	7
0	0	0	0	0	0	0	0
0.5	17.32	0.63	17.85	18.52	11.35	10.66	33.51
1	19.11	9.82	14.74	15.70	8.02	11.67	16.81
1.5	20.74	9.43	12.56	13.50	5.16	10.23	12.97
2	18.05	7.68	12.45	9.90	3.68	8.06	10.68
3	15.33	5.74	9.29	6.72	2.46	9.06	7.89
4	11.68	4.07	7.19	4.82	1.77	7.64	5.91
5	8.31	2.84	5.16	3.32	1.16	6.03	2.08
6	6.83	1.90	4.33	2.51	0.86	4.66	2.60
7	5.55	1.55	3.46	2.08	0.65	3.71	3.33
8	4.48	1.28	2.93	1.70	0.68	3.13	4.15
24	1.64	0.20	0.34	0.06	0.10	0.41	0.09

Appendix 2.33 Individual Plasma Paracetamol Concentrations Following Ingestion of a 20 mg kg^{-1} Body Weight Dose — Group D'

Time (hr)	Plasma Paracetamol Concentration (μg ml^{-1}) Group D' Subject							
	1	2	3	4	5	6	7	8
0	0	0	0	0	0	0	0	0
0.5	8.41	2.48	18.00	13.60	29.90	31.63	12.24	30.30
1	15.21	5.78	20.12	19.44	30.83	22.70	15.90	22.60
1.5	-	-	-	-	-	-	-	-
2	17.13	7.34	13.35	14.75	20.75	17.79	12.96	15.68
3	13.92	8.78	9.96	9.70	16.93	14.62	10.62	12.55
4	10.27	8.74	7.29	7.61	14.17	11.26	8.40	10.03
5	7.66	7.69	5.28	5.82	11.66	9.41	7.01	8.53
6	6.11	6.10	4.21	4.77	9.17	7.40	5.54	6.71
7	5.14	4.67	3.06	3.41	7.88	6.01	4.34	5.81
8	4.34	3.28	2.29	2.58	6.11	4.75	3.44	4.71
24	0.38	0.26	0.10	0.11	0.29	0.14	0.16	0.35

Appendix 2.34   Individual Plasma Paracetamol Glucuronide Concentrations Following Ingestion of a 20 mg kg^{-1} Body Weight Dose — Group A

Time (hr)	Plasma Paracetamol Glucuronide Concentration (μg ml^{-1})						
	Group A Subject						
	1	2	3	4	5	6	7
0	0.00	0.00	0.00	0.00	1.73	0.00	0.00
0.5	6.02	7.39	3.33	1.95	4.71	4.47	3.82
1	12.26	17.55	6.04	6.46	9.56	11.64	7.68
1.5	13.90	-	-	9.06	12.98	14.09	9.41
2	14.91	20.41	10.60	10.24	14.31	15.40	10.48
3	16.40	17.57	13.10	10.79	15.95	15.37	11.08
4	13.10	13.13	12.86	9.67	15.68	15.64	10.47
5	11.22	9.76	10.66	8.18	14.10	13.97	9.43
6	8.92	7.51	8.90	6.26	12.28	11.80	8.07
7	7.17	5.78	7.39	4.74	10.64	9.94	6.69
8	5.61	4.59	5.89	3.64	9.19	8.26	4.99
24	0.34	1.00	0.94	0.28	1.39	1.08	1.06

Appendix 2.35   Individual Plasma Paracetamol Sulphate Concentrations Following Ingestion of a 20 mg kg^{-1} Body Weight Dose — Group A

Time (hr)	Plasma Paracetamol Sulphate Concentration (μg ml^{-1}) Group A Subject						
	1	2	3	4	5	6	7
0	0.00	0.00	0.00	0.00	0.56	0.00	0.00
0.5	3.98	4.26	5.04	3.42	4.69	2.94	3.85
1	5.33	7.25	7.06	6.07	7.05	5.29	5.15
1.5	5.23	-	-	6.48	7.98	5.54	5.26
2	5.34	6.85	7.64	6.05	8.33	5.47	5.18
3	4.76	5.30	7.33	5.25	7.88	5.00	4.70
4	3.96	3.87	6.82	4.23	7.41	4.41	4.05
5	3.24	3.06	5.24	3.12	6.45	3.70	3.35
6	2.49	2.35	4.09	2.21	5.34	2.84	2.65
7	2.02	1.66	3.09	1.52	4.34	2.40	2.00
8	1.54	1.29	2.36	1.07	3.68	1.89	1.46
24	0.00	0.09	0.12	0.06	0.27	0.08	0.10

Appendix 2.36 Individual Plasma Paracetamol Cysteine Concentrations Following Ingestion of a 20 mg kg^{-1} Body Weight Dose — Group A

Time (hr)	Plasma Paracetamol Cysteine Concentration (μg ml^{-1})						
	Group A Subject						
	1	2	3	4	5	6	7
0	0.00	0.00	0.00	0.00	0.08	0.00	0.00
0.5	0.04	0.13	0.09	0.00	0.08	0.06	0.05
1	0.10	0.28	0.03	0.00	0.09	0.07	0.13
1.5	0.13	-	-	0.03	0.23	0.13	0.19
2	0.13	0.44	0.08	0.13	0.10	0.12	0.24
3	0.16	0.48	0.14	0.13	0.15	0.16	0.26
4	0.17	0.41	0.17	0.14	0.33	0.15	0.26
5	0.13	0.44	0.17	0.12	0.19	0.22	0.26
6	0.12	0.45	0.26	0.00	0.18	0.16	0.24
7	0.12	0.37	0.22	0.10	0.16	0.19	0.23
8	0.12	0.34	0.18	0.08	0.14	0.11	0.20
24	0.00	0.08	0.00	0.00	0.06	0.00	0.00

Appendix 2.37 Individual Plasma Paracetamol Glucuronide Concentrations
Following Ingestion of a 20 mg kg^{-1} Body Weight Dose — Group B

Time (hr)	Plasma Paracetamol Glucuronide Concentration (μg ml^{-1}) Group B Subject							
	1	2	3	4	5	6	7	8
0	0.00	0.00	0.00	0.00	0.00	0.00	0.00	0.00
0.5	4.30	2.37	3.66	3.67	7.44	3.73	2.72	3.59
1	13.23	6.24	5.97	16.64	13.06	9.56	5.24	9.59
1.5	18.37	8.88	6.51	30.51	14.28	12.03	-	18.55
2	19.02	10.70	7.00	30.52	14.48	13.97	6.65	17.50
3	18.37	13.98	7.19	26.53	13.54	14.15	7.75	17.03
4	15.95	13.51	6.51	20.29	11.97	14.15	8.38	14.20
5	12.15	12.26	5.55	14.51	9.34	13.02	7.62	11.11
6	9.43	11.12	5.16	9.60	7.49	11.05	6.28	8.60
7	6.85	10.23	4.61	7.95	5.49	9.16	5.81	6.78
8	5.27	8.36	3.68	4.70	4.21	8.85	4.45	5.53
24	0.00	0.73	0.20	0.26	0.43	0.65	0.25	0.25

Appendix 2.38   Individual Plasma Paracetamol Sulphate Concentrations Following Ingestion of a 20 mg kg^{-1} Body Weight Dose — Group B

Time (hr)	Plasma Paracetamol Sulphate Concentration (μg ml^{-1})							
	Group B Subject							
	1	2	3	4	5	6	7	8
0	0.00	0.00	0.00	0.00	0.00	0.00	0.00	0.00
0.5	3.25	1.53	1.85	2.50	4.61	3.47	4.36	1.12
1	6.06	3.41	2.54	6.46	6.00	5.83	7.19	2.15
1.5	5.66	3.70	2.60	7.57	6.22	6.59	-	3.59
2	5.06	3.85	2.72	6.46	5.96	6.76	8.33	3.38
3	4.03	4.05	2.65	4.77	5.49	5.74	8.05	3.64
4	3.06	3.29	2.19	3.28	4.76	6.08	7.41	2.97
5	2.10	2.62	1.96	2.24	3.79	5.55	6.28	2.53
6	1.42	2.17	1.83	1.48	2.73	4.38	5.01	1.96
7	0.97	1.86	1.38	1.17	1.99	3.52	4.43	1.53
8	0.71	1.53	1.12	0.66	1.51	3.19	3.38	1.26
24	0.00	0.15	0.09	0.03	0.00	0.23	0.23	0.00

Appendix 2.39   Individual Plasma Paracetamol Cysteine Concentrations Following Ingestion of a 20 mg kg^{-1} Body Weight Dose — Group B

Time (hr)	Plasma Paracetamol Cysteine Concentration ($\mu g\ ml^{-1}$)							
	Group B Subject							
	1	2	3	4	5	6	7	8
0	0.00	0.00	0.00	0.00	0.00	0.00	0.00	0.00
0.5	0.07	0.03	0.06	0.05	0.08	0.24	0.09	0.13
1	0.12	0.05	0.16	0.09	0.18	0.27	0.13	0.27
1.5	0.21	0.08	0.12	0.30	0.23	0.34	-	0.00
2	0.22	0.06	0.13	0.24	0.27	0.37	0.13	0.52
3	0.26	0.13	0.24	0.28	0.33	0.49	0.21	0.74
4	0.22	0.05	0.20	0.18	0.70	0.52	0.23	0.71
5	0.19	0.00	0.29	0.22	0.93	0.50	0.20	0.57
6	0.11	0.00	0.62	0.16	0.20	0.45	0.19	0.52
7	0.11	0.03	0.14	0.14	0.19	0.33	0.15	0.47
8	0.10	0.08	0.09	0.09	0.14	0.29	0.16	0.38
24	0.00	0.00	0.00	0.00	0.00	0.09	0.03	0.00

Appendix 2.40 Individual Plasma Paracetamol Glucuronide Concentrations Following Ingestion of a 20 mg kg^{-1} Body Weight Dose — Group C

Time (hr)	Plasma Paracetamol Glucuronide Concentration (μg ml^{-1})								
	Group C Subject								
	1	2	3	4	5	6	7	8	9
0	0.00	0.00	0.00	0.00	0.00	0.00	0.00	0.00	0.00
0.5	0.64	1.40	6.49	0.53	4.08	5.06	6.14	2.60	1.10
1	2.98	3.53	14.67	2.73	8.77	13.62	12.70	5.15	10.76
1.5	4.10	5.28	17.03	2.71	12.50	20.11	16.44	6.91	20.56
2	5.29	5.83	17.13	3.37	13.23	22.50	15.56	7.48	24.88
3	6.34	6.34	17.78	4.60	12.71	23.21	12.72	8.12	23.41
4	6.43	7.76	17.39	4.68	12.47	21.50	10.77	8.25	20.13
5	5.94	7.77	15.98	5.80	9.54	17.77	8.62	7.12	13.46
6	5.41	7.32	13.98	4.63	8.03	14.20	6.91	6.81	9.49
7	4.42	7.01	11.57	4.47	6.57	11.43	5.50	6.59	7.28
8	4.01	5.90	9.59	4.92	4.88	9.70	4.73	6.37	5.63
24	0.28	0.30	1.25	1.95	0.31	0.34	1.03	1.07	0.21

Appendix 2.41 Individual Plasma Paracetamol Sulphate Concentrations Following Ingestion of a 20 mg kg^{-1} Body Weight Dose — Group C

Time (hr)	Plasma Paracetamol Glucuronide Concentration (μg ml^{-1})								
	Group C Subject								
	1	2	3	4	5	6	7	8	9
0	0.00	0.00	0.00	0.00	0.00	0.00	0.00	0.00	0.00
0.5	1.38	1.04	3.13	0.49	3.75	1.94	4.98	1.24	0.70
1	3.34	2.33	5.12	1.97	5.71	7.24	3.38	2.11	4.82
1.5	3.86	2.96	5.57	1.93	5.92	4.44	6.59	2.55	6.84
2	4.20	3.20	5.30	2.11	5.48	4.20	5.81	2.63	7.16
3	3.91	3.39	4.77	3.02	4.96	3.52	4.55	2.69	5.48
4	4.32	4.05	3.84	2.87	4.16	2.86	3.77	3.05	4.57
5	3.80	4.16	3.20	3.71	3.31	2.36	2.92	2.83	2.95
6	2.99	3.90	2.59	2.83	2.68	1.77	2.35	2.58	2.09
7	2.45	3.56	2.01	2.47	2.08	1.43	1.86	2.56	1.54
8	2.33	3.04	1.64	2.39	1.56	1.12	1.51	2.47	1.30
24	0.00	0.46	0.00	0.88	0.00	0.00	0.09	0.48	0.13

Appendix 2.42   Individual Plasma Paracetamol Cysteine Concentrations Following Ingestion of a 20 mg kg^{-1} Body Weight Dose — Group C

Time (hr)	Plasma Paracetamol Glucuronide Concentration (μg ml^{-1})								
	Group C Subject								
	1	2	3	4	5	6	7	8	9
0	0.00	0.00	0.00	0.00	0.00	0.00	0.00	0.00	0.00
0.5	0.00	0.02	0.19	0.00	0.00	0.08	0.04	0.24	0.13
1	0.01	0.07	0.34	0.14	0.01	0.09	0.13	0.21	0.11
1.5	0.08	0.10	0.30	0.12	0.09	0.23	0.16	0.23	0.21
2	0.14	0.15	0.25	0.16	0.07	0.30	0.24	0.26	0.22
3	0.17	0.22	0.34	0.28	0.17	0.27	0.20	0.16	0.19
4	0.23	0.31	0.24	0.34	0.17	0.29	0.21	0.12	0.24
5	0.23	0.35	0.25	0.53	0.16	0.25	0.18	0.08	0.19
6	0.18	0.38	0.21	0.32	0.16	0.22	0.14	0.11	0.17
7	0.20	0.29	0.19	0.32	0.14	0.20	0.12	0.15	0.15
8	0.19	0.29	0.15	0.35	0.17	0.18	0.11	0.15	0.16
24	0.00	0.09	0.00	0.29	0.00	0.03	0.04	0.06	0.05

Appendix 2.43 Individual Plasma Paracetamol Glucuronide Concentrations Following Ingestion of a 20 mg kg^{-1} Body Weight Dose — Group D

Time (hr)	Plasma Paracetamol Glucuronide Concentration (μg ml^{-1})							
	Group D Subject							
	1	2	3	4	5	6	7	8
0	0.00	0.00	0.00	0.00	0.00	0.00	0.00	0.00
0.5	3.06	3.54	5.51	1.53	6.44	2.81	0.92	3.76
1	6.68	8.16	15.05	4.83	14.10	3.94	2.29	5.75
1.5	8.47	9.35	16.41	7.46	18.51	4.74	3.94	6.57
2	9.38	10.95	15.91	12.67	21.04	5.05	6.04	7.20
3	10.28	12.32	13.54	14.95	20.25	5.14	8.40	7.35
4	9.76	12.61	10.53	18.25	17.93	4.82	9.15	4.52
5	9.19	12.01	8.65	18.44	15.11	4.19	9.55	5.95
6	7.83	11.1	6.90	17.75	11.29	3.40	9.19	5.25
7	6.85	9.81	5.95	18.84	9.89	3.04	8.23	4.60
8	6.43	8.45	5.02	17.44	7.35	2.95	7.32	4.14
24	1.56	5.85	0.18	10.93	0.33	0.13	0.40	0.88

Appendix 2.44   Individual Plasma Paracetamol Sulphate Concentrations Following Ingestion of a 20 mg kg^{-1} Body Weight Dose — Group D

Time (hr)	Plasma Paracetamol Sulphate Concentration (μg ml^{-1}) Group D Subject							
	1	2	3	4	5	6	7	8
0	0.00	0.00	0.00	0.00	0.00	0.00	0.00	0.00
0.5	3.93	1.98	2.44	0.97	3.16	5.64	0.88	3.01
1	5.64	3.75	4.89	2.36	4.68	5.93	1.82	4.09
1.5	5.95	3.98	4.75	3.36	5.38	6.31	2.67	4.11
2	5.80	4.30	4.14	5.37	5.57	6.07	3.41	3.68
3	5.39	4.28	3.21	6.26	4.96	5.69	3.61	3.75
4	4.71	3.87	2.27	7.16	4.59	5.20	3.63	3.45
5	3.86	3.35	1.82	7.48	4.00	4.35	3.44	2.92
6	2.98	2.92	1.31	7.33	3.42	3.28	3.08	2.30
7	2.22	2.33	1.03	7.52	3.18	2.86	2.62	2.01
8	1.90	1.89	0.79	6.56	2.34	2.10	2.22	1.64
24	0.22	2.53	0.09	3.45	0.15	0.12	0.10	0.12

Appendix 2.45 Individual Plasma Paracetamol Cysteine Concentrations Following Ingestion of a 20 mg kg^{-1} Body Weight Dose — Group D

Time (hr)	Plasma Paracetamol Cysteine Concentration (μg ml^{-1})							
	Group D Subject							
	1	2	3	4	5	6	7	8
0	0.00	0.00	0.00	0.00	0.00	0.00	0.00	0.00
0.5	0.10	0.00	0.05	0.30	0.17	0.06	0.08	0.10
1	0.18	0.08	0.17	0.14	0.19	0.15	0.20	0.20
1.5	0.24	0.09	0.32	0.20	0.18	0.22	0.26	0.22
2	0.33	0.06	0.22	0.42	0.25	0.25	0.36	0.28
3	0.38	0.07	0.23	0.60	0.33	0.36	0.49	0.27
4	0.35	0.08	0.21	0.78	0.30	0.37	0.51	0.28
5	0.35	0.10	0.19	0.81	0.28	0.43	0.53	0.25
6	0.30	0.08	0.16	0.77	0.17	0.40	0.49	0.21
7	0.28	0.08	0.15	0.83	0.16	0.38	0.45	0.19
8	0.28	0.06	0.12	0.70	0.13	0.36	0.43	0.22
24	0.00	0.38	0.03	0.34	0.00	0.05	0.05	0.05

Appendix 2.46   Individual Plasma Paracetamol Glucuronide Concentrations
Following Ingestion of a 20 mg kg^{-1} Body Weight Dose — Group R

Time (hr)	Plasma Paracetamol Glucuronide Concentration (μg ml^{-1})						
	Group R Subject						
	1	2	3	4	5	6	7
0	0.00	0.00	0.00	0.00	0.00	0.00	0.00
0.5	2.70	2.60	5.10	7.62	7.05	2.73	5.63
1	4.91	8.53	10.85	15.37	15.51	6.98	13.14
1.5	9.01	12.99	15.36	18.97	18.67	11.29	15.70
2	11.17	16.26	19.08	24.17	18.69	15.41	18.32
3	15.64	20.85	23.59	28.32	18.76	20.88	20.77
4	18.40	21.17	26.17	29.93	18.03	26.22	20.68
5	22.47	19.66	27.26	29.24	15.21	28.30	14.31
6	24.04	18.85	27.94	27.64	13.51	29.97	15.96
7	24.78	18.46	26.52	26.13	11.80	29.95	17.56
8	24.66	16.83	25.63	24.16	10.08	29.35	18.55
24	19.14	4.98	7.30	6.19	1.10	11.51	1.97

Appendix 2.47 Individual Plasma Paracetamol Sulphate Concentrations
Following Ingestion of a 20 mg kg^{-1} Body Weight Dose — Group R

Time (hr)	Plasma Paracetamol Sulphate Concentration (μg ml^{-1})						
	Group R Subject						
	1	2	3	4	5	6	7
0	0.00	0.00	0.00	0.00	0.00	0.00	0.00
0.5	5.21	4.75	5.51	6.63	3.95	2.54	9.08
1	8.45	9.50	8.50	9.73	5.87	4.93	13.11
1.5	12.68	11.44	10.13	11.49	5.69	6.30	13.27
2	14.67	11.67	11.46	12.92	4.83	6.81	13.19
3	18.75	13.25	13.58	13.29	4.08	8.67	12.58
4	21.30	12.06	13.08	13.02	3.56	9.48	10.49
5	26.34	9.95	12.44	11.80	2.71	9.10	5.64
6	27.57	8.76	12.17	10.84	2.16	8.87	6.65
7	28.33	7.85	10.85	10.00	1.75	8.31	7.72
8	27.33	6.92	9.97	8.81	1.45	7.93	8.69
24	16.52	1.14	1.35	1.28	0.07	1.36	0.43

Appendix 2.48 Individual Plasma Paracetamol Cysteine Concentrations Following Ingestion of a 20 mg kg^{-1} Body Weight Dose — Group R

Time (hr)	Plasma Paracetamol Cysteine Concentration (μg ml^{-1}) Group R Subject						
	1	2	3	4	5	6	7
0	0.00	0.00	0.00	0.00	0.00	0.00	0.00
0.5	0.22	0.04	0.14	0.08	0.11	0.00	0.21
1	0.31	0.10	0.18	0.17	0.32	0.12	0.19
1.5	0.67	0.16	0.09	0.40	0.39	0.15	0.26
2	0.70	0.31	0.18	0.47	0.37	0.20	0.34
3	1.18	0.26	0.25	0.52	0.36	0.37	0.46
4	1.28	0.43	0.41	0.52	0.34	0.27	0.49
5	1.66	0.41	0.44	0.51	0.27	0.39	0.43
6	1.80	0.26	0.57	0.49	0.21	0.41	0.46
7	1.89	0.25	0.52	0.47	0.19	0.42	0.46
8	1.91	0.29	0.47	0.46	0.22	0.41	0.51
24	1.17	0.13	0.14	0.16	0.00	0.11	0.04

Appendix 2.49 Individual Plasma Paracetamol Glucuronide Concentrations Following Ingestion of a 20 mg kg^{-1} Body Weight Dose — Group D'

Time (hr)	Plasma Paracetamol Glucuronide Concentration (μg ml^{-1}) Group D' Subject							
	1	2	3	4	5	6	7	8
0	0.00	0.00	0.00	0.00	0.00	0.00	0.00	0.00
0.5	0.83	2.54	1.80	2.16	4.60	3.44	3.05	4.60
1	1.88	8.00	4.67	4.74	8.48	6.65	6.91	8.48
2	5.11	14.73	6.93	6.82	11.17	11.17	9.47	11.17
3	6.46	17.09	5.78	7.22	10.74	12.54	10.25	10.74
4	7.41	16.88	4.89	6.90	10.73	12.78	8.95	10.73
5	8.13	15.69	3.93	6.41	10.29	12.16	7.88	10.29
6	7.56	13.90	3.32	5.43	9.00	11.12	6.77	9.00
7	7.27	11.70	2.71	4.95	8.94	10.14	5.86	8.94
8	7.68	9.73	2.10	4.24	7.92	8.63	4.96	7.92
24	1.36	0.62	0.22	0.25	1.15	0.81	0.64	1.15

Appendix 2.50   Individual Plasma Paracetamol Sulphate Concentrations Following Ingestion of a 20 mg kg^{-1} Body Weight Dose — Group D'

Time (hr)	Plasma Paracetamol Sulphate Concentration (μg ml^{-1})							
	Group D' Subject							
	1	2	3	4	5	6	7	8
0	0.00	0.00	0.00	0.00	0.70	0.00	0.00	0.00
0.5	1.39	1.77	2.69	2.24	0.99	3.09	2.15	4.62
1	3.69	3.63	4.36	3.90	2.53	4.80	3.87	6.54
2	7.73	4.54	4.65	4.75	3.99	6.17	4.41	7.37
3	9.08	5.21	3.45	4.60	4.66	6.68	4.72	7.01
4	9.99	4.64	2.90	4.26	4.92	6.30	4.36	7.20
5	9.93	3.78	2.30	3.67	4.79	5.61	3.59	6.80
6	9.52	3.05	1.90	3.14	4.14	4.90	3.02	5.72
7	8.39	2.38	1.54	2.97	3.28	4.08	2.62	5.53
8	7.97	1.78	1.20	2.36	2.44	0.34	2.19	4.78
24	0.85	0.10	0.08	0.13	0.34	0.18	0.10	0.60

Appendix 2.51 Individual Plasma Paracetamol Cysteine Concentrations Following Ingestion of a 20 mg kg^{-1} Body Weight Dose — Group D'

Time (hr)	Plasma Paracetamol Cysteine Concentration (μg ml^{-1}) Group D' Subject							
	1	2	3	4	5	6	7	8
0	0.00	0.00	0.00	0.00	0.10	0.00	0.00	0.00
0.5	0.08	0.06	0.05	0.04	0.25	0.29	0.14	0.07
1	0.24	0.20	0.21	0.19	0.39	0.50	0.29	0.18
2	0.67	0.40	0.37	0.36	0.48	0.93	0.46	0.40
3	1.15	0.65	0.51	0.42	0.84	1.03	0.58	0.54
4	1.49	0.64	0.50	0.43	1.22	1.02	0.58	0.67
5	1.74	0.60	0.46	0.49	1.23	0.96	0.49	0.70
6	1.82	0.55	0.45	0.48	1.14	0.89	0.41	0.71
7	1.77	0.58	0.43	0.47	1.06	0.84	0.44	0.78
8	1.77	0.53	0.36	0.43	0.79	0.74	0.39	0.78
24	0.24	0.08	0.00	0.04	0.12	0.05	0.07	0.15

Appendix 2.52 Urinary Recovery of Paracetamol and Metabolites in Each Sample Following Ingestion of a 20 mg kg^{-1} Body Weight Dose — Group A

Time After Dosing	Urinary Recovery of Paracetamol and Metabolites in Individual Subjects (mg)						
	Group A Subject						
	1	2	3	4	5	6	7
Glucuronide							
0-4hr	279.42	0.00	214.48	296.05	161.07	371.60	305.64
4-8hr	281.74	410.35	295.76	216.28	177.43	283.44	112.89
8-24hr	172.81	166.00	134.57	108.87	155.37	224.79	182.22
0-24hr	733.98	576.36	644.81	621.20	493.87	879.83	600.76
Sulphate							
0-4hr	132.09	0.00	209.01	253.96	133.28	174.79	232.02
4-8hr	108.88	172.55	189.95	113.23	104.94	99.41	53.58
8-24hr	67.15	64.81	75.92	60.54	88.81	76.74	91.45
0-24hr	308.12	237.36	474.88	427.72	327.03	350.94	377.05
Cysteine							
0-4hr	4.76	0.00	5.52	6.49	3.41	5.54	15.56
4-8hr	6.66	17.13	10.69	8.98	4.98	7.51	7.17
8-24hr	9.56	15.53	14.23	11.60	8.99	10.56	17.07
0-24hr	20.97	32.66	30.44	27.06	17.38	23.61	39.80
Paracetamol							
0-4hr	21.47	0.00	21.00	15.20	18.34	49.24	24.25
4-8hr	14.40	24.98	14.74	11.27	11.09	10.08	6.89
8-24hr	12.82	13.45	9.58	9.90	8.83	9.47	14.30
0-24hr	48.69	38.44	45.32	36.38	38.27	68.79	45.44
Mercapturate							
0-4hr	6.17	0.00	4.65	5.87	4.21	7.93	12.53
4-8hr	10.25	21.46	12.22	6.62	5.92	9.32	4.89
8-24hr	9.21	22.70	11.20	6.88	9.37	12.39	8.34
0-24hr	25.63	44.16	28.07	19.38	19.50	29.64	25.76
Total							
0-4hr	443.92	0.00	454.66	577.57	320.32	609.09	590.00
4-8hr	421.92	646.48	523.36	356.37	304.36	409.76	185.42
8-24hr	271.55	282.49	245.49	197.80	271.38	333.95	313.38
0-24hr	1137.39	928.97	1223.51	1131.74	896.06	1352.80	1088.81

Appendix 2.53 Urinary Recovery of Paracetamol and Metabolites in Each Sample Following Ingestion of a 20 mg kg^{-1} Body Weight Dose — Group B

Time After Dosing	Urinary Recovery of Paracetamol and Metabolites in Individual Subjects (mg)							
	Group B Subject							
	1	2	3	4	5	6	7	8
Glucuronide								
0-4hr	356.19	44.97	154.40	45.18	404.16	103.02	248.96	150.74
4-8hr	248.71	83.78	160.41	652.93	204.80	153.58	119.67	472.95
8-24hr	100.65	231.21	142.57	147.44	102.50	138.64	86.48	168.67
0-24hr	705.55	359.96	457.38	845.54	711.46	395.24	455.10	792.36
Sulphate								
0-4hr	167.74	42.40	95.31	31.41	265.66	91.84	440.62	45.24
4-8hr	61.18	39.26	88.69	163.33	112.65	98.14	144.93	149.29
8-24hr	23.43	93.92	65.33	30.74	53.49	82.42	102.41	55.31
0-24hr	252.34	175.58	249.33	225.49	431.80	272.40	687.96	249.84
Cysteine								
0-4hr	8.45	1.73	8.87	0.86	12.99	6.38	14.17	12.00
4-8hr	8.19	3.35	10.86	11.71	9.31	10.05	8.37	55.90
8-24hr	5.13	14.23	10.00	5.69	6.00	19.33	8.43	21.43
0-24hr	21.76	19.31	29.72	18.27	28.31	35.75	30.97	89.33
Paracetamol								
0-4hr	11.16	5.59	10.00	4.50	18.07	10.73	16.30	7.53
4-8hr	7.60	5.43	17.56	14.37	14.74	15.44	7.67	13.73
8-24hr	6.73	18.89	14.62	7.40	13.55	18.16	7.24	5.21
0-24hr	25.49	29.91	42.19	26.28	46.37	44.33	31.22	26.47
Mercapturate								
0-4hr	8.81	1.93	10.60	0.75	11.89	4.83	10.34	5.79
4-8hr	8.20	3.67	14.02	21.78	9.97	10.76	6.17	32.26
8-24hr	4.78	13.56	16.25	9.86	8.12	22.96	4.01	12.68
0-24hr	21.79	19.16	40.87	32.38	29.99	38.55	20.52	50.73
Total								
0-4hr	552.34	96.61	279.18	82.69	712.78	216.80	730.39	221.30
4-8hr	333.88	135.48	291.54	864.12	351.47	287.96	286.81	724.12
8-24hr	140.72	371.82	248.76	201.14	183.68	281.51	208.57	263.30
0-24hr	1026.94	603.92	819.49	1147.95	1247.93	786.28	1225.77	1208.72

Appendix 2.54 Urinary Recovery of Paracetamol and Metabolites in Each Sample Following Ingestion of a 20 mg kg^{-1} Body Weight Dose — Group C

Time After Dosing	Urinary Recovery of Paracetamol and Metabolites (mg)								
	Group C Subject								
	1	2	3	4	5	6	7	8	9
Glucuronide									
0-4hr	91.26	89.61	251.32	30.33	245.33	487.84	318.02	76.50	641.13
4-8hr	148.24	114.96	283.84	75.97	127.93	279.60	34.12	199.23	344.47
8-24hr	145.92	144.19	161.31	193.84	86.11	293.64	143.46	301.77	189.07
0-24hr	385.41	348.76	696.47	300.14	459.37	1061.09	495.60	577.50	1174.66
Sulphate									
0-4hr	107.57	112.80	136.22	40.78	143.58	127.05	188.34	54.53	222.68
4-8hr	117.08	120.35	98.60	91.52	55.08	49.82	18.52	122.66	86.14
8-24hr	118.58	142.43	67.38	194.50	36.39	47.25	72.69	194.20	44.89
0-24hr	343.24	375.58	302.19	326.81	235.05	224.12	279.55	371.38	353.70
Cysteine									
0-4hr	4.00	6.11	9.25	3.53	6.48	11.38	9.22	2.15	8.72
4-8hr	10.55	11.69	8.89	11.80	3.97	6.59	1.21	7.33	7.68
8-24hr	24.33	21.46	9.82	48.63	8.68	14.23	10.53	19.54	7.06
0-24hr	38.88	39.26	27.96	63.96	19.12	32.19	20.96	29.02	23.46
Paracetamol									
0-4hr	18.45	15.30	14.79	4.31	24.31	38.14	14.79	6.43	25.03
4-8hr	28.66	16.27	15.09	10.25	8.65	13.56	1.79	11.26	10.32
8-24hr	19.58	26.83	13.43	33.68	5.20	13.63	11.19	28.21	9.51
0-24hr	66.68	58.40	43.32	48.24	38.16	65.33	27.77	45.90	44.87
Mercapturate									
0-4hr	4.61	3.18	6.74	2.34	4.49	8.61	8.84	1.85	11.78
4-8hr	14.67	8.06	6.86	8.69	4.36	5.88	1.26	9.69	10.36
8-24hr	26.69	11.61	4.55	38.10	8.18	12.54	8.85	23.25	8.77
0-24hr	45.97	22.84	18.15	49.13	17.04	27.02	18.95	34.79	30.91
Total									
0-4hr	225.90	226.99	418.32	81.28	424.19	673.03	539.22	141.47	909.33
4-8hr	319.19	271.33	413.27	198.24	199.99	355.44	56.90	350.16	458.97
8-24hr	335.10	346.51	256.49	508.75	144.57	381.28	246.72	566.97	259.30
0-24hr	880.19	844.83	1088.09	788.27	768.75	1409.75	842.84	1058.59	1627.60

Appendix 2.55 Urinary Recovery of Paracetamol and Metabolites in Each Sample Following Ingestion of a 20 mg kg^{-1} Body Weight Dose — Group D

Time After Dosing	Urinary Recovery of Paracetamol and Metabolites (mg)							
	Group D Subject							
	1	2	3	4	5	6	7	8
Glucuronide								
0-4hr	140.17	191.33	490.93	28.21	501.65	105.05	140.04	152.23
4-8hr	69.33	398.70	209.41	0.00	378.68	96.98	66.88	150.94
8-24hr	131.21	289.42	68.92	257.30	48.19	62.85	359.85	159.62
0-24hr	340.71	879.45	769.27	285.50	928.52	264.87	566.76	462.79
Sulphate								
0-4hr	203.41	146.61	304.13	20.65	180.67	210.46	75.27	208.68
4-8hr	62.45	213.50	85.95	0.00	132.69	141.81	33.76	138.55
8-24hr	97.96	128.42	24.43	160.25	16.62	92.35	137.89	135.40
0-24hr	363.82	488.53	414.52	180.90	329.99	444.63	246.91	482.63
Cysteine								
0-4hr	16.00	5.11	16.47	2.17	9.93	10.84	15.50	15.68
4-8hr	9.31	11.52	7.45	0.00	9.55	19.71	7.22	15.85
8-24hr	25.87	12.53	6.21	21.95	4.09	29.07	40.78	28.99
0-24hr	51.18	29.16	30.13	24.12	23.58	59.62	63.50	60.52
Paracetamol								
0-4hr	7.72	18.13	23.35	4.06	38.47	20.86	9.68	16.96
4-8hr	2.83	21.61	12.04	0.00	37.14	9.23	4.57	19.52
8-24hr	9.38	22.28	6.87	7.91	4.04	13.67	19.80	27.18
0-24hr	19.94	62.03	42.27	11.97	79.65	43.77	34.05	63.66
Mercapturate								
0-4hr	6.95	3.35	9.76	1.73	11.99	5.52	10.75	9.43
4-8hr	5.22	9.82	8.51	0.00	11.28	12.74	5.33	11.61
8-24hr	14.66	11.74	4.04	30.99	2.68	16.18	34.59	18.78
0-24hr	26.83	24.91	22.32	32.72	25.94	34.44	50.68	39.82
Total								
0-4hr	374.25	364.53	844.65	56.81	742.72	352.73	251.24	402.99
4-8hr	149.14	655.15	323.37	0.00	569.33	280.47	117.75	336.46
8-24hr	279.07	464.40	110.48	478.39	75.63	214.12	592.91	369.97
0-24hr	802.47	1484.08	1278.50	535.20	1387.68	847.32	961.90	1109.42

Appendix 2.56   Urinary Recovery of Paracetamol and Metabolites in Each Sample Following Ingestion of a 20 mg kg^{-1} Body Weight Dose — Group R

Time After Dosing	Urinary Recovery of Paracetamol and Metabolites (mg)					
	Group R Subject					
	1	2	3	4	5	6
Glucuronide						
0-4hr	5.62	92.00	4.35	12.26	42.84	61.96
4-8hr	34.77	145.81	171.82	53.99	95.14	448.90
8-24hr	98.15	330.01	210.49	336.23	236.21	254.98
0-24hr	138.54	567.82	386.66	402.48	374.20	765.84
Sulphate						
0-4hr	7.75	118.11	4.54	8.07	19.48	74.50
4-8hr	38.54	136.29	139.52	32.47	31.34	301.46
8-24hr	89.83	192.97	96.19	163.43	52.21	124.20
0-24hr	136.12	447.36	240.25	203.97	103.04	500.16
Cysteine						
0-4hr	1.08	2.75	0.02	1.01	2.48	4.55
4-8hr	4.34	5.32	7.60	2.61	5.25	24.45
8-24hr	10.58	12.65	11.95	11.38	13.02	15.30
0-24hr	16.00	20.72	19.57	15.00	20.75	44.31
Paracetamol						
0-4hr	3.31	9.98	0.38	2.62	1.90	7.56
4-8hr	5.35	5.78	5.73	4.54	3.26	18.95
8-24hr	5.32	12.80	6.66	15.30	8.98	12.81
0-24hr	13.98	28.56	12.77	22.46	14.14	39.32
Mercapturate						
0-4hr	0.39	2.50	0.08	0.25	1.88	2.21
4-8hr	3.22	4.68	7.05	1.80	4.54	25.82
8-24hr	12.70	10.22	10.78	12.00	8.51	15.66
0-24hr	16.31	17.39	17.91	14.06	14.93	43.69
Total						
0-4hr	18.15	225.33	9.37	24.22	68.58	150.78
4-8hr	86.22	297.88	331.72	95.41	139.54	819.58
8-24hr	216.58	558.64	336.07	538.34	318.93	422.95
0-24hr	320.95	1081.85	677.16	657.97	527.05	1393.31

Appendix 2.57 Urinary Recovery of Paracetamol and Metabolites in Each Sample Following Ingestion of a 20 mg kg^{-1} Body Weight Dose — Group D'

Time After Dosing	Urinary Recovery of Paracetamol and Metabolites (mg)							
	Group D' Subject							
	1	2	3	4	5	6	7	8
Gluc								
0-4hr	9.16	57.58	133.81	59.23	0.00	100.99	139.53	125.80
4-8hr	39.00	205.80	192.75	129.74	172.06	116.77	86.96	147.31
8-24hr	116.93	208.60	148.89	114.19	163.29	186.06	216.86	139.63
0-24hr	165.09	471.99	475.46	303.16	335.34	403.82	443.35	412.73
Sulp								
0-4hr	26.89	37.79	128.83	73.26	0.00	103.60	106.45	104.65
4-8hr	108.12	86.33	145.23	157.88	183.12	92.73	54.44	109.70
8-24hr	215.31	56.84	90.32	101.06	122.52	126.56	125.94	90.31
0-24hr	350.32	180.96	364.38	332.19	305.64	322.90	286.84	304.67
Cyst								
0-4hr	3.84	5.90	20.93	7.82	0.00	25.25	16.75	10.77
4-8hr	32.66	19.07	58.23	33.60	56.01	30.29	12.12	20.81
8-24hr	101.65	33.38	59.91	44.63	48.24	66.76	47.79	38.25
0-24hr	138.15	58.35	139.07	86.06	104.25	122.30	76.66	69.83
Para								
0-4hr	1.51	2.66	22.20	4.61	0.00	6.99	9.57	10.91
4-8hr	0.00	6.25	30.09	12.53	11.77	8.12	7.03	12.78
8-24hr	0.00	8.45	21.44	13.91	9.15	15.58	19.46	8.32
0-24hr	1.51	17.36	73.73	31.05	20.93	30.70	36.06	32.01
Merc								
0-4hr	1.58	2.81	9.47	4.47	0.00	16.43	8.19	6.73
4-8hr	15.96	20.65	33.61	20.32	28.63	22.67	7.48	15.30
8-24hr	44.93	27.05	42.08	32.27	31.16	47.31	19.52	26.30
0-24hr	62.46	50.51	85.16	57.06	59.79	86.41	35.19	48.33
Total								
0-4hr	42.97	106.74	315.24	149.39	0.00	253.26	280.50	258.86
4-8hr	195.73	338.10	459.92	354.08	451.59	270.59	168.04	305.90
8-24hr	478.83	334.32	362.64	306.05	374.36	442.28	429.57	302.80
0-24hr	717.53	779.16	1137.80	809.52	825.96	966.13	878.11	867.57

References

Adriaenssens PI (1980). Paracetamol metabolism in man. PhD Thesis, University of Edinburgh.

Adriaenssens PI & Prescott LF (1978). High performance liquid chromatographic estimation of paracetamol metabolites in plasma. British Journal of Clinical Pharmacology 6:87–8.

Aguilar MI, Hart SJ & Calder IC (1988). Complete separation of urinary metabolites of paracetamol and substituted paracetamols by reversed-phase ion-pair high-performance liquid chromatography. Journal of Chromatography Biomedical Applications 426:315–33.

Alkhayat A (1986). Modified enzymatic assay for acetaminophen [letter]. Clinical Chemistry 32(4):699–70.

Allcroft R & Carnaghan RRA (1966). Groundnut toxicity: An examination for toxin in human food products from animals fed toxic groundnut meal. Veterinary Record 75:259–63.

Alpert ME, Hutt MSR, Wogan GN & Davidson CS (1971). Association between aflatoxin content of food and hepatoma in Uganda. Cancer 28(253–60)

Ameer B, Divoll M, Abernethy DR, Greenblatt DJ & Shargel L (1983). Absolute and relative bioavailability of oral acetaminophen preparations. Journal of Pharmaceutical Sciences 72(8):955–8.

Andrews RS, Bond CC, Burnett J, Saunders A & Watson K (1976). Isolation and identification of paracetamol metabolites. Journal of International Medical Research 4 Suppl(4):34–9.

Aoyama T, Yamano S, Guzelian PS, Gelboin HV & Gonzalez FJ (1990). Five of 12 forms of vaccinia virus-expressed human hepatic cytochrome P450 metabolically activate aflatoxin B1. Proceedings of the National Academy of Sciences of the United States of America 87(12):4790–3.

Appleton BS, Goetchius MP & Campbell TC (1982). Linear dose-response curve for the hepatic macromolecular binding of aflatoxin B1 in rats at very low exposures. Cancer Research 42:3659–62.

Archer CT & Richardson RA (1980). An improved colorimetric method for the determination of plasma paracetamol. Annals of Clinical Biochemistry 17:45–6.

Armour A & Slater SD (1993). Paracetamol cardiotoxicity. Postgraduate Medical Journal 69:52–4.

Asao T, Buchi G, Abdel-Kader MM, Chang SB, Wick EL & Wogan GN (1965). The structures of aflatoxin B_1 and G_1. Journal of the American Chemical Society 87:882–6.

Austin H, Delzell E, Grufferman S, Levine R, Morrison AS, Stolley PD & Cole P (1986). A case-control study of hepatocellular carcinoma and the hepatitis B virus, cigarette smoking, and alcohol consumption. Cancer Research 46(2):962–6.

Autrup H, Essigmann JM, Croy RG, Trump BF, Wogan GN & Harris CC (1979). Metabolism of aflatoxin B_1 and identification of the major aflatoxin B_1-DNA adducts formed in cultured human bronchus and colon. Cancer Research 39:694–8.

Autrup H, Seremet T, Wakhisi J & Wasunna A (1987). Aflatoxin exposure measured by urinary excretion of aflatoxin B_1-guanine adduct and hepatitis B virus infection in areas with different liver cancer incidence in Kenya. Cancer Research 47(13):3430–3.

Autrup H, Seremet T & Wakhisi J (1990). Evidence for human antibodies that recognize an aflatoxin epitope in groups with high and low exposure to aflatoxins. Archives of Environmental Health 45(1):31–4.

Ayoola EA (1984). Synergism between hepatitis B virus and aflatoxin in hepatocellular carcinoma. In Williams AO, O'Connor GT, De-The GB & Johnson CA (Eds.), Virus-Associated Cancers in Africa. IARC Scientific Publications No. 63 (pp. 167–79). Lyon: International Agency for Research on Cancer.

Bailey DN (1982). Colorimetry of serum acetaminophen (paracetamol) in uremia. Clinical Chemistry 28(1):187–90.

Baraka OZ, Truman CA, Ford JM & Roberts CJC (1990). The effect of propranolol on paracetamol metabolism in man. British Journal of Clinical Pharmacology 29:261–4.

Bassir O & Emafo PO (1970). Oxidative metabolism of aflatoxin B1 by mammalian liver slices and microsomes. Biochemical Pharmacology 19:1681–7.

Beasley RP, Huang LY & Lin CC (1981). Hepatocellular carcinoma and hepatitis B virus. A prospective study of 22,707 men in Taiwan. Lancet ii:1129–32.

Beckett GJ, Chapman BJ, Dyson EH & Hayes JD (1985). Plasma glutathione S-transferase measurements after paracetamol overdose: evidence for early hepatocellular damage. Gut 26:26–31.

Blair D & Rumack BH (1977). Acetaminophen in serum and plasma estimated by high-pressure liquid chromatography: a micro-scale method. Clinical Chemistry 23(4):743–5.

Bland JM & Altman DG (1986). Statistical methods for assessing agreement between two methods of clinical measurement. Lancet i:307–10.

BNF (1993). British National Formulary.(25 ed.). British Medical Association and the Royal Pharmaceutical Society of Great Britain.

Boyd EM & Bereczky GM (1966). Liver necrosis from paracetamol. British Journal of Pharmacology 26:606–14.

Bréchot C, Degos F, Lugassy C, Thiers V, Zafrani S, Franco D, Bismuth H, Trepo C, Benhamou JP & Wands J (1985). Hepatitis B virus DNA in patients with chronic liver disease and negative tests for hepatitis B surface antigen. New England Journal of Medicine 312(5):270–6.

Bressac B, Kew M, Wands J & Ozturk M (1991). Selective G to T mutations of p53 gene in hepatocellular carcinoma from Southern Africa. Nature 350:429–31.

Briant RH, Dorrington RE, Cleal J & Williams FM (1976). The rate of acetaminophen metabolism in the elderly and the young. Journal of the American Geriatric Society 24:359–61.

Brodie BB & Axelrod J (1948). The fate of acetanilide in man. Journal of Pharmacology and Experimental Therapeutics 94:29–38.

Brodie BB & Axelrod J (1949). The fate of acetophenetidin (phenacetin) in man and methods for the estimation for acetophenetidin and its metabolites in biological material. Journal of Pharmacology and Experimental Therapeutics 97:58–67.

Brown SS, Campbell RS, Price CP, Rambohul E, Widdop B, Barbour HM, Roberts JG, Burnett D, Atkinson T, Scawen MD & Hammond PM (1983). Collaborative trial of an enzyme-based assay for the determination of paracetamol in plasma. Annals of Clinical Biochemistry 20:353–9.

Bulatao-Jayme J, Almero EM, Castro MCA, Jardeleza MTR & Salamat LA (1982). A case-control dietary study of primary liver cancer risk from aflatoxin exposure. International Journal of Epidemiology 11:112–9.

Buss P, Caviezel M & Lutz WK (1990). Linear dose-response relationship for DNA adducts in rat liver from chronic exposure to aflatoxin B_1. Carcinogenesis 11(12):2133–5.

Caldwell J, Davies S & Smith RL (1980). Inter-individual differences in the conjugation of paracetamol with glucuronic acid and sulphate. British Journal of Pharmacology 70:112P–3P.

Campbell TC, Caedo JP, Bulatao-Jayme J, Salamat L & Engel RW (1970). Aflatoxin M_1 in human urine. Nature 227:403–4.

Campbell TC & Hayes JR (1976). The role of aflatoxin metabolism in its toxic lesion. Toxicology and Applied Pharmacology 35:199–222.

Campbell TC, Chen JS, Liu CB, Li JY & Parpia B (1990). Nonassociation of aflatoxin with primary liver cancer in a cross-sectional ecological survey in the People's Republic of China. Cancer Research 50(21):6882–93.

Canalese J, Gimson AES, Davis M & William R (1981). Factors contributing to mortality in paracetamol-induced hepatic failure. British Medical Journal 282:199–201.

Chambers RE & Jones K (1976). Comparison of a gas chromatographic and colorimetric method for the determination of plasma paracetamol. Annals of Clinical Biochemistry 13:433–4.

Choo QL, Kuo G, Weiner AJ, Overby LR, Bradley DW & Houghton M (1989). Isolation of a cDNA clone derived from a blood-borne non-A, non-B viral hepatitis genome. Science 244:359–62.

Christopherson WM & Mays ET (1987). Risk factors, pathology, and pathogenesis of selected benign and malignant liver neoplasms. In Wanebo HJ (Eds.), Hepatic and Biliary Cancer (pp. 17–43). New York: Marcel Dekker, Inc.

Chu FS (1991). Mycotoxins: food contamination, mechanism, carcinogenic potential and preventive measures. Mutation Research 259:291–306.

Clark DWJ (1985). Genetically determined variability in acetylation and oxidation. Therapeutic implications. Drugs 29:342–75.

Clements JA & Prescott LF (1976). Data point weighting in pharmacokinetic analysis: intravenous paracetamol in man. Journal of Pharmacy and Pharmacology 28:707–9.

Clements JA, Heading RC, Nimmo WS & Prescott LF (1978). Kinetics of acetaminophen absorption and gastric emptying in man. Clinical Pharmacology and Therapeutics 24(4):420–31.

Clements JA, Critchley JAJH & Prescott LF (1984). The role of sulphate conjugation in the metabolism and disposition of oral and intravenous paracetamol in man. British Journal of Clinical Pharmacology 18:481–5.

Clissold SP (1986). Paracetamol and phenacetin. Drugs 32 Suppl(4):46–59.

Coles B, Meyer DJ, Ketterer B, Stanton CA & Garner RC (1985). Studies on the detoxication of microsomally-activated aflatoxin B_1 by glutathione and glutathione transferase *in vitro*. Carcinogenesis 5:693–7.

Coulter JBS, Lamplugh SM, Suliman GI, Omer MIA & Hendrickse RG (1984). Aflatoxins in human breast milk. Annals of Tropical Paediatrics 4:61–6.

Crespi CL, Penman BW, Steimel DT, Gelboin HV & Gonzalez FJ (1991). The development of a human cell line stably expressing human CYP3A4: role in the metabolic activation of aflatoxin B_1 and comparison to CYP1A2 and CYP2A3. Carcinogenesis 12(2):355–9.

Critchley JAJH, Cregeen RJ, Balali-Mood M, Pentland B & Prescott LF (1982). Paracetamol metabolism in heavy drinkers. British Journal of Clinical Pharmacology 13:276P–7P.

Critchley JAJH, Nimmo GR, Prescott LF & Woolhouse NM (1983). Ethnic differences in paracetamol metabolism: a comparative study in Scotland and Ghana. British Journal of Pharmacology 80:488P.

Critchley JAJH, Scott AM, Jarvie DR, Dyson EH & Prescott LF (1983). Effects of ethanol and cimetidine on the metabolic activation of paracetamol in man. British Journal of Pharmacology 80:485P.

Critchley JAJH, Dyson EH, Scott AM, Jarvie DR,& Prescott LF (1983). Is there a place for cimetidine or ethanol in the treatment of paracetamol poisoning? Lancet i:1375–6.

Critchley JAJH, Nimmo GR, Gregson CA, Woolhouse NM & Prescott LF (1986). Inter-subject and ethnic differences in paracetamol metabolism. British Journal of Clinical Pharmacology 22:649–57.

Crome P, Vale JA, Volan GN, Widdop B & Goulding R (1976). Oral methionine in the treatment of severe paracetamol (acetaminophen) overdose. Lancet ii:829–30.

Croy RG, Essigmann JM, Reinhold VN & Wogan GN (1978). Identification of the principle aflatoxin B_1-DNA adduct formed *in vivo* in rat liver. Proceedings of the National Academy of Science of the United States of America 75: 1745–9.

Dahlin DC, Miwa GT, Lu AYH & Nelson SD (1984). N-acetyl-p-benzoquinone imine: a cytochrome P-450-mediated oxidation product of acetaminophen. Proceedings of the National Academy of Science of the United States of America 81:1327–31.

Dechtiaruk WA, Johnson GF & Solomon HM (1976). Gas-chromatographic method for acetaminophen (N-acetyl-p-aminophenol) based on sequential alkylation. Clinical Chemistry 22(6):879–83.

Dalezios JI & Wogan GN (1972). Metabolism of aflatoxin B_1 in rhesus monkeys. Cancer Research 32:2297–302.

Davidson DGD & Eastham WN (1966). Acute liver necrosis following over-dosage of paracetamol. British Medical Journal 2:497–9.

Davis DC, Potter WZ, Jollow DJ & Mitchell JR (1974). Species differences in hepatic glutathione depletion, covalent binding and hepatic necrosis after acetaminophen. Life Sciences 14:2099–109.

Denning DW (1987). Aflatoxin and human disease. Advances in Drug Reactions and Accidental Poisoning Reviews 4:175–209.

Dirr HW & Schabort JC (1986). Aflatoxin B_1 transport in rat blood plasma. Binding to albumin *in vivo* and *in vitro* and spectrofluorimetric studies into the nature of the interaction. Biochimica et Biophysica Acta 881:383–90

Dougall JR, Cunningham B & Nimmo WS (1983). Paracetamol absorption from Paramax, Panadol and Solpadeine. British Journal of Clinical Pharmacology 15:487–9.

Dybing E, Holme JA, Gordon WP, Søderlund EJ, Dahlin DC & Nelson SD (1984). Genotoxicity studies with paracetamol. Mutation Research 138:21–32.

Eder H (1964). Chronic toxicity studies on phenacetin, N-acetyl-p-aminophenol (NAPA) and acetylsalicylic acid on cats. Acta Pharmacologica et Toxicologica 21:197–204.

Editorial (1984). Aflatoxins and kwashiorkor. Lancet ii:1133–4.

Essigmann JM, Croy RG, Nadzan AM, Busby Jr WF, Reinhold VN, Buchi G & Wogan GN (1977). Structural identification of the major DNA adduct formed by aflatoxin B_1 *in vitro*. Proceedings of the National Academy of Science of the United States of America 74:1870–4.

Federation of Medical Societies (1989). Medical Directory. (4th ed.). Hong Kong: The Federation of Medical Societies of Hong Kong.

Ferreira SH & Vane JR (1974). New aspects of the mode of action of non-steroidal anti-inflammatory drugs. Annual Review of Pharmacology 14:57–73.

Fleiss JL (1986). The Design and Analysis of Clinical Experiments. New York, U.S.A.: John Wiley & Sons, Inc.

Fletterick CG, Grove TH & Hohnadel DC (1979). Liquid-chromatographic determination of acetaminophen in serum. Clinical Chemistry 25(3):409–12.

Florén C, Thesleff P & Nilsson Å (1987). Severe liver damage caused by therapeutic doses of acetaminophen. Acta Medica Scandinavica 222:285–8.

Flower R (1974). Drugs which inhibit prostaglandin biosynthesis. Pharmacology Reviews 26:33–67.

Forrest JAH, Finlayson NDC, Adjepon-Yamoah KK & Prescott LF (1977). Antipyrine, paracetamol and lignocaine elimination in chronic liver disease. British Medical Journal 1:1384–7.

Forrest JAH, Adriaenssens P, Finlayson NDC & Prescott LF (1979). Paracetamol metabolism in chronic liver disease. European Journal of Clinical Pharmacology 15:427–31.

Forrest JAH, Clements JA & Prescott LF (1982). Clinical pharmacokinetics of paracetamol. Clinical Pharmacokinetics 7:93–107.

Forrester LM, Neal GE, Judah DJ, Glancey MJ & Wolf CR (1990). Evidence for involvement of multiple forms of cytochrome P-450 in aflatoxin B_1 metabolism in human liver. Proceedings of the National Academy of Sciences of the United States of America 87(21):8306–10.

Forrester LM, Henderson CJ, Glancey MJ, Back DJ, Park BK, Ball SE, Kitteringham NR, McLaren AW, Miles JS, Skett P & Wolf CR (1992). Relative expression of cytochrome P450 isoenzymes in human liver and association with the metabolism of drugs and xenobiotics. Biochemical Journal 281(2):359–68.

Gainsborough N, Maskrey VL, Nelson ML, Keating J, Sherwood RA, Jackson SHD & Swift CG (1993). The association of age with gastric emptying. Age and Ageing 22:37–40.

Galfrè G, Milstein C & Wright B (1979). Rat x rat hybrid myelomas and a monoclonal anti-Fd portion of mouse IgG. Nature 277:131–3.

Gan LS, Skipper PL, Peng XC, Groopman JD, Chen JS, Wogan GN & Tannenbaum SR (1988). Serum albumin adducts in the molecular epidemiology of aflatoxin carcinogenesis: correlation with aflatoxin B_1 intake and urinary excretion of aflatoxin M_1. Carcinogenesis 9(7):1323–5.

Garfinkel L (1980). Cancer mortality in non-smokers. Prospective study by the American Cancer Society. Journal of the National Cancer Institute 65:1169–73.

Garland WA, Hsiao KC, Pantuck EJ & Conney AH (1977). Quantitative determination of phenacetin and its metabolite acetaminophen by GLC-chemical ionization mass spectrometry. Journal of Pharmaceutical Sciences 66(3):340–4.

Garner C, Ryder R & Montesano R (1985). Monitoring of aflatoxins in human body fluids and application to field studies. Cancer Research 45:922–8.

Gazzard BG, Ford-Hutchinson AW, Smith MJH & Williams R (1973). The binding of paracetamol to plasma proteins of man and pig. Journal of Pharmacy and Pharmacology 25:964–7.

Geigy Scientific Tables (1982). Introduction to Statistics, Statistical Tables, Mathematical Formulae.(8th ed.). Basle, Switzerland: Ciba-Geigy Limited.

Gibson JB, Wu PC, Ho JCL & Lauder IJ (1980). Hepatitis B surface antigen, hepatocellular carcinoma and cirrhosis in Hong Kong: a necropsy study: 1963–1976. British Journal of Cancer 42:370–7.

Glynn JP & Kendal SE (1975). Paracetamol measurement [letter]. Lancet i:1147–8.

Goldblatt LA (1969). Introduction. In: Aflatoxin, Scientific Background Control and Implications. New York: Academic Press.

Goldfinger R, Ahmed KS, Pitchumoni CS & Weseley SA (1978). Concomitant alcohol and drug abuse enhancing acetaminophen toxicity. American Journal of Gastroenterology 70:385–88.

Gonzalez FJ (1989). The molecular biology of cytochrome P450s. Pharmacological Reviews 40(4):243–88.

Gonzalez FJ (1992). Human cytochromes P450: problems and prospects. Trends in Pharmacological Sciences 13:346–52.

Gorelick NJ (1990). Risk assessment for aflatoxin: I. Metabolism of aflatoxin B_1 by different species. Risk Analysis 10(4):539–59.

Gotelli GR, Kabra PM & Marton LJ (1977). Determination of acetaminophen and phenacetin in plasma by high-pressure liquid chromatography. Clinical Chemistry 23(6):957–9.

Groopman JD, Donahue PR, Zhu J, Chen J & Wogan GN (1985). Aflatoxin metabolism in humans: detection of metabolites and nucleic acid adducts in urine by affinity chromatography. Proceedings of the National Academy of Sciences of the United States of America 82:6492–96.

Groopman JD, Cain LG & Kensler TW (1988). Aflatoxin exposure in human populations: measurements and relationship to cancer. Critical Reviews in Toxicology 19(2):113–45.

Grove J (1971). Gas-liquid chromatography of N-acetyl-p-aminophenol (paracetamol) in plasma and urine. Journal of Chromatography 59:289–95.

Guengerich FP (1988). Roles of cytochrome P-450 enzymes in chemical carcinogenesis and cancer chemotherapy. Cancer Research 48:2946–54.

Hahn R, Wendel A & Flohé L (1978). The fate of extracellular glutathione in the rat. Biochimica et Biophysica Acta 539:324–37.

Hallworth MJ (1983). Enzymic method for acetaminophen adapted to a centrifugal analyzer [letter]. Clinical Chemistry 29(12):2123–4.

Hammond PM & Scawen MD (1981). Enzyme based paracetamol estimation. Lancet i:391–2.

Harris AL (1991). Telling changes of base. Nature 350:377–8.

Harris CC & Sun TT (1984). Multifactorial etiology of human liver cancer. Carcinogenesis 5(6):697–701.

Harris CC, Laveck G, Groopman J, Wilson VL & Mann D (1986). Measurement of aflatoxin B_1, its metabolites, and DNA adducts by synchronous fluorescence spectrophotometry. Cancer Research 46:3249–53.

Harrison JC & Garner RC (1991). Immunological and HPLC detection of aflatoxin adducts in human tissues after an acute poisoning incident in S.E. Asia. Carcinogenesis 12(4):741–3.

Harrison PM, Keays R, Bray GP, Alexander GJM & Williams R (1990). Improved outcome of paracetamol-induced fulminant hepatic failure by late administration of acetylcysteine. Lancet 335:1572–3.

Heading RC, Nimmo J, Prescott LF & Tothill P (1973). The dependence of paracetamol absorption on the rate of gastric emptying. British Journal of Pharmacology 47:415–21.

Hendrickse RC (1984). The influence of aflatoxins on child health in the tropics with particular reference to Kwashiorkor. Transactions of the Royal Society of Tropical Medicine and Hygiene 78:427–35.

Hendrickse RG & Maxwell SM (1988). Heroin addicts, AIDS and aflatoxins [letter]. British Medical Journal 296:1257.

Hepler B, Weber J, Sutheimer C & Sunshine I (1984). Homogeneous enzyme immunoassay of acetaminophen in serum. American Journal of Clinical Pathology 81(602–10)

Herd B, Wynne H, Wright P, James O & Woodhouse K (1991). The effect of age on glucuronidation and sulphation of paracetamol by human liver fractions. British Journal of Clinical Pharmacology 32:768–70.

Hertzog PJ, Smith JRL & Garner RC (1982). Production of monoclonal antibodies to guanine imidazole ring-opened aflatoxin B_1 DNA, the persistent DNA adduct *in vivo*. Carcinogenesis 3(7):825–8.

Ho JCI, Wu PC & Mak TK (1981). Liver cell dysplasia in association with hepatocellular carcinoma, cirrhosis and hepatitis B surface antigen in Hong Kong. International Journal of Cancer 28:571–4.

Hong Kong Government (1990). Harmful Substances in Food Regulations. Chapter 132 subsidiary legislation, Public Health and Municipal Service Ordinance. The Government Printer, Hong Kong

Horai Y & Ishizaki T (1988). Pharmacogenetics and its clinical implications Part II. Oxidation polymorphism. Rational Drug Therapy 22(6):1–8.

Horvitz RA & Jatlow PI (1977). Determination of acetaminophen concentrations in serum by high-pressure liquid chromatography. Clinical Chemistry 23(9): 1596–8.

Howie D, Adriaenssens PI & Prescott LF (1977). Paracetamol metabolism following overdosage: application of high performance liquid chromatography. Journal of Pharmacy and Pharmacology 29:235–7.

Hsieh LL, Hsu SW, Chen DS & Santella RM (1988). Immunological detection of aflatoxin B_1-DNA adducts formed *in vivo*. Cancer Research 48:6328–31.

Hsu IC, Metcalf RA, Sun T, Welsh JA, Wang NJ & Harris CC (1991). Mutational hotspot in the p53 gene in human hepatocellular carcinoma. Nature 350:427–8.

Huggett A & Blair IA (1983). The mechanism of paracetamol-induced hepatotoxicity: implications for therapy. Human Toxicology 2:399–405.

IARC (1976). IARC Monographs on the Evaluation of Carcinogenic Risk of Chemicals to Man. Volume 10.ed.). Lyon, France: International Agency for Research on Cancer.

IARC (1987). IARC Monographs on the Evaluation of the Carcinogenic Risk of Chemicals to Humans: Aflatoxins. Suppl 7.ed.. Lyon, France: International Agency for Research on Cancer.

Idle JR, Mahgoub A, Sloan TP, Smith RL, Mbanefo CO & Bababunmi EA (1981). Some observations on the oxidation phenotype status of nigerian patients presenting with cancer. Cancer Letters 11:331–8.

Idle JR (1989). Cytochrome P450 IIID phenotypes and human cancer risk. Cancer Detection and Prevention 14(2):275–80.

Insel PA (1992). Analgesic-antipyretics and antiinflammatory agents: drugs employed in the treatment of rheumatoid arthritis and gout. In Gilman AG, Rall TW, Nies AS & Taylor P (Eds.), The Pharmacological Basis of Therapeutics (pp. 638–81). New York: McGraw-Hill.

Jackson AA & Golden MHN (1987). Severe malnutrition. In Weatherall DJ, Ledingham JGG & Warrell DA (Eds.), Oxford Textbook of Medicine (pp. 8.12–8.28). Oxford: English Language Book Society/Oxford University Press.

Jacqz E, Hall SD & Branch RA (1986). Genetically determined polymorphisms in drug oxidation. Hepatology 6(5):1020–32.

James O, Lesna M, Roberts SH, Pulman L, Douglas AP, Smith PA & Watson AJ (1975). Liver damage after paracetamol overdose. Comparison of liver-function tests, fasting serum bile acids, and liver histology. Lancet ii:579–81.

Janes J & Routledge PA (1992). Recent developments in the management of paracetamol (acetaminophen) poisoning. Drug Safety 7(3):170–7.

Jayasinghe KSA, Roberts CJC & Read AE (1986). Is biliary excretion of paracetamol significant in man? British Journal of Clinical Pharmacology 22: 363–6.

Jollow DJ, Mitchell JR, Potter WZ, Davis DC, Gillette JR & Brodie BB (1973). Acetaminophen-induced hepatic necrosis. II. Role of covalent binding *in vivo*. Journal of Pharmacology and Experimental Therapeutics 187(1):195–202.

Jollow DJ, Mitchell JR, Potter WZ, Davis DC, Gillette JR & Brodie BB (1973). Acetaminophen-induced hepatic necrosis. II. Role of covalent binding *in vivo*. Journal of Pharmacology and Experimental Therapeutics 187(1):195–202.

Jollow DJ, Thorgeirsson SS, Potter WZ, Hashimoto M & Mitchell JR (1974). Acetaminophen-induced hepatic necrosis. VI. Metabolic disposition of toxic and nontoxic doses of acetaminophen. Pharmacology 12:251–71.

Josting D, Winne D & Bock KW (1976). Glucuronidation of paracetamol, morphine and 1-naphthol in the rat intestinal loop. Biochemical Pharmacology 25:613–6.

Kamali F, Thomas SHL & Ferner RE (1993). Paracetamol elimination in patients with non-insulin dependent diabetes mellitus. British Journal of Clinical Pharmacology 35:58–61.

Keays AT, Gove C, Forbes A, Alexander CJM & Williams R (1989). Use of late N-acetylcysteine in severe paracetamol overdose. Gut 30:A1512.

Keegan C, Smith C, Ungemach F & Simpson J (1984). A fluorescence polarisation immunoassay for the quantitation of acetaminophen [abstract]. Clinical chemistry 30(6):1025.

Kensler TW, Egner PA, Trush MA, Bueding E & Groopman JD (1985). Modification of aflatoxin B_1 binding to DNA *in vivo* in rats fed phenolic antioxidants ethoxyquin and a dithiothione. Carcinogenesis 6(5):759–63.

Klutch A, Levin W, Chang RL, Vane F & Conney AH (1978). Formation of a thiomethyl metabolite of phenacetin and acetaminophen in dogs and man. Journal of Clinical Pharmacology and Therapeutics 24(3):287–93.

Knox HG & Jurand J (1977). Determination of paracetamol and its metabolites in urine by high-performance liquid chromatography using reversed-phased bonded supports. Journal of Chromatography 142:651–70.

Knox JH & Jurand J (1978). Determination of paracetamol and its metabolites in urine by high-performance liquid chromatography using ion-pair systems. Journal of Chromatography 149:297–312.

Korduba CA & Petruzzi RF (1984). High-performance liquid chromatographic method for the determination of trace amounts of acetaminophen in plasma. Journal of Pharmaceutical Sciences 73(1):117–9.

Krishnamachari KAVR, Bhat RV, Nagarajan V & Tilak TBG (1975). Hepatitis due to aflatoxicosis. Lancet i:1061–3.

Lam KC, Yu MC, Leung JWC & Henderson BE (1982). Hepatitis B virus and cigarette smoking: risk factors for hepatocellular carcinoma in Hong Kong. Cancer Research 42:5246–8.

Lau JY & Lai CL (1990). Hepatocarcinogenesis. Tropical Gastroenterology 11(1):9–24.

Lauterburg BH & Velez ME (1988). Glutathione deficiency in alcoholics: risk factor for paracetamol hepatotoxicity. Gut 29:1153–7.

Lee HS, Ti TY, Koh YK & Prescott LF (1992). Paracetamol elimination in

Chinese and Indians in Singapore. European Journal of Clinical Pharmacology 43:81–4.

Lee HS, Sarosi I & Vyas GN (1989). Aflatoxin B_1 formamidopyrimidine adduct in human hepatocarcinogenesis: a preliminary report. Gastroenterology 97:1281–7.

Leung NWY & Critchley JAJH (1991). Increased oxidative metabolism of paracetamol in patients with hepatocellular carcinoma. Cancer Letters 57:45–48.

Levitt RC, Fysh JM, Jensen NM & Nebert DW (1979). The *Ah* locus: biochemical basis for genetic differences in brain tumor formation in mice. Genetics 92:1205–10.

Levy G & Yamada H (1971). Drug biotransformation interactions in man III: Acetaminophen and salicylamide. Journal of Pharmaceutical Sciences 60(2):215–21.

Lin L, Yang F, Ye Z, Xu E, Yang C, Zhang C, Wu D & Nebert DW (1991). Case-control study of cigarette smoking and primary hepatoma in an aflatoxin-endemic region of China: a protective effect. Pharmacogenetics 1:79–85.

Ling KH, Wang JJ, Wu R, Tung TC, Lin CK, Lin SS & Lin TM (1967). Intoxication possibly caused by aflatoxin B_1 in the mouldy rice in Shaung-Chih township. Journal of the Formosan Medical Association 66:517–25.

Linsell A (1987). Primary liver cancer: epidemiology and etiology. In Wanebo HJ (Eds.), Hepatic and Biliary Cancer (pp. 3–15). New York: Marcel Dekker, Inc.

Liu YH, Miller CR, Taylor JA, Nagorney D, Lucier G & Thompson CL (1990). Glutathione S-transferase activity in human liver and lymphocytes and its role in regulating carcinogen-derived DNA adduct formation. The Toxicologist 10: 579.

London WT (1981). Primary hepatocellular carcinoma — Etiology, pathogenesis and prevention. Human Pathology 12:1085–97.

Lowenthal DT, Øie S, Van Stone JC, Briggs WA & Levy G (1976). Pharmacokinetics of acetaminophen elimination by anephric patients. Journal of Pharmacology and Experimental Therapeutics 196(3):570–8.

Lowry OH, Rosenbrough NJ, Farr AL & Randall LJ (1951). Protein measurement with the Folin phenol reagent. Journal of Biological Chemistry 193:265–75.

Maddern G, Miners J, Collins PJ & Jamieson GG (1985). Liquid gastric emptying assessed by direct and indirect techniques: radionuclide labelled liquid emptying compared with a simple paracetamol marker method. Australian and New Zealand Journal of Surgery 55:203–6.

Maddrey WC (1987). Hepatic effects of acetaminophen. Journal of Clinical Gastroenterology 9(2):180–5.

Makarananda K (1989). Immunological detection of human exposure to aflatoxins. PhD Thesis, University of Surrey.

Malan J, Moncrieff J & Bosch E (1985). Chronopharmacokinetics of paracetamol in normal subjects. British Journal of Clinical Pharmacology 19:843–5.

Mandel HG, Manson MM, Judah DJ, Simpson JL, Green JA, Forrester LM, Wolf CR & Neal GE (1987). Metabolic basis for the protective effect of the antioxidant ethoxyquin on aflatoxin B_1 hepatocarcinogenesis in the rats. Cancer Research 47:5518–23.

Martin U, Temple RM, Winney RJ & Prescott LF (1991). The disposition of paracetamol and the accumulation of its glucuronide and sulphate conjugates during multiple dosing in patients with chronic renal failure. European Journal of Clinical Pharmacology 41:43–6.

Masri MS, Haddon WF, Lundin RE & Hsieh DPH (1974). A newly identified major metabolite of aflatoxin B_1 in monkey liver. Journal of Agricultural and Food Chemistry 22:512–5.

McGilveray IJ & Mattok GL (1972). Some factors affecting the absorption of paracetamol. Journal of Pharmacy and Pharmacology 24:615–9.

Medical and Health Department Hong Kong Government (1984). Cancer Registry 1984.

Melbye M, Skinhoj P, Nielsen HN, Vestergaard BF, Ebbesen P, Hansen JP & Biggar RJ (1984). Virus-associated cancers in Greenland: frequent hepatitis B virus infection but low primary hepatocellular carcinoma incidence. Journal of the National Cancer Institute 73(6):1267–72.

Merrill AH & Campbell TC (1974). Preliminary study of *in vitro* aflatoxin B_1 metabolism by human liver. Toxicology and Applied Pharmacology 27:210–3.

Metcalfe SA, Colley PJ & Neal GE (1981). A comparison of the effects of pretreatment with phenobarbitone and 3-methylcholanthrene on the metabolism of aflatoxin B_1 by rat liver microsomes and isolated hepatocytes *in vitro*. Chemico-Biological Interactions 35:145–57.

Metcalfe SA & Neal GE (1983). The metabolism of aflatoxin B_1 by hepatocytes isolated from rats following the in vivo administration of some xenobiotics. Carcinogenesis 4(8):1007–12.

Miles JS & Wolf CR (1991). Developments and perspectives on the role of cytochrome P450s in chemical carcinogenesis. Carcinogenesis 12(12):2195–9.

Miller RP, Roberts RJ & Fischer LJ (1976). Acetaminophen elimination kinetics in neonates, children and adults. Clinical Pharmacology and Therapeutics 19(3):284–94.

Minamide Y, Horie T & Awazu S (1992). High molecular weight protein aggregates formed in the liver of the rat following large doses of paracetamol. Journal of Pharmacy and Pharmacology 44:932–4.

Miners DJ & Kissinger PT (1979). Evidence for the involvement of N-acetyl-p-quinoneimine in acetaminophen metabolism. Biochemical Pharmacology 28:3285–90.

Miners JO, Attwood J & Birkett DJ (1983). Influence of sex and oral contraceptive steroids on paracetamol metabolism. British Journal of Clinical Pharmacology 16(503–9)

Miners JO, Attwood J & Birkett DJ (1984). Determinants of acetaminophen metabolism: effect of inducers and inhibitors of drug metabolism on acetaminophen's metabolic pathways. Clinical Pharmacology and Therapeutics 35(4):480–6.

Miners JO, Robson RA & D.J. B (1986). Paracetamol metabolism in pregnancy. British Journal of Clinical Pharmacology 22:359–62.

Miners JO, Osborne NJ, A.L. T & Birkett DJ (1992). Perturbation of paracetamol urinary metabolic ratios by urine flow rate. British Journal of Clinical Pharmacology 34:359–62.

Mitchell JR, Jollow DJ, Potter WZ, Davis DC, Gillette JR & Brodie BB (1973a). Acetaminophen-induced hepatic necrosis. I. Role of drug metabolism. Journal of Pharmacology and Experimental Therapeutics 187(1):185–94.

Mitchell JR, Jollow DJ, Potter WZ, Gillette JR & Brodie BB (1973b). Acetaminophen-induced hepatic necrosis. IV. Protective role of glutathione. Journal of Pharmacology and Experimental Therapeutics 187(1):211–7.

Mitchell JR, Thorgeirsson SS, Potter WZ, Jollow DJ & Keiser H (1974). Acetaminophen-induced hepatic injury: protective role of glutathione in man and rationale for therapy. Clinical Pharmacology and Therapeutics 16(4):676–84.

Morris ME & Levy G (1984). Renal clearance and serum protein binding of acetaminophen and its major conjugates in humans. Journal of Pharmaceutical Sciences 73(8):1038–41.

Moss EJ, Neal GE & Judah DJ (1985). The mercapturic acid pathway metabolites of a glutathione conjugate of aflatoxin B_1. Chemico-Biological Interactions 55: 139–55.

Moss EJ & Neal GE (1985). The metabolism of aflatoxin B_1 by human liver. Biochemical Pharmacology 34:3193–7.

Mowat AP (1987). Liver disorders in infancy and childhood. In Weatherall DJ, Ledingham JGG & Warrell DA (Eds.), Oxford Textbook of Medicine (pp. 12.265). Oxford: English Language Book Society/Oxford University Press.

Mrochek JE, Katz S, Christie WH & Dinsmore SR (1974). Acetaminophen metabolism in man, as determined by high-resolution liquid chromatography. Clinical Chemistry 20(8):1086–96.

Mucklow JC, Fraser HS, Bulpitt CJ, Kahn C, Mould G & Dollery CT (1980). Environmental factors affecting paracetamol metabolism in London factory and office workers. British Journal of Clinical Pharmacology 10:67–74.

Nakatsuru Y, Qin X, Masahito P & Ishikawa T (1989). Immunological detection of *in vivo* aflatoxin B_1-DNA adduct formation in rats, rainbow trout and coho salmon. Carcinogenesis 11(9):1523–6.

Nash RM, Stein L, Penno MB, Passananti GT & Vesell ES (1984). Sources of interindividual variations in acetaminophen and antipyrine metabolism. Clinical Pharmacology and Therapeutics 36(4):417–30.

Nayak NC, Dhar A, Sachdeva R, Mittal A, Seth HN, Sudarsanam D, Reddy B, Wagholikar UL & Reddy CR (1977). Association of human hepatocellular carcinoma and cirrhosis with hepatitis B virus surface and core antigens in the liver. International Journal of Cancer 20(5):643–54.

Neal GE (1987). Influences of metabolism: Aflatoxin metabolism and its possible relationships with disease. In Watson DH (Eds.), Natural Toxicants in Food: Progress and Prospects. Chichester: Ellis Horwood Ltd.

Neal GE, Judah DJ, Stripe F & Patterson DSP (1981). The formation of 2,3-dihydroxy-2,3-dihydro-aflatoxin B_1 by the metabolism of aflatoxin B_1 by liver microsomes isolated from certain avian and mammalian species and the possible role of this metabolite in the acute toxicity of aflatoxin B_1. Toxicology and Applied Pharmacology 58:431–7.

Neal GE, Judah DJ & Green JA (1986). The *in vitro* metabolism of aflatoxin B_1 catalyzed by hepatic microsomes isolated from control or 3-methylcholanthrene-stimulated rats and quail. Toxicology and Applied Pharmacology 82:454–60.

Nebert DE, Atlas SA, Guenthner TM & Kouri RE (1978). The *Ah* locus: genetic regulation of the enzymes which metabolize polycyclic hydrocarbons and the risk for cancer. In Ts'o POP & Gelboin HV (Eds.), Polycyclic Hydrocarbons and Cancer: Chemistry, Molecular Biology and Environment (pp. 345–90). New York: Academic Press.

Nebert DW (1981). Genetic differences in susceptibility to chemically induced myelotoxicity and leukemia. Environmental Health Perspectives 39:11–22.

Nebert DW, Nelson DR, Coon MJ, Estabrook RW, Feyereisen R, Fujii-Keriyama Y, Gonzalez FJ, Guengerich FP, Gunsalus IC, Johnson EF, Loper JC, Sato R, Waterman MR & Waxman DJ (1991). The P450 gene superfamily: update on new sequences, gene mapping, and recommended nomenclature. DNA and Cell Biology 10:1–14.

Nelson SD (1982). Metabolic activation and drug toxicity. Journal of Medicinal Chemistry 25(7):753–65.

Nesbitt BF, O'Kelly J, Sargeant K & Sheridan A (1962). Toxic metabolites of *Aspergillus flavus*. Nature 195:1062–3.

Ngindu A, Johnson BK, Kenya PR, Ngira JA, Ocheng DM, Nandwa H, Omondi TN, Jansen AJ, Ngare W, Kaviti JN, Gatei D & Siongok TA (1982). Outbreak of acute hepatitis caused by aflatoxin poisoning in Kenya. Lancet i: 1346–8.

Nimmo J, Heading RC, Tothill P & Prescott LF (1973). Pharmacological modification of gastric emptying: effects of propantheline and metoclopromide on paracetamol absorption. British Medical Journal 1:587–9.

Nimmo WS, Heading RC, Wilson J, Tothill P & Prescott LF (1975). Inhibition of gastric emptying and drug absorption by narcotic analgesics. British Journal of Clinical Pharmacology 2:509–13.

Notarianni LJ, Oldham HG & Bennett PN (1987). Passage of paracetamol into breast milk and its subsequent metabolism by the neonate. British Journal of Clinical Pharmacology 24:63–7.

Okuda K, Isaburo F, Hanai A & Urano Y (1987). Changing incidence of hepatocellular carcinoma in Japan. Cancer Research 47:4967–72.

Olson LC, Bourgeois CH, Cotton RB, Harikal S, Grossman RA & Smith TJ (1971). Encephalopathy and fatty degeneration of the viscera in northeastern Thailand. Clinical syndrome and epidemiology. Pediatrics 47:707–16.

Olubuyide IO, Makarananda K, Judah DJ & Neal GE (1991). Investigation of the assay of AFB_1-albumin adducts using proteolysis products in ELISA. International Journal of Cancer 48(3):468–72.

Osborne NJ, Tonkin AL & Miners JO (1991). Interethnic differences in drug glucuronidation: a comparison of paracetamol metabolism in caucasians and chinese. British Journal of Clinical Pharmacology 32:765–67.

Oshima A, Tsukuma H, Hiyama T, Fujimoto I, Yamano H & Tanaka M (1984). Follow-up study of HBsAg-positive blood donors with special references to effect of drinking and smoking on development of liver cancer. International Journal of Cancer 34:775–9.

Patterson DSP & Roberts BA (1971). The *in vitro* reduction of aflatoxins B*1* and B2 bysoluble avian liver enzymes. Food and Cosmetics Toxicology 9:829–37.

Patterson DSP & Roberts BA (1972). Aflatoxin metabolism in duck liver homogenates: the relative importance of reversible cyclopentenone reduction and hemiacetal formation. Food and Cosmetic Toxicology 10:501–12.

Peers FG, Gilman GA & Linsell CA (1976). Dietary aflatoxin and human liver cancer. International Journal of Cancer 17:167–76.

Peers F, Bosch X, Kaldor J, Linsell A & Pluijmen M (1987). Aflatoxin exposure, hepatitis B virus infection and liver cancer in Swaziland. International Journal of Cancer 39(5):545–53.

Peers FG & Linsell CA (1973). Dietary aflatoxins and liver cancer — a population based study in Kenya. British Journal of Cancer 27:473–84.

Perucca E & Richens A (1979). Paracetamol disposition in normal subjects and in patients treated with antiepileptic drugs. British Journal of Clinical Pharmacology 7:201–6.

Plummer S, Boobis AR & Davies DS (1986). Is the activation of aflatoxin B_1 catalysed by the same form of cytochrome P-450 as that 4-hydroxylating debrisoquine in rat and/or man? Archives of Toxicology 58:165–70.

Popper H, Roth L, Purcell RH, Tennant BC & Gerin JL (1987). Hepatocarcinogenicity of the woodchuck hepatitis virus. Proceedings of the National Academy of Science of the United States of America 84:886–90.

Potter WZ, Davis DC, Mitchell JR, Jollow DJ, Gillette JR & Brodie BB (1973).

Acetaminophen-induced hepatic necrosis. III. Cytochrome P-450 mediated covalent binding *in vitro*. Journal of Pharmacology and Experimental Therapeutics 187(1):203–10.

Potter WZ, Thorgeirsson SS, Jollow DJ & Mitchell JR (1974). Acetaminophen-induced hepatic necrosis V. correlation of hepatic necrosis, covalent binding and glutathione depletion in hamsters. Pharmacology 12:129–43.

Potter DW & Hinson JA (1986). Reactions of N-acetyl-p-benzoquinone imine with reduced glutathione, acetaminophen and NADPH. Molecular Pharmacology 30:33–41.

Prescott LF (1971). The gas-liquid chromatography estimation of phenacetin and paracetamol in plasma and urine. Journal of Pharmacy and Pharmacology 23:111–5.

Prescott LF (1974). Gastrointestinal absorption of drugs. Medical Clinics of North America 58(5):907–16.

Prescott LF (1980). Kinetics and metabolism of paracetamol and phenacetin. British Journal of Clinical Pharmacology 10:291S–8S.

Prescott LF (1982). Analgesic nephropathy. Drugs 23:75–149.

Prescott LF (1983). Paracetamol overdosage. Pharmacological considerations and clinical management. Drugs 25:290–314.

Prescott LF & Wright N (1973). The effects of hepatic and renal damage on paracetamol metabolism and excretion following overdosage. A pharmacokinetic study. British Journal of Pharmacology 49:602–13.

Prescott LF, Wright N, Roscoe P & Brown SS (1971). Plasma paracetamol half life and hepatic necrosis in patients with paracetamol overdosage. Lancet i:519–22.

Prescott LF, Newton RW, Swainson CP, Wright N, Forrest ARW & Matthew H (1974). Successful treatment of severe paracetamol overdosage with cysteamine. Lancet i:588–92.

Prescott LF, Park J & Proudfoot AT (1976). Cysteamine, L-methionine and D-penicillamine in paracetamol poisoning. Journal of International Medical Research 4(Suppl 4):112–7.

Prescott LF, Ballantyne A, Park J, Adriaenssens P & Proudfoot AT (1977). Treatment of paracetamol (acetaminophen) poisoning with N-acetylcysteine. Lancet ii:432–4.

Prescott LF, Illingworth RN, Critchley JAJH, Stewart MJ, Adam RD & Proudfoot AT (1979). Intravenous N-acetylcysteine: the treatment of choice for paracetamol poisoning. British Medical Journal 2:1097–100.

Prescott LF, Critchley JAJH, Balali-Mood M & Pentland B (1981). Effects of microsomal enzyme induction on paracetamol metabolism in man. British Journal of Clinical Pharmacology 12:149–53.

Prescott LF & Critchley JAJH (1983). The treatment of acetaminophen poisoning. Annual Review of Pharmacology and Toxicology 23:87–101.

Prescott LF, Speirs GC, Critchley JAJH, Temple RM & Winney RJ (1989). Paracetamol disposition and metabolite kinetics in patients with chronic renal failure. European Journal of Clinical Pharmacology 36:291–7.

Price CP, Hammond PM & Scawen MD (1983). Evaluation of an enzymic procedure for the measurement of acetaminophen. Clinical Chemistry 29(2):358–61.

Quinn BA, Crane TL, Kocal TE, Best SJ, Cameron RG, Rushmore TH, Farber E & Hayes MA (1990). Protective activity of different hepatic cytosolic glutathione S-transferases against DNA-binding metabolites of aflatoxin B_1. Toxicology and Applied Pharmacology 105:351–63.

Quinn PS, Gamble M & Judah JD (1975). Biosynthesis of serum albumin in rat liver. Isolation and probable structure of 'proalbumin' from rat liver. Biochemical Journal 146:389–93.

Ramsdell HS & Eaton DL (1990a). Mouse liver glutathione S-transferase isoenzyme activity toward aflatoxin B_1-8, 9-epoxide and benzo[a]pyrene-7, 8-dihydrodiol-9, 10-epoxide. Toxicology and Applied Pharmacology 105: 216–25.

Ramsdell HS & Eaton DL (1990b). Species susceptibility to aflatoxin B_1 carcinogenesis: comparative kinetics of microsomal biotransformation. Cancer Research 59:615–20.

Ramsdell HS, Parkinson A, Eddy AC & Eaton DL (1991). Bioactivation of aflatoxin B_1 by human liver microsomes: role of cytochrome P450 IIIA enzymes. Toxicology and Applied Pharmacology 108:436–47.

Raucy JL, Lasker JM, Lieber CS & Black M (1989). Acetaminophen activation by human liver cytochromes P450IIE1 and P450IA2. Archives of Biochemistry and Biophysics 271(2):270–83.

Rawlins MD, Henderson DB & Hijab AR (1977). Pharmacokinetics of paracetamol (acetaminophen) after intravenous and oral administration. European Journal of Clinical Pharmacology 11:283–6.

Renwick AG, Ahsan CH, Challenor VF, Daniels R, Macklin BS, Waller DG & George CF (1992). The influence of posture on the pharmacokinetics of orally administered nifedipine. British Journal of Clinical Pharmacology 34:332–6.

Reye RDK, Morgan G & Baral J (1963). Encephalopathy and fatty degeneration of the viscera. A disease entity in childhood. Lancet ii:749–52.

Richter A & Smith SE (1974). Bioavailability of different preparations of paracetamol. British Journal of Clinical Pharmacology 1:495–8.

Roberts DW, Bucci TJ, Benson RW, Warbritton AR, McRae TA, Pumford NR & Hinson JA (1991). Immunohistochemical localization and quantification of the 3-(cystein-S-yl)-acetaminophen protein adduct in acetaminophen hepatotoxicity. American Journal of Pathology 138(2):359–71.

Roebuck BD & Wogan GN (1977). Species comparison of *in vitro* metabolism of aflatoxin B_1. Cancer Research 37:1649–56.

Rogers SM, Back DJ & Orme ML (1987a). Intestinal metabolism of ethinyloestradiol and paracetamol in vitro: Studies using Ussing Chambers. British Journal of Clinical Pharmacology 23:727–34.

Rogers SM, D.J. B, Stevenson PJ, Grimmer SFM & Orme ML (1987b). Paracetamol interaction with oral contraceptive steroids: increased plasma concentrations of ethinyloestradiol. British Journal of Clinical Pharmacology 23:721–5.

Sabbioni G (1990). Chemical and physical properties of the major serum albumin adduct of aflatoxin B_1 and their implications for the quantification in biological samples. Chemico-biological Interactions 75(1):1–15.

Sabbioni G, Skipper PL, Büchi G & Tannenbaum SR (1987). Isolation and characterization of the major serum albumin adduct formed by aflatoxin B_1 *in vivo* in rats. Carcinogenesis 8(6):819–24.

Sabbioni G, Ambs S, Wogan GN & Groopman JD (1990). The aflatoxin-lysine adduct quantified by high-performance liquid chromatography from human serum albumin samples. Carcinogensis 11(11):2063–6.

Sabbioni G & Wild CP (1991). Identification of an aflatoxin G_1-serum albumin adduct and its relevance to the measurement of human exposure to aflatoxins. Carcinogenesis 12(1):97–103.

Salhab AS & Edwards GS (1977). Comparative *in vitro* metabolism of aflatoxicol by liver preparations from animals and humans. Cancer Research 37:1016–21.

Sato C, Matsuda Y & Lieber CS (1981). Increased hepatotoxicity of acetaminophen after chronic ethanol consumption in the rat. Gastroenterology 80:140–8.

Seeff LB, Cuccherini A, Hyman MPH, Zimmerman J, Adler E & Benjamin SB (1986). Acetaminophen hepatotoxicity in alcoholics: a therapeutic misadventure. Annals of Internal Medicine 104:399–404.

Serck-Hanssen A (1970). Aflatoxin-induced fatal hepatitis? Archives of Environmental Health 20:729–31.

Shank RC, Bourgeois CH, Reschamras N & Chandavimol P (1971). Aflatoxins in autopsy specimens from Thai children with an acute disease of unknown aetiology. Food and Cosmetics Toxicology 9:501–7.

Shank RC & Wogan GN (1972a). Dietary aflatoxins and human liver cancer. I. Toxigenic moulds in foods and foodstuffs of Tropical South-East Asia. Food and Cosmetics Toxicology 10:51–60.

Shank RC & Wogan GN (1972b). Dietary aflatoxins and human liver cancer. II. Aflatoxins in market foods and foodstuffs of Thailand and Hong Kong. Food Cosmetics Toxicology 10:61–9.

Shargel L & Yu ABC (1993). Applied Biopharmaceutics and Pharmacokinetics. (3rd ed.). Connecticut, U.S.A.: Appleton & Lange.

Shaulsky G, Johnson RL, Shockcor JP, Taylor LEC & Stark AA (1990). Properties of aflatoxin-DNA adducts formed by photoactivation and characterization of the major photoadduct as aflatoxin-N^7-guanine. Carcinogenesis 11(4):519–27.

Shimada T & Guengerich FP (1989). Evidence for cytochrome P-450$_{NF}$, the nifedipine oxidase, being the principal enzyme involved in the bioactivation of aflatoxins in human liver. Proceedings of the National Academy of Science of the United States of America 86:462–5.

Shiu W, Dewar G, Leung N, Leung WT, Chan M, Tao M, Lui C, Chan CL, Lau WY, Metreweli C (1990). Hepatocellular carcinoma in Hong Kong: clinical study on 340 cases. Oncology 47(3):241–5.

Shively CA & Vesell ES (1975). Temporal variations in acetaminophen and phenacetin half-life in man. Clinical Pharmacology and Therapeutics 18(4): 413–24.

Siegers CP, Rozman K & Klaassen CD (1983). Biliary excretion and enterohepatic circulation of paracetamol in the rat. Xenobiotica 13(10):591–6.

Siegers CP, Loeser W, Gieselmann J & Oltmanns D (1984). Biliary and renal excretion of paracetamol in man. Pharmacology 29:301–3.

SIMED (1991). Siphar User's Manual, Version 4.0. Créteil, Cedex, France: SIMED, Centre d'Études et de Recherches en Statistiques et Informatique Médicales.

Siraj MY, Hayes AW, Unger PD, Hogan GR, Ryan NJ & Wray BB (1981). Analysis of aflatoxin B$_1$ in human tissues with high-pressure liquid chromatography. Toxicology and Applied Pharmacology 58:422–30.

Sizaret P, Malaveille C, Montesano R & Frayssinet C (1982). Detection of aflatoxins and related metabolites by radioimmunoassay. Journal of the National Cancer Institute 69(6):1375–80.

Smilkstein MJ, Knapp GL, Kulig KW & Rumack BH (1988). Efficacy of oral N-acetylcysteine in the treatment of acetaminophen overdose. New England Journal of Medicine 319:1557–62.

Speirs GC (1989). The disposition of paracetamol N-acetyl-D-L-methionate in healthy subjects and renally impaired patients. PhD Thesis, University of Edinburgh.

Spooner RJ, Reavey PC & Mcintosh L (1976). Rapid estimation of paracetamol in plasma. Journal of Clinical Pathology 29:663.

Spooner JB & Harvey JG (1976). The history and usage of paracetamol. Journal of International Medical Research 4 Suppl(4):1–6.

Stemhagen A, Slade J, Altman R & Bill J (1983). Occupational risk factors and liver cancer. A retrospective case-control study of primary liver cancer in New Jersey. American Journal of Epidemiology 117(4):443–54.

Stewart MJ & Willis RG (1975). Simplified gas chromatographic assay for paracetamol. Annals of Clinical Biochemistry 12:4–8.

Stewart MJ, Adriaenssens PI, Jarvie DR & Prescott LF (1979). Inappropriate methods for the emergency determination of plasma paracetamol. Annals of Clinical Biochemistry 16:89–95.

Stewart MJ & Watson ID (1987). Analytical reviews in clinical chemistry:

methods for the estimation of salicylate and paracetamol in serum, plasma and urine. Annals of Clinical Biochemistry 24:552–65.

Street HV (1975). Estimation and identification in blood plasma of paracetamol (N-acetyl-p-aminophenol) in the presence of barbiturates. Journal of Chromatography 109:29–36.

Strubelt O, Obermeier F & Siegers CP (1978). The influence of ethanol pretreatment on the effects of nine hepatotoxic agents. Acta Pharmacologica et Toxicologica 43:211–8.

Sun TT & Chu YY (1984). Carcinogenesis and prevention strategy of liver cancer in areas of prevalence. Journal of Cellular Physiology (suppl) 3:39–44.

Suzanger M, Emami A & Barnett R (1976). Aflatoxin contamination of village milk in Isfahan, Iran. Tropical Science 18:155–9.

Swenson KH, Miller EC & Miller JA (1974). Aflatoxin B_1-2,3-oxide. Evidence for its formation in rat liver *in vivo* and by human liver microsomes *in vitro*. Biochemical and Biophysical Research Communications 60:1036–43.

Swenson DH, Lin JK, Miller EC & Miller JA (1977). Aflatoxin B_1-2,3-oxide as a probable intermediate in the covalent binding of aflatoxin B_1 and B_2 to rat liver DNA and ribosomal RNA *in vivo*. Cancer Research 37:172–81.

Tabor E & Kobayashi K (1992). Hepatitis C virus, a causative infectious agent of non-A, non-B hepatitis: prevalence and structure — summary of a conference on hepatitis C virus as a cause of hepatocellular carcinoma. Journal of the National Cancer Institute 84(2):86–90.

Teschke R, Stutz G & Strohmeyer G (1979). Increased paracetamol-induced hepatotoxicity after chronic alcohol consumption. Biochemical and Biophysical Research Communications 91:368–74.

Thomson JS & Prescott LF (1966). Liver damage and impaired glucose tolerance after paracetamol overdosage. British Medical Journal 2:506–7.

Trenti T, Bertolotti M, Castellana CN, Ferrari A, Pini LA & Sternieri E (1992). Plasma glutathione level in paracetamol daily abuser patients. Changes in plasma cysteine and thiol groups after reduced glutathione administration. Toxicology Letters 64/65:757–61.

Triggs EJ, Nation RL, Long A & Ashley JJ (1975). Pharmacokinetics in the elderly. European Journal of Clinical Pharmacology 8:55–62.

Tsuboi S, Nakagawa T, Tomita M, Seo T, Ono H, Kawamura K & Iwamura N (1984). Detection of aflatoxin B_1 in serum samples of male Japanese subjects by radioimmunoassay and high-performance liquid chromatography. Cancer Research 44:1231–4.

Vale JA, Meredith TJ & Goulding R (1981). Treatment of acetaminophen poisoning: The use of oral methionine. Archives of Internal Medicine 141:394–6.

van Rensburg SJ, Cook-Mozaffari P, van Schalkwyk DJ, van der Watt JJ, Vincent TJ & Purchase IF (1985). Hepatocellular carcinoma and dietary aflatoxin in Mozambique and Transkei. British Journal of Cancer 51:713–26.

Viña J, Perez C, Furukawa T, Palacin M & Viña JR (1989). Effect of oral glutathione on hepatic glutathione levels in rats and mice. British Journal of Nutrition 62:683–91.

Wang CJ, Wang SW, Shiah HS & Lin JK (1990). Effect of ethanol on hepatotoxicity and hepatic DNA-binding of aflatoxin B_1 in rats. Biochemical Pharmacology 40(4):715–21.

Wiener K (1977). Paracetamol estimation: comparison of a quick colorimetric method with a standard spectrophotometric method. Annals of Clinical Biochemistry 14:55–8.

Wiener K & Longlands MG (1977). Plasma paracetamol estimation. Journal of Clinical Pathology 30:91.

Wild CP, Garner RC, Montesano R & Tursi F (1986). Aflatoxin B_1 binding to plasma albumin and liver DNA upon chronic administration to rats. Carcinogenesis 7(6):853–8.

Wild CP, Pionneau FA, Montesano R, Mutiro CF & Chetsanga CJ (1987). Aflatoxin detected in human breast milk by immunoassay. International Journal of Cancer 40(3):328–33.

Wild CP, Jiang YZ, Allen SJ, Jansen LA, Hall AJ & Montesano R (1990a). Aflatoxin-albumin adducts in human sera from different regions of the world. Carcinogenesis 11(12):2271–4.

Wild CP, Jiang YZ, Sabbioni G, Chapot B & Montesano R (1990b). Evaluation of methods for quantitation of aflatoxin-albumin adducts and their application to human exposure assessment. Cancer Research 50(2):245–51.

Wild CP, Montesano R, Van Benthem J, Scherer E & Den Engelse L (1990c). Intercellular variation in levels of adducts of aflatoxin B_1 and G_1 in DNA from rat tissues: a quantitative immunocytochemical study. Journal of Cancer Research and Clinical Oncology 116:134–40.

Wilkinson AP, Denning DW & Morgan MRA (1988). Analysis of UK sera for aflatoxin by enzyme-linked immunosorbent assay. Human Toxicology 7:353–6.

Wolf CR, Smith CAD, Gough AC, Moss JE, Vallis KA, Howard G, Carey FJ, Mills K, McNee W, Carmichael J & Spurr NK (1992). Relationship between the debrisoquine hydroxylase polymorphism and cancer susceptibility. Carcinogenesis 13(6):1035–8.

Wood ML, Smith JRL & Garner RC (1988). Structural characterization of the major adducts obtained after reaction of an ultimate carcinogen aflatoxin B_1-dichloride with calf thymus DNA *in vivo*. Cancer Research 48:5391–6.

World Health Organization Task Group on Environmental Health Criteria for Mycotoxins (1979). Mycotoxins. Environmental Criteria No.11. Geneva, Switzerland: United Nations Environment Programme and the World Health Organization.

Wu PC (1978). Detection of hepatitis B surface antigen in liver biopsies from 655 Chinese patients in Hong Kong. Asian Journal of Infectious Diseases 2:223–9.

Wyllie TD & Morehouse LG (1977). Mycotoxic Fungi. Mycotoxins. Mycotoxicosis. AnEncyclopedic Handbook. Volume I. Mycotoxic fungi and chemistry of mycotoxins. Marcel Dekker, Inc.

Wynne HA, Cope LH, Herd B, Rawlins MD, James OFW & Woodhouse KW (1990). The association of age and fertility with paracetamol conjugation in man. Age and Ageing 19:419–24.

Yeh FS, Yu MC, Mo CC, Luo S, Tong MJ & Henderson BE (1989). Hepatitis B virus, aflatoxins, and hepatocellular carcinoma in southern Guangxi, China. Cancer Research 49(9):2506–9.

Zaman SN, Melia WM, Johnson RD, Portman BC, Johnson PJ & Williams R (1985). Risk factors in development of hepatocellular carcinoma in cirrhosis: prospective study of 613 patients. Lancet i:1357–9.

Zhang YJ, Chen CJ, Haghighi B, Yang GY, Hsieh LL, Wang LW & Santella RM (1991). Quantitation of aflatoxin B_1-DNA adducts in woodchuck hepatocytes and rat liver tissue by indirect immunofluroescence analysis. Cancer Research 51:1720–5.

Zuckerman AJ (1974). Viral hepatitis, the B antigen and liver cancer. Cell 1:65–7.